TEACHING
EVIDENCE-BASED
PRACTICE IN NURSING

A Guide for Academic
and Clinical Settings

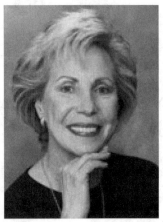

Dr. Rona F. Levin, PhD, RN, is Professor and Project Director for the Joan M. Stout, RN Evidence-Based Practice Initiative at the Lienhard School of Nursing, Pace University, and is Visiting Faculty Member at the Visiting Nurse Service of New York. She is Professor Emeritus at Felician College, Lodi, New Jersey, where she was director of the division of nursing and subsequently director of the division of health sciences. She received her AAS degree in nursing from Queens College, her BS and MS degrees from Adelphi University, and her PhD from New York University. During her career Dr. Levin has held positions as staff nurse, head nurse, educator, researcher, and educational administrator. She has conducted and published research on pain management, nursing diagnoses, and diagnostic competencies of nurses, and has written on a wide variety of nursing research and educational issues. She presents locally, regionally, nationally, and internationally on evidence-based practice (EBP) in relation to curriculum development and research on mentoring nurses to integrate EBP into their clinical practice.

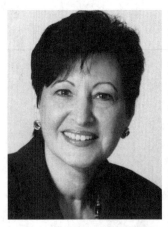

Harriet R. Feldman, PhD, RN, FAAN, is dean and professor of the Lienhard School of Nursing, Pace University. She received her BS and MS degrees from Adelphi University, and PhD from New York University. She has held positions in administration, teaching, and clinical practice. From 1997 to 2005, she was the editor of *Nursing Leadership Forum*. Her book *Nurses in the Political Arena: The Public Face of Nursing*, coauthored with Sandra Lewenson in 2000, received an AJN Book of the Year and Sigma Theta Tau International Nursing Print Media awards. Recent edited books are *The Nursing Shortage: Strategies for Recruitment and Retention in Clinical Practice and Education* (2003) and with Martha J. Greenberg, *Educating Nurses for Leadership* (2005). Dr. Feldman holds the following appointments: Board of the Commission on Collegiate Nursing Education; Public Policy Chair of the Greater New York/Nassau/Suffolk Organization of Nurse Executives; and Health Advisory Committee to US Representative Nita Lowey. She is a Fellow of the American Academy of Nursing and Fellow of the New York Academy of Medicine.

TEACHING EVIDENCE-BASED PRACTICE IN NURSING

A Guide for Academic and Clinical Settings

Rona F. Levin, PhD, RN

and

Harriet R. Feldman, PhD, RN, FAAN

Editors

SPRINGER PUBLISHING COMPANY
New York

Springer Publishing Company, Inc.
11 West 42nd Street
New York, NY 10036

Acquisitions Editor: Ruth Chasek
Production Editor: Sara Yoo
Cover design: Joanne Honigman
Composition: International Graphic Services, Newtown, PA

06 07 08 / 4 3 2

Library of Congress Cataloging-in-Publication Data

Teaching evidence-based practice in nursing: a guide for academic and clinical settings / [edited by] Rona F. Levin and Harriet R. Feldman.
    p. ; cm.
    Includes bibliographical references and index.
    ISBN 0-8261-3155-7
    1. Nursing—Study and teaching. 2. Evidence-based medicine.
[DNLM: 1. Nursing Education Research—education. 2. Evidence-Based Medicine—education. 3. Nursing Education Research—methods. WY 18 T2516 2006] I. Levin, Rona F. II. Feldman, Harriet R.
RT71.T335 2006
610.73'071'1—dc22   2005022198

Printed in the United States of America by Bang Printing.

For Sebastian Bryce, Tyler Reardon, and Emerson Rae with love and my hope that you will become all that you want to be.

"Mimi"

To my family, who keeps me grounded in reality yet encourages me to dream, and especially to my husband, Ron, and mother, Florence, who are always supportive and take pride in all that I do.

Harriet

Contents

Part 3 Teaching/Learning Evidence-Based Practice
in the Academic Setting

Part 4   Teaching/Learning Evidence-Based Practice
in the Clinical Setting

Contributors

Janet Allan, PhD, RNC, FAAN
Dean and Professor
University of Maryland School of
   Nursing
Baltimore, Maryland

Michael J. Barnes, PhD
Associate Professor
Clinical Psychology
Hofstra University
Hempstead, New York

**Diná de Almeida Lopes Monteiro
   da Cruz, PhD**
Nurse and Associate Professor
University of São Paulo School of
   Nursing
São Paulo, Brazil

**Cibele Andrucioli de Mattos
   Pimenta, MNSc, PhD**
Professor
University of São Paulo School of
   Nursing
São Paulo, Brazil

**Linda Q. Everett, PhD, RN,
   CNAA, BC**
Associate Director, University of
   Iowa Hospitals and Clinics
Director, Nursing Services and
   Patient Care/Chief Nursing
   Officer
University of Iowa Hospitals and
   Clinics
Iowa City, Iowa

Ellen Fineout-Overholt, PhD, RN
Director, Center for Advancement
   of Evidence-Based Practice
Associate Professor, Clinical
   Nursing
Arizona State University College
   of Nursing
Tempe, Arizona

Jeanne T. Grace, RNC, PhD
Associate Professor of Clinical
   Nursing
Chair Biomedical Board 03,
   RSRB
University of Rochester
Rochester, New York

Judith Haber, PhD, RN, FAAN
New York University College of
   Nursing
Professor & Director of
   Master's & Post-Master's
   Programs
New York, New York

Barbara Krainovich-Miller, EdD,
   RN, APRN, BC
Coordinator, Nursing Education
   Master's and Post-Master's
   Certificate Programs
New York University College of
   Nursing
New York, New York

Helen T. Lane, MLS
Instructional Services Librarian
Pace University, Lienhard School
   of Nursing
New York, New York

Sandra B. Lewenson, PhD, RN
Associate Dean for Academic
   Affairs
Pace University, Lienhard School
   of Nursing
Pleasantville, New York

Margaret Lunney, RN, PhD
Professor
College of Staten Island, City
   University of New York
Staten Island, New York

Bernadette Mazurek Melnyk,
   PhD, RN, CPNP/NPP, FAAN,
   FNAP
Dean and Distinguished
   Foundation Professor in
   Nursing
Arizona State University College
   of Nursing
Tempe, Arizona

Jamesetta A. Newland, PhD, RN
Director, Primary Health Care
   Associates
Pace University, Lienhard School
   of Nursing
University Health Care
New York, New York

Teresa L. Panniers, PhD, RN
Associate Professor
Assistant Dean for Graduate
   Nursing Programs
George Mason University College
   of Nursing and Health Science
Fairfax, Virginia

Patricia Quinlan, RN, MPA,
   CPHQ
Director of Nursing Education,
   Quality, and Research
Hospital for Special Surgery,
   Department of Nursing
New York, New York

Ellen R. Rich, PhD, RN
Associate Professor and Director
  of the Center for Nursing
  Research & Scholarly Practice
Molloy College, Department of
  Nursing
Huntington Station, New York

Relinie Rosenberg, BS, RN

**Lillie M. Shortridge-Baggett,
  EdD, RN, FAAN**
Professor and Codirector of
  International Affairs
Pace University, Lienhard School
  of Nursing
New York, New York
Visiting Professor, Utrecht
  University (The Netherlands)
Adjunct Professor, Queensland
  University of Technology
  (Australia)
Visiting Professor, University of
  Antwerp (Belgium)

Joanne K. Singleton, PhD, RN
Professor
Pace University, Lienhard School
  of Nursing
New York, New York

**Marita G. Titler, PhD, RN,
  FAAN**
Director, Research, Quality, and
  Outcomes Management
University of Iowa Hospitals and
  Clinics, Department of Nursing
  Services and Patient Care
Iowa City, Iowa

**Marie Truglio-Londrigan, PhD,
  RN**
Associate Professor
Pace University, Lienhard School
  of Nursing
Pleasantville, New York

**Theresa M. Valiga, EdD, RN,
  FAAN**
Chief Program Officer
National League for Nursing
New York, New York

**Priscilla Sandford Worral, PhD,
  RN**
Coordinator for Nursing
  Research
University Hospital
Adjunct Associate Professor
State University of New York/
  Upstate Medical University
Syracuse, New York

Preface

In this book, we present a compilation of innovative, useful strategies for educators to teach evidence-based practice (EBP), both in academic and in clinical settings. Many of our practicing nurses have not yet had the necessary education to use EBP; this book was written to help nurse educators fill this gap. It was also written to encourage faculty to include EBP in the academic curriculum.

We believe that all professional nurses, regardless of educational preparation, need to be able to practice evidence-based nursing. Foremost, this begins with the ability to ask searchable and answerable clinical questions—in other words, to question one's practice. In order to do this, the following skills and characteristics need to be developed: constant curiosity, knowledge of basic research principles, knowledge of and experience in how to ask relevant questions and the ability to search for and critique the evidence to answer these questions, the application of relevant evidence to practice, and the evaluation of its effectiveness. Anything less is inadequate at this point in our professional evolution. Part of the questioning process is to assess the validity of nursing protocols and procedures that each clinical agency develops to standardize practice. Upon what types of evidence, if any, are they based? At the master's level, students need to learn not only how to assess protocols, but also how to develop them for advanced nursing practice. Knowing how to access, critique, and use the best evidence to do this job is crucial.

This book provides readers with practical strategies from more than 20 distinguished educators who are experienced in teaching EBP to nurses. Part 1 introduces EBP in nursing and our philosophy of teaching it. Part 2 covers the teaching of core principles of EBP for nurses, which can be used in both academic and clinical settings. Parts 3 and 4 describe specific strategies for the academic and clinical settings, respectively.

We hope you find the book a handy and meaningful guide and welcome your feedback.

Rona F. Levin, PhD, RN
Harriet R. Feldman, PhD, RN, FAAN

Acknowledgments

Family, friends, and colleagues have contributed in countless ways to the writing of this book, and I wish to thank them all. My husband, Roy, deserves an award for his constant support and encouragement. He never complained about the hours he spent alone when I was thinking and writing. I owe special thanks to my children, Sherry and Robert, for encouraging me to pursue my professional as well as my maternal career. In addition to my birth children, I wish to thank my new children (Sherry's and Robert's spouses), Cliff and Laura, for always appreciating my work. I am grateful to my parents, Ruth and Martin Kaufman, who I know are watching from the stars. Your unconditional love and belief in me when I was growing up are what give me courage to create.

Finally, I owe a special note of appreciation to my dear friend and coeditor, Harriet Feldman, for believing in the idea for this book and agreeing to work with me to help make that idea a reality.

Rona F. Levin

So many people played a role in my scholarly and professional work and I would like to express my gratitude to them. My husband, Ron, has been an amazing cheerleader for all of my efforts, professional and otherwise. Our children, Craig, Jaime, Debbie, and Arlene, and their families—Frank, Devon, Ford, Bill, and Lindsay—and especially my mother, Florence Martin, and my brothers and their respective families have always been both supportive and proud of the work that I do. The tremendous support I have received from family, friends, and my colleagues at Pace University has also helped me to pursue these and other professional projects.

Partnering with Rona Levin on a number of past projects as well as the current one has been a treat. This book made a number of turns as the pieces came together, but we were always ready to listen to each other and debate, as necessary, to make changes. Having a sense of humor did not hurt either!

Harriet R. Feldman

We are all familiar with the popular expression "it takes a village." Although this is Rona's first book for Springer, it is Harriet's seventh. Yet, we both know the meaning of cooperation and collaboration well. The many contributors not only shared their work with us but they also helped to shape the flow of the book and its chapters. And so we would like to thank them for sharing their experience and expertise toward creating a book we can all be proud of. Students past and present also helped to stimulate our thinking about what was important to include.

We would also like to thank Ursula Springer for listening to Rona's rough idea for a book and thinking it had potential. She has always been a risk taker and we both value that very much. Although she has since left Springer for another venture, we would like to acknowledge our editor at Springer, Ruth Chasek, for her insightful comments, hands-on approach, and easygoing style.

Last, but certainly not least, we are grateful to the Hugoton Foundation for funding the Joan M. Stout, RN Evidence-Based Practice Initiative at the Lienhard School of Nursing. This project could not have been possible without the continued interest and support of Joan K. Stout. The project helped to spur many of the ideas and works described in the chapters of this book.

Rona and Harriet

Foreword

Although evidence-based practice (EBP) is now recognized as the gold standard framework for implementing clinical decision making and delivering high-quality care, only a small percentage of nurses and interdisciplinary health professionals are using this approach to their practices. Evidence from several studies indicates that the slow paradigm shift to EBP is attributable to multiple factors, such as perceived lack of time, lack of administrative support and mentorship, as well as inadequate search and critical appraisal skills. Another major barrier to advancing EBP is that educators in many institutions across the country continue to teach research courses in baccalaureate and master's programs in the traditional manner (e.g., detailed emphasis on strategies necessary for the generation of evidence instead of the use and application of evidence, and a lengthy critique process of single studies versus rapid critical appraisal of a body of evidence designed to answer a clinical question). One result of teaching research the traditional way is that students often acquire a negative attitude toward research and leave their professional programs with little desire to continue to read, critique, use, and apply evidence from research.

In order for the paradigm shift to accelerate, educators need to teach students an EBP approach to clinical care that facilitates a "spirit of inquiry" long after graduation from their educational programs. Aside from core courses in EBP, it is necessary to integrate evidence-based decision-making processes throughout all courses in baccalaureate and master's programs in order to facilitate this lifelong approach to learning and high-quality clinical practice.

In their outstanding book, Rona Levin and Harriet Feldman draw upon several years of educational experience to capture creative approaches for teaching EBP. This book includes comprehensive and unique strategies for teaching EBP for all types of learners across a variety of educational and clinical practice settings. The concrete examples of teaching assignments provided in the book bring the content alive and serve as a useful, detailed guide for how to incorporate this material into meaningful exercises for learners. Levin and Feldman's book is a truly wonderful and necessary resource for educators working in all health care professional programs as well as clinical settings. Use of the strategies highlighted in their book no doubt will play an important role in accelerating the paradigm shift to EBP that will lead to a higher quality of care being delivered by health care professionals.

Bernadette Mazurek Melnyk, PhD, RN, CPNP/NPP, FAAN, FNAP
Dean and Distinguished Foundation Professor in Nursing
Arizona State University College of Nursing
Associate Editor, *Worldviews on Evidence-Based Nursing*

Part 1

Setting the Stage

Introduction to Part 1

Harriet R. Feldman

As we said in the Preface, this book is about sharing *useful strategies for educators to teach evidence-based practice* (EBP*) and facilitating the work of faculty to develop curricula that incorporate EBP and the work of nurses in the clinical setting to implement EBP. In order to learn from and implement these strategies, however, it is critical to have the foundation or mind-set for a different kind of teaching, one that is focused mainly on the learner and not on the teacher. How best can we facilitate our students' learning? What are the attitudes and values inherent in this new approach? What are the skills that students need to question their practice and ultimately make changes in the way they deliver care?

Part 1 provides this foundation so that you can better understand the important tools for teaching and learning EBP in nursing within an evolving paradigm shift. Following the recommendation of the Institute of Medicine's landmark report, *Health Professions Education: A Bridge to Quality,* in chapter 1 Levin makes the case for educating students and practicing nurses in using an EBP framework to stay abreast of the knowledge explosion in health and medicine and provide high-quality patient care. This chapter—*EBP in Nursing: What Is It?*—provides a primer to the language and skills of EBP; the importance of identifying answerable questions from either clinical, educational, or administrative perspectives; where to look for evidence; how to appraise the validity of

---

Note: This is the only instance in the book where the term "evidence-based practice" is spelled out. Throughout the book, evidence-based practice is referred to as EBP; the words are not spelled out in each chapter prior to use of this abbreviation.

evidence; ways to integrate the evidence, including the perspectives of others; the importance of conducting self-evaluation as part of one's professional role; and differentiation of EBP from research utilization.

In chapter 2, Feldman and Levin go into more depth about the need for a different approach to teaching and learning by engaging students firmly in the learning process. The notion of student centeredness has been bandied about for quite some time and has existed in a number of iterations, starting with Socrates. Why has it become so popular at this point? Many colleges and universities have adopted this orientation, as evidenced by the language on their Web sites and in their catalogues, but what does it really mean? Many colleagues have complained about the attitude of consumerism that students often display; that is, they expect that a tailored product will be delivered and that they are "entitled" to various services. This is not the way we view student centeredness; to us it means that students are partners in, rather than consumers of, the business of learning. This value is set forth in the presentation of philosophical foundations for teaching and learning, where the idea of collaborative learning is introduced. So in this interest we advocate for students working in mentoring relationships with their faculty and together with peers to achieve shared goals. This approach to learning fits well with EBP in that it is an active process requiring multiple perspectives, group work, and procedures for setting objectives and evaluating outcomes. Besides, as the chapter states, the collaborative approach to learning is itself based on evidence.

Chapter 1

Evidence-Based Practice in Nursing: What Is It?

Rona F. Levin

> You can't depend on your judgment when your imagination is out of focus.
>
> —Mark Twain

Once upon a time there was a nurse and a wizard who were great friends. They did everything together—went on long walks and discussed philosophies of life, encouraged the king in Wherever Land to provide health care for all its citizens, and created healing spas for the body, soul, and especially the imagination. Often when the wizard needed healing, he preferred the nurse's touch to any magical potion he could create. And when the nurse needed answers to clinical questions, the wizard provided them.

On one particular day the nurse and the wizard planned to go for a walk in the forest. The nurse was excited about this outing as she had been working very hard and needed answers to some burning clinical questions. She waited and waited and waited but the wizard never showed up. The nurse went to his home to find out what had happened to him. She was devastated when she learned that his time had come to go to wizard heaven. Of course, she would miss her dear friend very much.

When her grief lessened, she began to think about her profession and wondered how she would ever be able to find the answers to her burning questions now that the wizard, her mentor, was gone. Luckily for the nurse, evidence-based practice was on the way to Wherever Land.

WHAT IS EVIDENCE-BASED PRACTICE?

Evidence-based practice is a framework for clinical practice that incorporates the best available scientific evidence with the expertise of the clinician and the patient's preferences and values to make decisions about health care. [An excellent history of EPB in medicine is provided in chapter 11 (Table 11.2)]. EBP has been introduced as a model for decision making or problem solving in clinical nursing practice, and begins with asking "burning" questions about clinical practices. Although this book emphasizes how to teach nursing students and nurses the EBP model for decision making in clinical practice, it also addresses the importance of using an evidence-based approach to the teaching and administration of nursing.

When teaching students essential tools to use in clinical practice, we propose an approach, borrowed from evidenced-based medicine (Sackett, Straus, Richardson, Rosenberg, & Haynes, 2000), that incorporates how to: (a) ask clinical questions that can be answered through research and other evidence sources; (b) find the best evidence to answer these clinical questions; (c) appraise the validity of the evidence to support answers to clinical questions; (d) integrate the evidence with clinical expertise and patients' perspectives; and (e) evaluate the effectiveness of carrying out all of the above. You can see how these same skills can also be applied to educational and administrative questions in nursing. Instead of the clinician's expertise, we may substitute the expertise of the educator and administrator; and instead of considering patient preference and values when asking educational or administrative questions, we may substitute student and nurse values, respectively.

This model is flexible and dynamic, not linear. Though we need to know what we are looking for before we start searching for answers to questions, we should be prepared to go back and forth between asking questions and finding answers in the literature; between the answers found in the literature and their application to the population and setting with which we are concerned; and between application of this process and evaluation of EBP strategies we use. Questions may need to be altered if they do not lead us down the right path; for example, the available research evidence may not agree with patients' perspectives or be applicable to a particular clinical setting.

Asking Answerable Clinical Questions in Nursing

To date, most evidence-based literature sources in medicine and nursing focus on clinical questions about the effectiveness of interventions, whether discussing treatment for an actual problem or measures for prevention, and they use what is called a PICO format for asking such questions (Melnyk & Fineout-Overholt, 2004; Sackett et al., 2000). The acronym stands for population, intervention, comparison intervention, and outcome. One example of this type of question would be, What is the effect of clean versus sterile urinary catheter insertion on urinary tract infections in women who have undergone gynecologic surgery? This is a treatment, therapy, or intervention question. There are also questions of secondary prevention, prognosis, and harm (Sackett et al., 2000; Thornton & Mangino, 2003). Examples of these types of clinical questions are as follows:

- In a population of older adults living independently in a community, does the availability of nursing case-management services decrease unplanned visits to primary care providers and hospital emergency departments? (secondary prevention)

- In a population of menopausal women, what is the likelihood of cardiac events in those who take hormone replacement therapy (HRT) compared to women who do not take HRT? (prognosis)

- In a population of adult male patients undergoing cardiac catheterization, does the application of continuous pressure postcatheterization increase the incidence of pain at the catheter insertion site? (harm)

Less attention has been paid to how to ask and answer diagnostic questions in nursing. In order to facilitate this, Levin, Lunney, and Krainovich-Miller (2004) devised an acronym for framing diagnostic questions, the *PCD format*. P refers to the patient population; C refers to the cues or cue clusters; and D refers to differential diagnosis (see Box 1.1).

For the PCD question in Box 1.1, possible diagnoses to consider would be: sleep pattern disturbance, ineffective coping, hopelessness, powerlessness, fear and/or anxiety, cognitive impairment, and others. After reviewing the evidence that is available on these diagnoses, the nurse might ask the following questions: What is the strength of the cues in relation to the possible diagnoses? Based on the evidence, which of the possible diagnoses represents the best match with the cues? Does the patient validate the nurse's interpretation (Levin et al., 2004)?

**Box 1.1
Example: PCD Question**

In adult critical care patients (**population**) who exhibit angry out-
bursts, complaints about treatments that interfere with sleep/
rest, and irritable behavior (**cue cluster**), what are the possible
nursing diagnoses to consider (**differential diagnosis**)?

Asking Answerable Questions About Education and Administration in Nursing

In this book we are taking EBP a step beyond where it has been to include
educational and administration decision making. After all, if we are teaching current and future nurses to base their practice on the best evidence,
should we not as nursing educators and nursing service administrators
do the same?

Education

The types of questions educators need to ask concern best teaching practices for achieving learning outcomes as well as questions related to
the clinical content they are teaching. Below are examples of focused,
answerable questions about teaching practices:

- What is the effect of collaborative versus didactic teaching strategies on course and teacher evaluations in a population of generic
  baccalaureate students, master's degree students, etc.? (a question
  of intervention)

- Does the introduction of an EBP approach to clinical decision
  making improve NCLEX scores, student satisfaction/employer
  satisfaction in a population of generic baccalaureate students/
  graduates? (questions of prognosis)

- What is the effect of didactic versus experiential learning on the
  critical thinking scores of RN completion students? (a question
  of intervention)

Administration

By now we are sure you are getting the hang of asking focused, searchable,
answerable questions. And those concerning system-wide initiatives or
management practices are no different. Examples are as follows:

- What is the effect of involving staff nurses in developing nursing protocols versus professional development and administrative development of such protocols on the job satisfaction and retention rate of nurses as well as specified and protocol-related patient outcomes? (a question of intervention)

- What characteristics or cue clusters are able to predict nurse burnout and turnover of staff nurses working in an acute care institution? (a question of diagnosis and prognosis.)

Finding the Evidence

In order to find the evidence to answer burning clinical, educational, or administrative questions, nurses need to possess knowledge of the databases available and the most appropriate databases to search for answers to their specific questions. Good sources for this knowledge are CINHAL, MEDLINE, ERIC, and PSYCHINFO, to name a few.

Diagnostic research in nursing is in its infancy. As such it may be necessary to look to other than nursing databases or sources for evidence. For example, when asking a treatment question, one may go to the Cochrane Library database (www.cochrane.org, see chapter 4) to find systematic reviews (summaries of single studies) on a particular topic. The type of diagnostic research in nursing we are discussing does not currently have such a database, so one needs to review the individual studies on a diagnosis of interest. One important source of such studies is the *NANDA International Journal* and proceedings of NANDA (North American Nursing Diagnosis Association) and National Nursing Network (NNN) conferences over the past 30 years.

Appraising the Validity of the Evidence

Once the evidence is uncovered, the next step is to read it with a critical eye. This is the step that makes use of the critiquing skills learned in a basic nursing research course, except that there are only three major questions you need to answer: What is validity of the evidence you have uncovered? Are the results of these studies clinically, educationally, and administratively significant or important? Is the evidence usable with my population of patients, students or nurses in the setting in which I practice? Several chapters, for example 3, 4, 5, 15, and 20, deal with strategies to teach critical analysis of evidence.

Integrate the Evidence With Nurses' Experience and Patient Perspective

And let us not forget the perspectives of the students we are teaching and the nurses we are leading!

An EBP framework includes using our own expert judgment and the patient's unique perspective and value system when applying the research or evidence in our practice. The clinical expertise of the nurse refers to his or her assessment of the client's condition through subjective history-taking and in conjunction with the objective findings of physical examination and laboratory reports. Of course, the nurse's previous education and experience is of paramount importance in determining level of expertise.

Patients' unique perspectives include their value and belief system, that is, what they live for and their self-determined choices, which include treatment options. In relation to nursing diagnoses, this means we share the diagnosis we formulate (based on the best available evidence) with our patient and validate our impressions with him or her. In relation to students, it means we constantly ask for their feedback about our educational practices. And for administrators and managers it means we always consider the nurses we are leading when making decisions that concern them.

Conduct Self-Evaluation of Use of EBP

Self-evaluation is an inherent part of being a professional. As with any of our practices, it behooves us to ask ourselves if we have done a good job of asking the appropriate question, finding and appraising the most relevant evidence with which to answer our question, and integrating this evidence with our own expertise and the patient's, student's, or nurse's perspective in arriving at our answers and solutions. In addition, we need to ask ourselves what we have done with the answers to our "burning questions." Did we apply innovation in our practice? If so, did we evaluate its effect on predetermined outcomes? Was the innovation successful in achieving desired results? If so, how are we diffusing that innovation (Rogers, 2003)?

The Qualitative Versus Quantitative Debate

Because EBP started with the discipline of medicine, very little attention was given to qualitative data as evidence, although Sackett et al. (2000) do give lip service to such evidence. In fact, in most EBP rating systems (see chapter 11), qualitative evidence is at the low end of scale for level and quality ratings. We need to consider, however, that in the discipline of nursing we sometimes ask questions for which quantitative data do not provide answers. One example of such questions is, What is the experience like for children with cancer? (See chapter 6 for a discussion of how to teach the use of qualitative research as evidence.) The point here is that in order to find the appropriate evidence, you must ask the right question. The question will determine the type of evidence (quantitative or qualitative) that is most relevant and has the greatest potential to provide an answer.

How Does EBP Differ From Research Utilization?

EBP is a broader concept than research utilization. Research utilization considers research as the only source of evidence whereas EBP considers the findings of research as one source of evidence. Other sources include clinical guidelines produced by expert panels, theoretical evidence, and case reports. Also, as described above, EBP integrates the clinician's expertise and client preferences when applying the best evidence to practice. Although both EBP and research utilization involve the critical appraisal of research reports, EBP addresses the critical appraisal of all existing evidence. Finally, research utilization is focused primarily on whether or not an innovation is ready for application to practice. This has to do with whether or not an appropriate and valid research base is available for use. In contrast, EBP addresses the assessment of current protocols and practices as well as the introduction of new innovations (see Box 1.2).

Why Do EBP?

One of the reasons we really need to be teaching our students how to ask and answer clinical questions is because of the increasing rate at which knowledge is being accumulated and disseminated. We can no longer rely on textbooks to provide the latest and best information to guide our practice. Books are often outdated by the time they are

Box 1.2
EBP vs. Research Utilization (RU)

EBP	RU
Broader concept	Component of EBP
Evidence other than research	Only research accepted as evidence
Critical appraisal of all evidence	Critical appraisal of research reports

published (Sackett et al., 2000). For example, I usually ask my graduate research students to tell me their favorite site for giving an intramuscular injection. The majority of them still respond that they give the injection in the buttocks and many continue to use the four-quadrant method to locate the injection site. Some say they use the dorsogluteal site instead of the buttocks, but still may use the four-quadrant method to locate the site rather than using anatomical landmarks. Rarely do students mention the ventrogluteal site for giving an IM injection, which is the safest (away from nerves) and most accessible site to use. In addition, when nurses say they use the dorsogluteal site, I ask how they position the patient. Most respond that they ask patient to lie on his or her side. Since the late seventies and early eighties, research has supported the prone position as the most comfortable for the patient when giving an IM in this site. My burning question then is, Why do we continue to teach students how to practice based on tradition and not the best evidence?

The latest Institute of Medicine (IOM) report (2003) contains the following vision statement: "All health professionals should be educated to deliver patient-centered care as members of an interdisciplinary team, emphasizing *evidence-based practice*, quality improvement approaches and informatics" (p. 3). Only through teaching students and practicing nurses how to practice using an EBP framework can we hope to keep up with the knowledge explosion and provide the highest quality of care to our patients. And it is up to the educators and administrators in our discipline to bring EBP to their lands.

And so we come to the moral of the story.

> As time went by, the wizard's health professional protégés in Wherever Land began to teach students of all health disciplines how to use an EBP framework to ask and answer their own burning questions about their practice so they no longer had to rely on wizardry. The nurse realized as she was learning how to answer her own questions that the wizard had taught her the most important lesson of all—how to ask a question. For that is where the whole process begins.

REFERENCES

Institute of Medicine of the National Academies. (2003). *Health professions education: A bridge to quality*. Washington, DC: National Academies Press.

Levin, R. F., Lunney, M., & Krainovich-Miller, B. (2004, March). *Diagnostic accuracy and evidence-based practice*. Paper presented at the NNN 2004 Conference, Chicago, IL.

Melnyk, B. M., & Fineout-Overholt, E. (Eds.). (2004). *Evidence-based practice in nursing and health care: A guide to best practice.* Hagerstown, MD: Lippincott Williams & Wilkins.

Rogers, E. M. (2003). *Diffusion of innovations* (5th ed.). New York: Free Press.

Sackett, D. L., Straus, S. E., Richardson, W. S., Rosenberg, W., & Haynes, R. B. (2000). *Evidence-based medicine: How to teach and practice EBM* (2nd ed.). Edinburgh, Scotland: Churchill Livingston.

Thornton, Y., & Mangino, C. (2003). *Evidence-based practice toolkit.* Unpublished manuscript, Center for Research and Evidence-based Practice, University of Rochester School of Nursing.

Chapter 2

Our Approach to Teaching/ Learning EBP: The Talking Head Versus the Dancing Feet

Harriet R. Feldman and Rona F. Levin

> Tell me and I'll listen. Show me and I'll understand. Involve me and I'll learn.
>
> —Teton Lakota Indian Proverb

How do you engage a class of learners to make the right connections? This is an age-old question. As a teacher you want to turn students on, make learning exciting and not anxiety-provoking, and help them draw relevance from both the content and the experience. Our philosophy is briefly introduced in the preface to this book. In this chapter we delve further into the concept of student centeredness, philosophical foundations of teaching and learning, ideas of "fit" for teaching EBP, and how you can take the lead as a faculty member to guide students toward an appreciation for, and knowledge of, EBP.

SETTING THE CONTEXT: STUDENT CENTEREDNESS

Is the notion of student centeredness the current rage or a value system that has waxed and waned over time? Socrates was student centered as he helped his pupils explore ideas and concepts. The Socratic method calls for the teacher to profess ignorance in terms of the topic to be learned, followed by dialogue aimed at discovery on the part of the learner. Through the approach of question and answer, truths are uncovered. Critique, not of people but of concepts and ideas, is also part of the experience to get at the truth, in some ways like peeling an onion where the layers are removed to examine the center. The Socratic method is both inductive and deductive, in that a problem or issue is critiqued to find truth and tested to understand consequences. According to Samples (n.d.), "the definitional method of Socrates is a real contribution to the logic of philosophical inquiry. It inspired the dialectical method of Plato and exerted a not inconsiderable influence on the logic of Aristotle" (p. 2). Socrates focused on the contributions of the learner; the teacher is present to facilitate the development of the learners' skills of inquiry.

Many colleges and universities have adopted the term "student centered" as part of their mission or statement of values. For example, Capital University (n.d.) discusses the "Journey of the Student" in the description of its assessment initiative. To capture the image of the journey it uses the metaphor of a spiral staircase as a "visual representation to illuminate the components and stages of growth and development [that are] inherent" (p. 1). Florida Coastal School of Law (n.d.) describes student centeredness as a

> state of mind that manifests itself in how our priorities are ordered. This ethos . . . assumes . . . that a student will receive clear answers to his or her questions, reasoned explanation of any decision affecting him or her, and timely access to those persons who are in administrative or academic responsibility. (p. 1)

It states further that students are "interacted with as learning partners" and that learning will take place in a "supportive learning environment." Last, Salisbury University (n.d.) identifies student centeredness among its values, stating that "our students are the primary reason for our existence. Our focus is on their academic and individual success. . . . We are committed to helping students learn to make reasoned decisions and to be accountable for the outcomes of the decisions they have made" (p. 1).

In summary, we believe that the learning experience should be respectful, cognizant of differences and talents among learners, challenging, thoughtful, and focused on the learner rather than on the teacher. Being a "talking head" is antithetical to the idea of student centeredness in that it does not engage students in the learning process. Faculty with "dancing feet" on the other hand, who are active in drawing students out, reflect the values and principles of Socrates.

One further note on the topic of Socratic method is that it is not exclusive to the teaching of adults. An interesting article by Russell Yates (n.d.) describes his teaching experiences with students who are 8 to 11 years of age. He reports that

> Learning and not teaching is the focus in my classroom. This simple statement is filled with implications. If teaching is the focus of a classroom, then control over student academic, social, and behavioral actions becomes the job of the teacher. . . . This type of classroom supports a "culture of silence" . . . a programming of conformity if looked at on a societal scale. It is also, as I see it, a Behaviorist way of managing instruction in which management of learning is reliant on forces external to the child, including reinforcement and an emphasis on consequences administered by the teacher. In contrast, a learning focused classroom, as I see it, puts the primary emphasis on the process of learning and the use of knowledge. The teacher's job is then one of helping students acquire learning skills and the practicing of those skills in ways that are useful and meaningful to the student. The teacher does not act as some sort of all-important filter of information . . . but rather becomes more of a guide. (p. 1)

Because adults are the focus of the learning of EBP, it is germane to mention the work of Malcolm Knowles (n.d., 1975) in this section on context. Knowles was a strong proponent of andragogy, or adult learning. According to him, andragogy is based on at least five assumptions about adult learners: self-concept, experience, readiness to learn, orientation to learning, and internal motivation to learn (2004). He describes self-directed learning as a process "in which individuals take the initiative, with or without the help of others, in diagnosing their learning needs, formulating learning goals, identifying human and material resources for learning, choosing and implementing appropriate learning strategies, and evaluating learning outcomes" (1975, p. 18). This process has guided our approach to teaching/learning for many years and continues to be relevant to today's learner.

PHILOSOPHICAL FOUNDATIONS
FOR TEACHING AND LEARNING

It is within the context of the roots of Socrates and Knowles that we approach the notion of cooperative (collaborative) learning. According to Johnson, Johnson, and Smith (1991), cooperative learning is a strategy that actively involves students in the learning process. Not altogether a new idea, "as early as the first century, Quintilian argued that students could benefit from teaching one another" (p. 4). This approach enables faculty to "increase students' achievement, create positive relationships among students and promote students' healthy psychological adjustment to school" (p. iii). Cooperative learning offers a way to structure learning situations so that "students work together to achieve shared goals" (p. iii). Students collaborate (student-student interaction) to foster learning, rather than approaching learning in isolation. Cooperative learning uses the concept of small groups working together to enrich the learning experience.

There are three strategies that may be used: formal learning groups, informal learning groups, and cooperative base groups. Johnson and colleagues (1991) describe formal cooperative learning groups as those used to teach specific content; informal cooperative learning groups as those that "ensure active cognitive processing of information during a lecture;" and cooperative base groups as those providing "long-term support and assistance for academic progress" (p. 9). In the formal group the teacher shares concepts, principles, and strategies that students must understand and apply. The informal group focuses on specific materials that must be learned, and may consist of focused group discussions prior to or following a lecture. Cooperative base groups "provide each student with the support, encouragement, and assistance he or she needs to progress academically" (p. 10). So, cooperative learning involves students working together to achieve an understanding of course content, search for new meaning, solve related problems, or create a product. This approach is student centered where responsibility for learning is shared by student and teacher for governance and evaluation of the learning effort. The group or team embraces both content and process in this effort.

[Please note that collaborative and cooperative are often identified as though they were identical; however, they are at opposite ends of the structure continuum of learning. Collaborative learning is least structured and cooperative learning is most structured.]

WHAT IS THE FIT WITH EBP?

Using the idea of cooperative learning, then, learning is viewed as active, requires challenge, is illuminated by multiple perspectives, is a social activity, and is a shared experience between students and teacher. Conditions necessary for its success include positive interdependence; promotive interaction, responsibility, and accountability; interpersonal and group skills; and processing or group functioning. The role of the teacher is to involve the student in the learning experience. To do this, the teacher needs to establish a structure for learning that includes setting objectives, assigning group membership, communicating purpose, monitoring group process (and providing guidance for this), and evaluating process and outcome. Expected outcomes are facilitation of peer collaboration (which simulates the world of work), promotion of respect for peers, awakening of new ideas, and reinforcement of learning.

WHY USE THIS APPROACH TO LEARNING?

Because it is based on solid evidence. Examples are a meta-analysis of cooperative learning studies with college students (Johnson & Johnson, 1993), meta-analysis on the effects of cooperative learning on students of all ages (Bossert, 1988), and a comprehensive longitudinal study of college students (Astin, 1993). Research has supported the premises that students who participate in cooperative learning groups attain higher academic achievement, develop more positive peer relations, and experience healthier psychosocial adjustment than do students who participate solely in competitive or individualistic learning (Johnson et al., 1991).

Important strengths to consider in response to the question of why to use cooperative learning are because it fosters the sharing of ideas so that varied perspectives on issues and problems are examined; it is socially positive and the sharing of work creates a bonding experience; trust is built when people must rely on each other's strengths and support each other's limitations; and confidence is built in "what I know" when learning is reinforced. There are also drawbacks to the cooperative learning experience. For example, if groups meet outside of class, timing and other commitments may be an issue. More time may be needed to complete an assignment. Peer assessment can be controversial whether or not it factors into one's grade. In terms of assessment, the teacher will need to consider whether or not peer input and review belong in the course evaluation, whether group process as well as product should be evaluated, and whether group members should be involved in developing their own criteria for assessment. Furthermore, should grades be individual or by group and how does this decision get made?

In teaching EBP, it is implicit that students will have at least a beginning base of nursing knowledge from which to draw. That base can be built upon through cooperative learning groups. For example, a group of students is assigned to establishing a basis for a particular nursing protocol by looking at the evidence through literature search, interviews of nursing staff, and other means developed by group members. A time frame is established, perhaps 3 weeks, to gather the information and develop a presentation of findings. Students work together to find the evidence that supports or refutes the protocol. Some group members may work on the literature and others may interview selected nursing staff, such as the in-service educator or a member of the research team. Others may review protocols on the same topic that are used in different health care facilities. The group sets the framework for completing the first part of this learning activity—finding the evidence. The next part might consist of the group's coming together to discuss their findings, determine whether or not the assignment has been completed, and decide on the manner of presenting the information to the class.

TAKING THE LEAD: NEXT STEPS FOR FACULTY

Johnson and colleagues (1991) identify five parts of the instructor's role when using formal cooperative learning groups:

1. Specifying the objectives for the lesson;
2. Making decisions about placing students in learning groups before the lesson is taught;
3. Explaining the task and goals structure to the students;
4. Monitoring the effectiveness of the cooperative learning groups and intervening to assist with tasks (such as answering questions and teaching skills) or to increase students' interpersonal and group skills; and
5. Evaluating students' achievement and helping students discuss how well they collaborated with each other (pp. 59–60).

Being familiar with these parts is essential to the success of the teacher with dancing feet. Though it is tempting to be the talking head to impart knowledge (teacher is the messenger and student is the recipient), this approach of passive learning instead stifles critical inquiry and students may become lost in the subject matter. Looking for evidence implies that the learner is active, discerning, and thoughtful. If a teacher is to prepare students to apply clinical evidence to the care of patients, families, and groups, there must be a commitment to facilitating problem solving through active learning experiences.

There are many strategies for implementing cooperative learning to teach EBP. First, the teacher must consider how a learning group should be formed. It is important that the students and teacher collaborate on team membership. Is diversity of academic ability a factor of importance? Should you consider student interest in a particular problem or project? Do the schedules of group members play a role in their participation? What size should the group be? Second, you need to decide what strategies to use to develop and support group functioning. For example, members can identify commonalities and differences among team members to facilitate bonding. The team could come up with a name to establish camaraderie. There are also games that help people learn about each other. Reading about group behavior and team building will help the teacher understand and facilitate group development and process.

Third, group functioning depends on active participants. Members must agree on the methods they will use to assure participation. For example, everyone should come prepared to group meetings, be given an opportunity to present his or her opinion and ask questions, and focus on listening carefully to each other, offering constructive criticism of ideas and giving positive feedback when appropriate. Fourth, the issue of evaluation of group work must be addressed. The teacher may decide not to grade group work, and this should be stated at the outset. On the other hand, the teacher may decide that group products, for example, papers or presentations, will be evaluated based on specific criteria, also stated at the outset. Also, a decision needs to be made about an individual versus a group grade. Perhaps some aspects of the assignment may receive a group grade and others an individual grade. If consensus is not reached on a particular problem or issue, it may be appropriate to separately grade the "minority opinion."

Teaching EBP is at the very least challenging, but it is also extremely rewarding to see students get it. Faculty development is critical to this effort, because cooperative learning strategies often represent a new way of teaching. The remainder of the book focuses on varied strategies to use with students and clinicians that will help to support this development. Our mission as educators is not about teaching. It is about helping students to learn and understand the relevance of that learning to their chosen path in life. And so we need to bring life to what we teach with our dancing feet, not with our talking heads.

REFERENCES

Astin, A. W. (1993). *What matters in college: Four critical years revisited.* San Francisco: Jossey-Bass.

*Bossert, S. T. (1988). Cooperative activities in the classroom. *Review of Educational Research, 15*, 225–250. [meta-analysis]

Capital University Assessment. (n.d.). Retrieved December 9, 2004, from http://www.capital.edu/acad/academic-affairs/assessment.html

Florida Coastal School of Law. (n.d.). Retrieved December 9, 2004, from http://www.fcsl.edu/admissions/centeredness/index.asp

*Johnson, D. W., & Johnson, R. T. (1993, Spring). What we know about cooperative learning at the college level. *Cooperative Learning, 13*(3), 17–18.

Johnson, D. W., Johnson, R. T., & Smith, K. A. (1991). *Cooperative learning: Increasing college faculty instructional productivity.* ASHE-ERIC Higher Education Report No. 4. Washington, DC: George Washington University, School of Education and Human Development.

Knowles, M. S. (1975) *Self-directed learning. A guide for learners and teachers.* Englewood Cliffs, NJ: Prentice-Hall/Cambridge.

Malcolm Knowles, informal adult education, self-direction, and andragogy. (n.d.). Retrieved December 9, 2004, from http://www.infed.org/thinkers/et-knowl.htm

Salisbury University. (n.d.). Retrieved December 9, 2004, from http://www.salisbury.edu/Info/values.html

Samples, K. (n.d.). Retrieved December 9, 2004, from http://www.str.org/free/studies/socrates.htm

Yates, R. (n.d.). *My teaching philosophy.* Retrieved December 9, 2004, from http://www.multiage-education.com/russportfolio/teachingphilosophy2.html

---

*References marked with an asterisk indicate studies included in a meta-analysis.

Part 2

The Basics of Teaching/Learning Evidence-Based Practice

Introduction to Part 2

Harriet R. Feldman

The chapters in this section represent the core skills needed for EBP in any setting. In chapter 3 Levin describes how to teach the formulation of the clinical question. Asking the question starts the EBP process rolling, and it's not as simple as it sounds. Chapter 4 describes the basic skill of searching the literature, primarily by using the Internet. Levin is joined by librarian Helen Lane in writing this chapter. Chapter 5, also by Levin, covers the basics of synthesizing evidence or analyzing the results of many studies to come up with coherent themes and trends in evidence that point toward ways to improve practice. The following chapters provide two different ways to teach students to understand and critically appraise systematic reviews of evidence, based on qualitative (chapter 6) and quantitative (chapter 7) approaches. In chapter 6, Panniers addresses the vexing issue of how to summarize evidence derived from qualitative studies. She makes the case that while meta-analysis has been an effective approach to summarizing quantitative studies, the voices of the patient, clinicians, consumer interest groups, and others have not been heard. Until recently the rich information that comes from qualitative studies largely has been excluded from the decision-making process; however, meta-synthesis has begun to change that. Because of this approach to summarizing evidence, qualitative research is beginning to inform nursing practice.

In chapter 7 Barnes and Levin advocate for meta-analysis as an important way to summarize evidence from quantitative studies. They share experiences they have had teaching research to nursing students and clinicians, as they endeavor to make the complex concepts of meta-analysis understandable to these learners. They have achieved some success using the age-old advice of meeting the students where they are, using either mathematical or conceptually oriented ways to convey the material. By using numerous clinical examples when presenting content on the method of meta-analysis, and involving learners in the interactive critique of studies on topics that interest them, the authors have been able to facilitate the learning of this complex topic.

The next two chapters look at protocols from two aspects: creation and assessment. Rich and Newland, two experienced nurse practitioners who have developed numerous protocols for clinical practice, emphasize the process of evidence-based clinical protocol development for teaching advanced practice nurses. They use the Apgar score used at infant birth to make the point that it is important to develop clinical protocols that will lead to the most favorable outcome—a 10. In chapter 9, Levin and Shortridge-Baggett share their experiences in teaching the appraisal of extant practice protocols in order to determine whether they are evidence-based. Although similar in intent, the learning activities described are differentiated between undergraduate and graduate students. The authors further detail the range of outcomes, both expected and unanticipated, in teaching research using an EBP approach.

Finally, Fineout-Overholt does not disappoint us in her discussion in chapter 10 of measuring educational outcomes. She says that "evaluation of outcomes is integral to best practice," and we could not agree more with that statement. How else will you know if you are successful in your teaching and that the learner has learned? Fineout-Overholt describes levels of evaluation, the infrastructure needed to support evaluation, and how to plan for evaluation from the beginning. She then discusses three areas of evaluation: educator, learner, and program. Sound familiar? Educators have been doing this forever, yet how often do we take the time to review evaluation instruments for continued fit with our philosophy and mission? How well do we use the outcomes to inform our practice as educators? If we don't know how we are having impact on the learning process, how can we improve what we do? These kinds of questions are addressed in this chapter. Last, five examples of evaluation instruments are shared.

Chapter 3

Teaching Students to Formulate Clinical Questions: Tell Me Your Problems and Then Read My Lips

Rona F. Levin

> Instruction begins when you the teacher learn from the learner;
> put yourself in his place so that you may understand . . . what
> he learns and the way he understands it.
> —Soren Kierkegaard

The literature on EBP does a wonderful job of helping students and clinicians to formulate focused clinical questions (e.g., Nolan, Fineout-Overholt, & Stephenson, 2004; Sackett, Straus, Richardson, Rosenberg, & Haynes, 2000). When teaching the novice about clinical problems, however, we need to meet the students where they are at the moment, that is, in their practice settings and not necessarily knowing how to identify the problems that exist. We also need to keep in mind as teachers that although it may be easy for us to put clinical problems in the format of a focused, searchable question, this is a skill that takes nurturing and practice. Therefore, I believe there are at least two steps of cognitive activities that need to occur prior to asking students to formulate focused, searchable clinical questions: identification and clarification. We can form a teaching trajectory or process to teach this material, which leads eventually to the focused, searchable question. The steps are:

- Problem identification

- Problem clarification

- Problem focus

PROBLEM IDENTIFICATION

Somewhere along the path of my teaching career, I came across a principle that I am sure we have all happened upon: Start where you find the student! I cannot remember where or when I heard or read it or who authored the saying but I have always put it to good use. In terms of helping students to identify clinical problems, it means letting them tell you what is on their minds about their clinical experience in their own words as a first step in formulating a focused, searchable question.

Engaging students in a discussion of problems they are encountering in the practice setting creates the practical link between the content you are teaching and how that content relates to students' daily clinical experience. Thus, this is where we begin. As part of an introductory class or as an out-of-class assignment, depending on the length of class, have students describe in a paragraph a clinical problem they are experiencing in their setting. (The exercise may also be done as an online teaching strategy using a discussion board with students and instructor or via e-mail with the instructor.) This activity allows students to first describe their clinical problem in their own words, an easy first step in the identification-clarification-focus format. Such an exercise also helps you as the instructor to assess students' current thinking about clinical problems and how much time needs to be devoted to helping them clarify their clinical problems, which is the next step.

Several years ago, one of my service colleagues attended the class I taught on identifying clinical problems. Each student had written a paragraph describing a problematic situation in their practice for homework and was now reading it aloud to the rest of the class. My service colleague was quite impressed with the students' ability to describe practice problems "in their own words." And while the students themselves had thought about what they wrote in the past, they never took pen to paper to articulate their thinking—a first and necessary step preceding clarification and focus.

PROBLEM CLARIFICATION

Once students are able to describe a clinical problem, the next step is to clarify their thinking about it. One of the ways to approach the clarification task is through Socratic dialogue between student and teacher. An abbreviated example of the use of this approach is as follows:

> I recently had the opportunity of introducing EBP to nurses in a hospital setting as part of a pilot study to test the success of EBP educational interventions. Using the Socratic method, I asked the nurses to describe what they considered a problem on their unit. One of the nurses replied, "Patient satisfaction." I then asked, "How is patient satisfaction a problem?" The nurse went on to say that patients complained about noise on the unit. "Ah," I said, "are you having a problem with noise on the unit?" "Yes," she responded, "noise is the problem." Once noise was identified as the problem, we could proceed to looking at patient outcomes that noise was affecting, patient satisfaction being one. Other outcomes we discussed were sleep/rest patterns and pain. The focused, searchable question was evolving.

Another way to approach the task of clarifying the clinical problem is through group discussion, whether face-to-face or electronically through interactive dialogue. An electronic interactive assignment might include students' providing a transcript of the dialogue they have had with at least one other classmate or colleague about their identified clinical problem, providing the focused question that results from that dialogue.

PROBLEM FOCUS

Now it is time to help students formulate the focused, clinical question that will guide the search for evidence. In their chapter "Asking Compelling Clinical Questions" (see Box 3.1), Nollan, Fineout-Overholt, and Stephenson (2004) do a wonderful job of providing question templates for asking PICO questions (i.e., population, intervention, comparison intervention, and outcome; see chapter 1) related to therapy, etiology diagnostic tools, prevention, prognosis, and harm. Their chapter also includes clinical scenarios, which may be used as an exercise to give

Box 3.1
Question Templates for Asking PICO Questions

THERAPY

In _____, what is the effect of _____ on _____ compared with _____?

ETIOLOGY

Are _____ who have _____ at _____ risk for/of _____ compared with _____?

DIAGNOSIS OR DIAGNOSTIC TEST

Are (Is) _____ more accurate in diagnosing _____ compared with _____?

PREVENTION

For _____ does the use of _____ reduce the future risk of _____ compared with _____?

PROGNOSIS

Does _____ influence _____ in patients who have _____?

MEANING

How do _____ diagnosed with _____ perceive _____?

From R. Nollan, E. Fineout-Overholt, & P. Stephenson, 2004, p. 31.

students practice in formulating focused questions before they tackle their own. Of course, depending on the students' clinical focus or nurses' current practice specialties, you may wish to develop your own clinical scenarios so that they are more relevant for your particular audience. Once students have clarified their clinical problem and are able to articulate the intervention or diagnosis of interest, the outcome or outcomes in which they are interested, and the population in which the problem exists, I then challenge them to put all this information in the appropriate PICO or PCD (see Boxes 3.1 and 3.2) format.

To review, the PICO format includes the client *population* of interest; the *intervention*, which can be a treatment, exposure to disease or risk

Box 3.2
Question Template for PCD Questions

In _____ who exhibit _____ what are the possible
nursing diagnoses to consider?

From R. F. Levin, M. Lunney & B. Miller, 2005.

behavior, or prognostic variable; a *comparison,* which may include an
alternate or standard therapy, absence of risk or prognostic factor, or
alternate prognostic variable; and the *outcome* of interest. The PCD
format stands for *population* of interest, the observed *cues* or *cue cluster,*
and the *differential* diagnoses (see chapter 1 for an explanation of these
terms). Box 3.3 and Box 3.4 provide sample exercises for developing
questions in a PICO format in an acute care setting and a home-care
setting, respectively. To view a sample clinical scenario, for developing
a PCD question, please refer to chapter 15.

As I introduce the question templates to students, I say, "Read my
lips!" At one time, I thought that by using this approach students would
simply be able to fill in the blanks and immediately have a beautifully
focused, searchable question. I have learned, however, that not everyone
is able to lip-read; apparently that is also a skill to be learned. Sometimes
it takes several conversations or electronic dialogues before students have
the appropriate question to guide their evidence search. Therefore, I have
students submit their focused clinical question by e-mail or on a discussion
board to obtain instructor and peer feedback prior to the next class or
before beginning an evidence search. As you can see, another of the
principles on which I base my teaching is that students need to master
the foundation before they can build the house. Using this approach,
students should be able to have a focused clinical question, which will
lead them to the next step in the EBP process, in 1 or 2 weeks.

The teaching trajectory and strategies for helping students learn how
to identify, clarify, and focus clinical questions is especially important if
their work on formulating questions is a prelude to a term paper or
assignment, which includes synthesizing evidence on a clinical question
and coming to a conclusion about its application in practice. In my
experience unless students have the appropriate and guiding question,
they may get lost along the way. More often than I would like to admit,
students have retrieved studies that do not belong in the same evidence
base or retrieved irrelevant studies. Therefore, before students proceed
with the next steps of EBP, they must have developed the focused, searchable question, the foundation from which to build their house of answers.

Box 3.3
Evidence-Based Practice Exercise: Formulating Searchable, Answerable Clinical Questions (Acute Care)

Scenarios and Question Templates for Asking PICO Questions*

Purpose: To practice formulating various types of clinical questions in order to locate evidence that will provide answers.

Questions of Therapy

"Urinary tract infection is the most common hospital acquired infection" (Brosnahan, Jull, & Tracy, 2004). You note that the number of UTIs in patients who have had urethral catheters for short-term voiding problems on your unit is 20% over the benchmark. The protocol for catheter insertion and care includes use of sterile technique for catheter insertion and hygienic procedures. You have read that there are a variety of catheters available and wonder if one kind is better than another for reducing the incidence of infection. You decide to search the literature to find the best evidence to answer this question.

In _____, what is the effect of _____ on _____ compared with _____?

Questions of Secondary Prevention

Recent quality assurance studies show that the percentage of falls in your hospital has increased steadily over the passed year. You know that falls are particularly prevalent in patients over the age of 65. The protocol for fall prevention in your agency includes such precautions as keeping side rails up at specific times with specific clients, referral to physical therapy (PT) by a physician when indicated, and explaining to patients when and how to use the call button when necessary. You wonder if there are other preventative nursing measures you can provide to your patients that would decrease falls, especially among elderly patients. You decide to search the literature to determine if there is evidence to support the effectiveness of a program of risk assessment and intervention and what that might include.

For _____, does the introduction of _____ reduce the risk of _____ compared with _____?

Box 3.3 (continued)

Questions of Prognosis

One of your patients is a 55-year-old woman who recently had a myocardial infarction. She smokes at least one pack of cigarettes a day. Although she has been admonished by her primary care physician to stop smoking, she has not stopped. You know you have an obligation to discuss smoking cessation with your patient and its effects on her health status and want to provide the best evidence to her of the relationship between smoking and heart disease.

Does _____ **influence** _____ **in clients who** _____?

*Adapted from R. Nollan, E. Fineout-Overholt, & P. Stephenson, 2005.
Prepared by Rona F. Levin, PhD, RN, for a presentation to nursing staff in an acute care setting, December 8, 2004.

Box 3.4
Evidence-Based Practice Exercise: Formulating Searchable, Answerable Clinical Questions (home care)

Scenarios and Question Templates for Asking PICO Questions*

Purpose: To practice formulating various types of clinical questions in order to locate evidence that will provide answers.

Questions of Therapy

You pay a home visit to a 75-year-old woman who has an indwelling catheter. A home health aide comes in every week day to assist this woman with her ADLs. Her daughter, who is a practical nurse, visits at least every 3 days at which time she changes the catheter. Over the past month this woman has had two urinary tract infections, which have been treated with courses of antibiotics. You wonder whether frequent catheter change may be responsible for the infections and decide to search the literature to find the best evidence to answer this question.

In _____, what is the effect of _____ on _____ compared with _____?

Questions of Secondary Prevention

Recent OASIS reports show that the percentage of falls in your region of the long-term-care division has increased steadily over the past year. You have read that at least 30% of people over 65 who live independently in the community fall each year (Gillespie, Gillespie, Robertson, Lamb, Cumming, & Rowe, 2003). You know there is a protocol for fall prevention in your agency, which mainly involves referral to physical therapy (PT) by a physician. You wonder if there are preventative nursing measures you can provide to your clients other than referral to PT. You decide to search the literature to determine if there is evidence to support the effectiveness of a program of home hazard assessment and modification and what that might include.

For _____, does the introduction of _____ reduce the risk of _____ compared with _____?

Box 3.4 (continued)

Questions of Prognosis

One of your clients is a 55-year old woman who recently had a myocardial infarction. She smokes at least one pack of cigarettes a day. Although she has been admonished by her primary care physician to stop smoking, she has not stopped. You know that you have an obligation to discuss smoking cessation with your client and its effects on her health status and want to provide the best evidence to her of the relationship between smoking and heart disease.

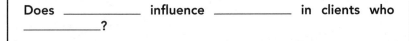

Does _____ **influence** _____ **in clients who** _____?

---

*Adapted from R. Nollan, E. Fineout-Overholt, & P. Stephenson, 2005.
Prepared by Rona F. Levin, PhD, RN, for presentation to nursing staff at the Visiting Nurse Service of New York, October 25, 2004.

REFERENCES

Brosnahan, J., Jull, A., & Tracy, C. (2004). Types of urethral catheters for management of short-term voiding problems in hospitalized adults. *The Cochrane database of systematic reviews 2004*, Issue 1, Art. No. CD004013.pub2. DOI: 10.1002/14651858.CD004013.pub.2.

Gillespie, L. D., Gillespie, W. J., Robertson, M. C., Lamb, S. E., Cumming, R. G., & Rowe, B. H. (2004). Interventions for preventing falls in elderly people (Cochrane Review). *Cochrane Library*, Issue 3. Chichester, UK: Wiley.

Levin, R. F., Lunney, M., & Krainovich-Miller, B. (2004, October–December). Improving diagnostic accuracy using an evidence-based nursing model. *International Journal of Nursing Terminologies and Classification, 15*(4), 114–122.

Nollan, R., Fineout-Overholt, E., & Stephenson, P. (2004). Asking compelling clinical questions. In B. M. Melnyk & E. Fineout-Overholt (Eds.), *Evidence-based practice: A guide to best practice* (pp. 25–37). Philadelphia: Lippincott Williams & Wilkins.

Sackett, D. L., Straus, S. E., Richardson, W. S., Rosenberg, W., & Haynes, R. B. (2000). *Evidence-based medicine* (2nd ed.). Edinburgh, Scotland: Churchill Livingstone.

Chapter 4

Strategies to Teach Evidence Searching: It Takes a Library

Rona F. Levin and Helen T. Lane

> I never teach my pupils; I only attempt to provide the conditions in which they can learn.
> —Albert Einstein

Directions for using electronic search engines abound. Shouldn't everyone, therefore, be able to follow instructions and complete their search for evidence? The answer to this question is no. Even the first author, as an experienced researcher and evidence searcher, needed help to understand fully and negotiate the electronic university databases in order to complete the most successful search. So, maybe the first principle for teaching this material is: No matter what your level of education or sophistication with the research process, you do not know as much about how to search for the answers to your questions as an instructional or reference librarian does. Thus the ideal approach to facilitate students' learning how to search for evidence is to collaborate with your instructional or reference librarian to develop the content and approach to teaching this content and process. Even better, ask an instructional or reference librarian to conduct the class with you. We have done this and the feedback from students, both in academic and clinical settings, has been positive. In fact, several nurses with master's degrees whom we have taught in their clinical settings have said they wished they had this class while they were in school working toward their degrees. And so with this introduction in mind, here are some basic strategies we use to teach nursing students and clinical nurses how to find the evidence to answer their burning clinical questions.

WHAT TO LOOK FOR FIRST

One of the espoused advantages of using an evidence-based approach to practice is that it saves time. One of the ways it saves time is that practitioners are taught to look for systematic reviews of evidence first, that is, before searching for primary single studies. Systematic reviews include meta-analyses (see chapter 7), meta-syntheses (see chapter 6) and integrative reviews of the literature. Systematic reviews are considered the best type of evidence if, of course, they meet the criteria for validity and source reliability. (See chapters 6 and 7 for guides on how to critique meta-syntheses and meta-analyses.) The point to make with students is that systematic reviews are the types of evidence to look for first. There is no need for the busy practitioner to search for and synthesize the findings of primary studies when a reputable and reliable source (e.g., the Cochrane Collaboration) has already done this. Of course, if a systematic review of evidence on the topic of interest does not exist, we then move to a search for other levels of evidence.

USING A FOCUSED, CLINICAL QUESTION TO GUIDE THE SEARCH

Rather than simply tell or show-and-tell students about available databases and how to access them, using a focused clinical question to guide a real search makes the class come alive. This learning activity is like going on a treasure hunt. And when a jewel or a piece of evidence turns up, so does the excitement. The initial question that guides the search should be one the educator and librarian have researched previously and that is related to the audience's practice area. In other words, those presenting the class know exactly where the jewels are hidden.

For example, we have used the following questions to show students how to access and search databases for a systematic review, knowing that there are meta-analyses to address them:

- In a population of older adults living in the community, does the introduction of a fall risk assessment and fall prevention program reduce the incidence and severity of falls?

- In a population of adult hospitalized patients, what is the effectiveness of silver-nitrate-impregnated urinary catheters compared with antibiotic-impregnated urinary catheters on the incidence of urinary tract infections?

A sample question for which no systematic review exists also may be used to help students access and negotiate databases for a more complicated search of other types of evidence.

CONNECTING TO THE INTERNET

There is no substitute for teaching search strategies using an Internet connection to an electronic library. The interaction this allows makes the search in real time much more interesting for students than showing PowerPoint slides of what databases look like or distributing handouts of Web pages. An added value is that students actually go through the specific steps they need to take to conduct a search. Using this strategy, we have found that students get involved in the process by offering suggestions for trying different terms or phrases to limit or expand the search.

If you have an electronic classroom in your institution where each student has his or her own computer, this is the ideal setting in which to conduct the class on searching for evidence. Not only can students follow the sample search being conducted by the instructor more easily, but they also can try out their own skills at searching. That is, after the formal part of class, give them a different focused question they can use to do their own search. We have found the formal presentation takes about an hour. If a 2-hour block of time is devoted to this content, then students can engage in the practice search independently during the second hour and share their findings with each other in a summary discussion.

FOCUSING ON MAJOR DATABASES

Knowing the best tools to use in searching for evidence is crucial to quality EBP, especially with the growing options (both reliable and unreliable) that exist on the Web and via online subscription databases.

We generally limit the introduction to databases during the sample search to what we call the big three: The Cochrane Database of Systematic Reviews, MEDLINE, and CINAHL. These are well-used resources that provide access to a range of useful evidence, including systematic reviews. Furthermore, your students are likely to encounter these databases no matter where their careers take them.

Although there are several other useful and trusted databases and organizations that are regularly used to search for evidence (see Box 4.1), we choose to limit our introductory presentation to the above three in order to provide more depth in the how-to of searching specific databases. Providing students with handouts of the other good sources for finding evidence or referring them to other written sources (e.g., Fineout-Over-holt, Nollan, Stephenson, & Sollenberger, 2005) that describe these data-bases works well and saves valuable class time. Our goal is to help students learn the search process in detail. For this they need a walk-through demonstration. Once students learn how to negotiate databases, all they need is a list of reliable evidence sources and Web sites to begin the treasure hunt.

If you are teaching a class for students in a formal academic program, they will have access to their school's electronic library and the databases to which their school's library subscribe. On the other hand, if you are teaching nurses or other health care providers in their home institution or at a continuing education conference, it is more helpful to show the audience how to navigate their own library's system. For example, at one continuing-education presentation we gave at a hospital, the second author contacted the medical librarian of that institution to find out what vendors and databases were available there and connected to that library for the class.

Many of your students will already be very familiar with searchable periodical indexes (aka, databases) such as MEDLINE. Even so, confusion can arise because most periodical databases exist in a variety of formats and computer interfaces, depending on the platform provided by the database vendor. For example, MEDLINE is available as a subscription database via EBSCO, ProQuest, and Ovid and also exists on the Web as PubMed. Students will frequently refer to a database by the name of the vendor. For example, they might say, "I found these articles searching OVID," rather than using the name of the database (e.g., CINAHL). Sometimes they are completely unaware of what databases they searched using the OVID or other similar platforms.

Having a frank discussion with your students regarding their research habits and knowledge, and discussing this with the librarian prior to any

Box 4.1
Useful Web Sites for Evidence Searching*

Database or Organization Web Site

CINAHL	http://www.cinahl.com
Cochrane Collaboration	http://www.cochrane.org
Embase	http://embase.com
Clinical Evidence	http://clinicalevidence.com
National Guidelines Clearinghouse (NGC)	http://www.guideline.gov
National Library of Medicine	http://www.nlm.nih.gov
PsycInfo	http://www.apa.org/psycinfo/
PubMed, MEDLINE	http://www.ncbi.nih.gov/entrez/query.fcgi
The Joanna Briggs Institute	http://www.joannabriggs.edu.au/pubs/best practice.php

Meta-Search Engines

Prime Evidence	http://www.primeanswers.org
TRIP+	http://www.tripdatabase.com
SUMSearch	http://sumsearch.uthscsa.edu

---

*Some of these databases are not searchable without a personal or library subscription. Others are free to search, but full-text articles are "pay-per-view." Without a personal or library subscription, only citations or abstracts may be available, not full text articles. With some databases, full text articles may be available for a fee to those who do not have a subscription.

hands-on workshop he or she is planning, will help the librarian prepare more fully for the specific group of students that will be taught. Most people have a tendency to stay within their comfort zone when doing research. Some questions you might ask your students are:

- When was the last time you did a substantial amount of research?

- What search tools or search engines did you use?

- How did you access these search tools or databases?

TEACHING SEARCH STRATEGIES AND TERMINOLOGY

With their "burning" clinical questions written out in PICO or PCD format (see chapter 1), students may be tempted to simply use the concepts in the question as the search terms. After all, isn't it best to be specific when looking for evidence? The answer is both yes and no.

The purposes of a PICO or PCD format for stating clinical questions is to help clarify and focus the question in one's own mind, and to create a clear picture of the evidence needs. Asking the right question is integral to database searching; however, it's a different story when communicating these needs to a computer and may entail using a different language.

Database search engines are very literal. The search terms you plug in are the only terms the search engine looks for. Moreover, as a rule, database search engines default to a search for *all* of your terms within the limits of the title, author, abstract, and subject headings of the articles indexed by that database. Therefore, if so much as one of your search terms is missing from *any* of these areas, you will receive no results from your search. This is true even if the term is used frequently within the text of the article. The Cochrane Library via Wiley is the exception to this rule because it defaults to searching the complete text.

In a piece she wrote for the journal *Evidence-Based Nursing*, Fleming (1998) suggests that in order to come up with a focused, searchable question, sometimes it is necessary to do a broader background search. We couldn't agree more. Our advice is to start with a broad search, and either narrow or expand it depending on the number of results you receive from your initial query. As the second author often advises when leading the library instruction workshops: "If you're fishing in unfamiliar waters, you should cast wide a net before you bait your line." In other words, see what's out there first, then go for what you really want.

Here are some tips on how to do this without sacrificing accuracy:

1. You can use the PICO-formatted question to generate a simpler, broader question. Do this by reducing the query to the intervention and the outcome alone. So, if the original PICO question is, *In adult patients with short-term voiding problems what is the effect of urethral catheter design compared with standard latex cathe-*

ters on the rate of urinary tract infection? the simplified question would be, *What is the effect of urethral catheter design on the rate of urinary tract infection?*

2.   Use this simple question and identify and generate search words by reducing it again to its main nouns. From the above example, your search words would be *urethral catheters* and *urinary tract infections*. These two phrases will comprise your initial, wide-net search. (The nouns *design* and *rate* are qualifying nouns.)

3.   Next, think of all the ways a person might write about these things. Someone writing about *urethral catheters* might refer to *urinary catheterization* or *indwelling catheters. Urinary tract infections* frequently are referred to as *UTIs.* Come up with as many synonymous or related terms and phrases as possible. Keep these on hand just in case your original search words don't bring back sufficient results.

4.   On the other hand, if your query results in too many database hits, then begin to narrow it by adding qualifying search terms. For instance, from the example above, you might add the term "design" or the phrase "short-term voiding."

5.   Take note of the database's preset limiters or refiners. Most databases offer the option to limit your results to certain types of publications and documents. For example, the Cochrane Library allows you to limit your results to reviews from the Cochrane Database of Systematic Reviews. MEDLINE allows you to limit to the document type, meta-analysis.

The following is an example of our teaching strategy using the Cochrane Library from Wiley InterScience, and a search within The Cochrane Database of Systematic Reviews using the suggestions above. (Please note that if you have access to the Cochrane databases via OVID, your search screen will look very different from the screen shots shown below.)

First, we advise students to go directly to the Advanced Search tool, and not let the word "advanced" fool them into thinking it will be difficult to use. The advanced search actually offers more guidance than the simple search, as well as more options for searching (see Figure 4.1). Enter each search word (or phrase) in a separate box, connected by AND. From the example above, the two main search phrases are "urethral catheters" and "urinary tract infections" (see Figure 4.2). Scroll down and take a look at the preset limiters. Under "Restrict Search by Product, select The Cochrane Database of Systematic Reviews (see Detail 1 of Figure 4.2). After you hit the search button, your results page should appear. In this particular search, we received 31 results (in Figure 4.3). This is certainly

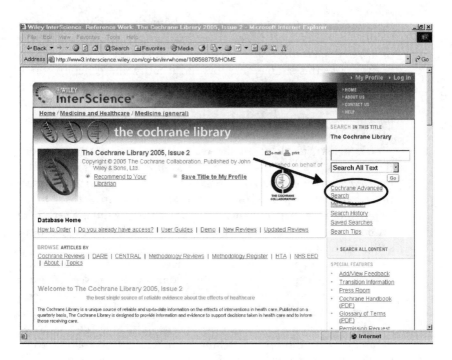

FIGURE 4.1   Cochrane Library Home Page via Wiley Interscience

a small enough number that you easily could browse the results to find if there is a meta-analysis that fits your query.

For the sake of demonstration, however, let's add a qualifying search term or phrase, like "design" or "short-term voiding." Note that the problem searching with a word like "design," is that it is a common word with multiple uses and meanings, and therefore like to bring back inaccurate results. Unfortunately, so are the synonymous terms "models" and "types." As a general rule, avoid such words when using search engines. In order to add more words to your search, click on "Edit Search," circled in Figure 4.3. This will take you back to the Advanced Search page. Enter the phrase "short-term voiding" in the next box down. Use the drop-down menu to select "Search All Text" (see Figure 4.4). The new list of results has only 19 articles, which easily can be browsed (see Figure 4.5). It is important to note that no matter what database search engine you use, the more search terms you connect with AND, the fewer results you will receive. A systematic review relevant to the clinical question appears in the middle of the first page of results (see Figure 4.6). We found our treasure!

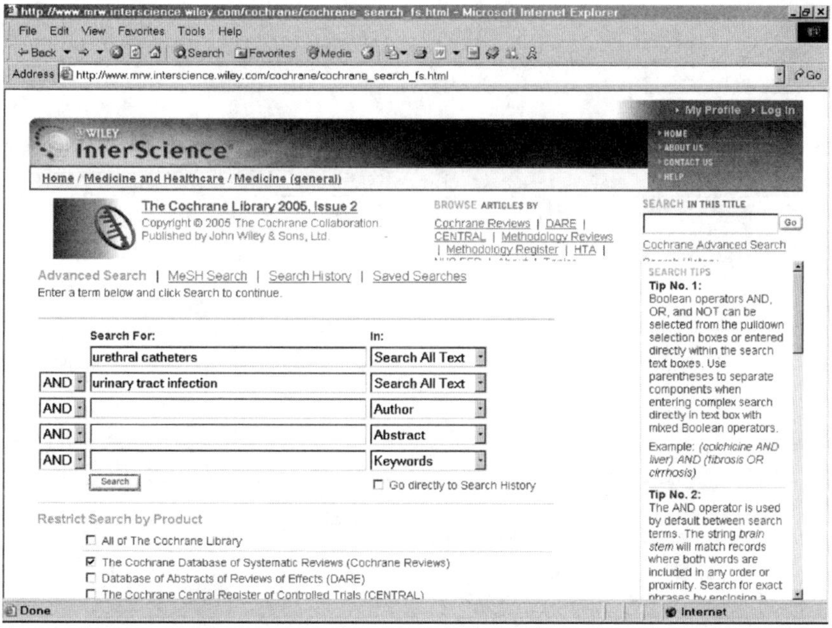

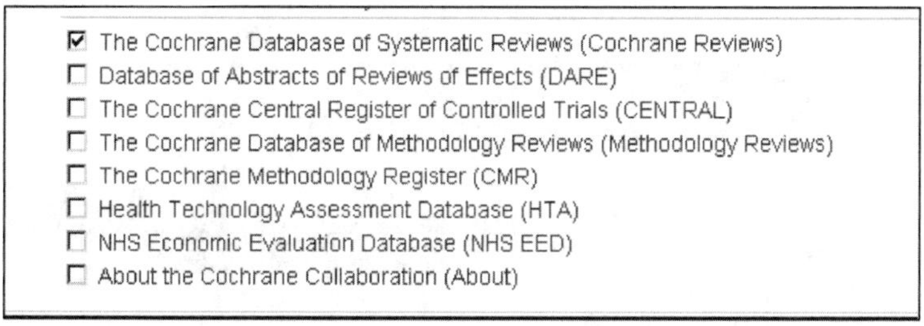

Figure 4.2, detail 1

FIGURE 4.2   Beginning an Advanced Search in Cochrane

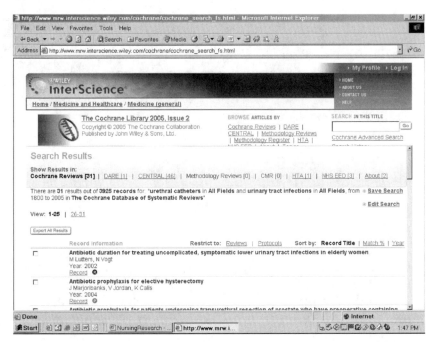

FIGURE 4.3 List of Studies Using Two Main Phrases from Clinical Question

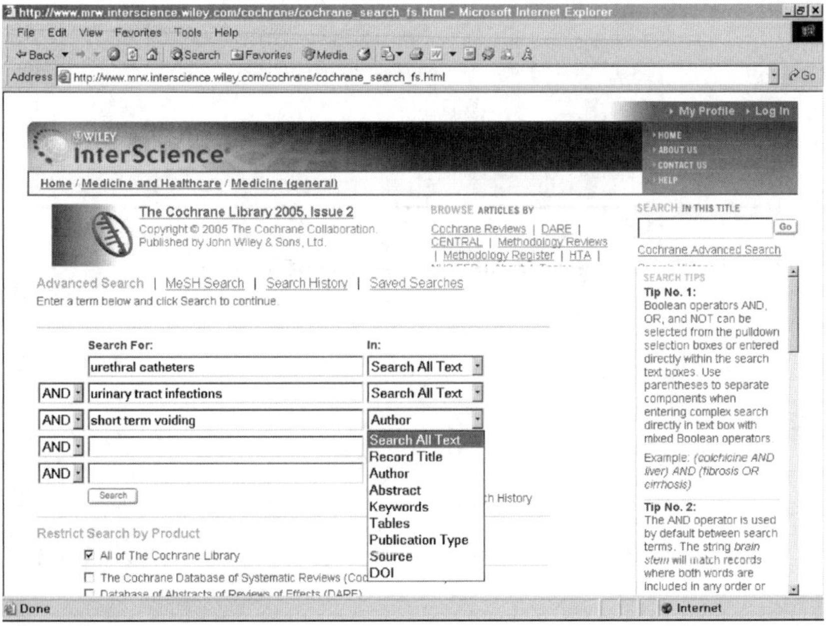

FIGURE 4.4 Advanced Search Using a Qualifying Term

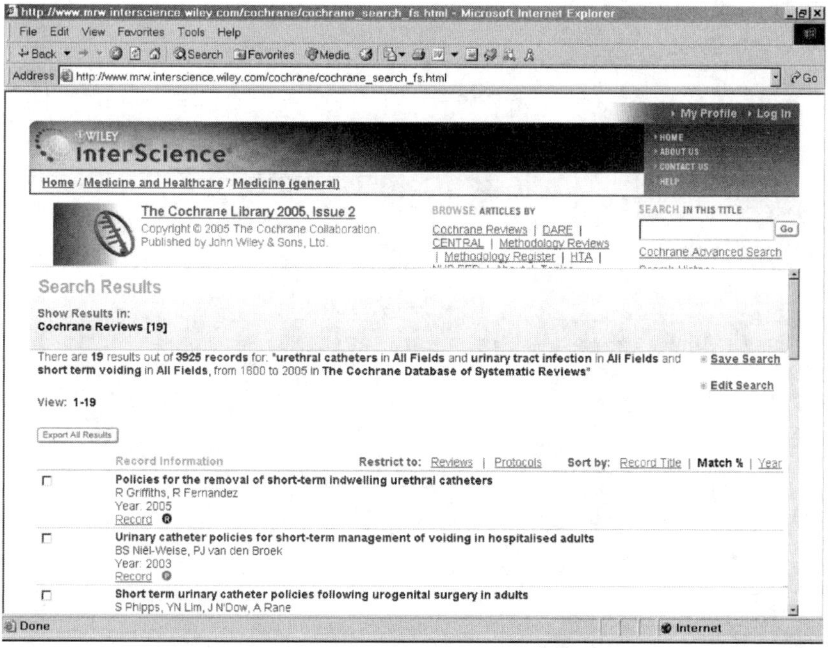

FIGURE 4.5   List of Studies Retrieved Adding a Qualifying Term

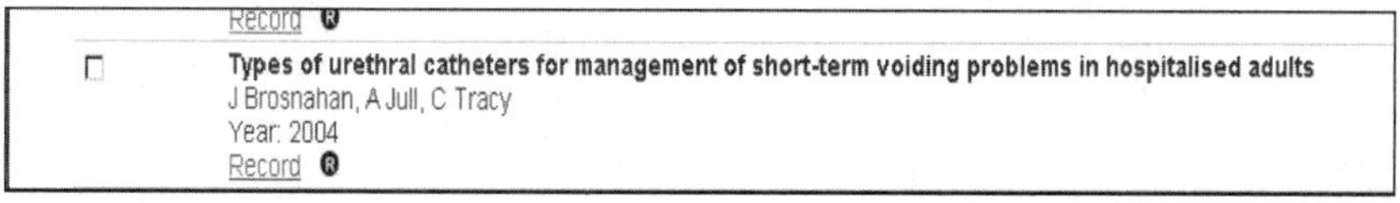

FIGURE 4.6   The Treasure Found

REFERENCES

Fineout-Overholt, E., Nollan, R., Stephenson, P., & Sollenberger, J. (2005). Finding relevant evidence. In B. M. Melnyk & E. Fineout-Overholt (Eds.), *Evidence-based practice in nursing and healthcare: A guide to best practice* (pp. 39–69). Philadelphia: Lippincott Williams & Wilkins.

Fleming, K. (1998). Notebook: Answering answerable questions. *Evidence-Based Nursing, 1*(2), 36–37.

Chapter 5

Synthesizing Evidence and Separating Apples From Oranges

Rona F. Levin

The one real object of education is to have a [person] in the
condition of continually asking questions.
—Bishop Mandell Creighton

Synthesizing evidence to answer a burning clinical question is a difficult
task for many of us, particularly students. So one of the first assignments
I give students in a graduate research course is to formulate a burning
clinical question and then find a sample of evidence that bears on this
question.

A major challenge we face as faculty is helping students to think
critically. The task of deciding whether or not research studies belong in
the same evidence-base, that is, are relevant to the clinical question being
asked, is a daunting one for many students. They seem to have particular
trouble identifying the specific protocol of an intervention (what we used
to call the operational definition) and the outcome variables of interest. When I started teaching a graduate research course from an EBP

perspective, I thought this learning task would be one of the simpler ones. I was wrong.

I realized the error of my thinking when students began showing me articles to approve for an assignment on finding evidence that was relevant to their clinical question. More often than not, neither the independent (e.g., intervention, prognostic factor, risk factor) nor dependent (outcome) variables in several studies matched. Many students went through this process several times before they understood that if one is trying to find related articles on treatment effectiveness, at the very least the treatment needed to be the same in all of the studies.

After students learn how to identify clinical problems and focus clinical questions, they need to find the evidence that bears on that clinical question. The first step is for students to access the abstracts of the studies they find. Based on the abstract, they are to determine whether or not the dependent or outcome variables and independent or treatment variables in the studies are the same, similar, or not related at all. If they determine the latter to be the case, then they know the study is not relevant and there is no need to access the entire study.

I ask them to show me three abstracts they believe are relevant to their clinical question. If I approve the abstract, then they retrieve the full study. If I see that the abstract is not relevant to their question, I direct them to search further. This is an essential first step to point students in the right direction for finding the appropriate evidence for their clinical question. If students do not complete this portion of the assignment correctly, they cannot possibly write a coherent paper synthesizing the relevant evidence on a clinical problem and determining its readiness for application to practice.

LEARNING ACTIVITY 1:
APPLES OR APPLES AND ORANGES?

As part of a class prior to directing students to find evidence on a clinical problem, I use the following interactive exercise to help them determine whether or not studies belong in the same evidence base, that is, to differentiate apples from apples and oranges. Students read the abstracts of two studies in class. I choose to have them read the abstracts in class because when I previously assigned two entire studies for students to read prior to class, they rarely completed the assignment. By using the abstracts only, students are able to read the material in 5 to 10 minutes during break or class time. You may use either the abstracts of actual studies, write your own abstracts of actual studies, or create fictional abstracts. I have found that using the latter two approaches allows you to incorporate all the relevant details needed for students to judge the comparability of studies. Also, I choose two abstracts that do not belong in the same evidence base.

After reading the abstracts, I ask students to identify the following components for each study:

- Clinical problem as identified by the author(s)

- Dependent variable(s) or outcome variable(s)

- Independent variable(s) or interventions/prognostic factors/risk factors

- Population being studied

Next, I ask students to make judgments about similarities and differences for each of these components by asking the following questions:

- Are the dependent or outcome variable(s) in each study the same, similar, or different? If similar, describe the variations.

- Are the independent variable(s) in each study the same, similar, or different? If similar, describe the variations.

- Is the population the same in each study?

- Is the clinical problem in each study the same, similar, or different?

After answering the first three questions, students are prepared to answer the last question in a PICO format, which I require them to do. Having the clinical question for each study in such a format makes the final question of the exercise much easier to answer: Do studies 1 and 2 belong in the same evidence base? Students should now be prepared to develop their own clinical questions and look for relevant, related evidence.

LEARNING ACTIVITY 2: ANSWERING A CLINICAL QUESTION

Before embarking on a full-blown synthesis of evidence, a product many faculty members require in a nursing research or other nursing course, students need to master the process. In order to do so, they need practice in synthesizing evidence on a small scale. Therefore, the first graded assignment in a nursing research course could consist of sampling three studies on a particular clinical question and learning how to critique an evidence base (i.e., critique the three studies as a whole rather than individually). Box 5.1 provides readers with the actual assignment I have used to accomplish this learning goal. As stated in the beginning of this chapter, students do not proceed with the assignment until they have (a) developed and I have approved their clinical question, and (b) accessed three studies that we have agreed are indeed all apples. Of course, they could all be oranges as well.

In addition to providing practice in learning the basic skills needed to develop a successful synthesis paper, I provide students with a sample paper demonstrating how to critique an evidence base. In the past I have used a paper I developed for this purpose. Currently, a colleague who teaches the graduate research course uses a synthesis paper written by Garrelts and Melnyk (2001), which is an excellent example of this type of paper (refer to Appendix A for the full article).

To summarize, the main purposes of this learning exercise are to help students develop skill in (1) finding the evidence to answer a burning clinical question; (2) critiquing an evidence base; and (3) determining whether or not the evidence justifies a change in practice. Providing students with learning exercises that give them practice in the above skills builds confidence in their ability and thus facilitates successful completion of a synthesis paper.

Box 5.1
Synthesizing Evidence on a Clinical Problem

Student Assignment

1. Select a *clinical nursing problem.*
   Example. You are working on a surgical unit and observe that patients who undergo certain types of surgical procedures are not achieving effective pain relief with regularly prescribed pain medication. What nursing interventions, other than administering analgesics, can be used to achieve effective pain relief in postoperative patients?
2. Identify the *outcome variable* of interest (dependent variable).
   In the above clinical problem, the outcome variable is postoperative pain.
3. Conduct a *literature search* focusing on research that addresses the effects of nursing interventions on postoperative pain.
4. Choose *at least three studies* that have a *similar problem* or *purpose.*
   An example is, "What is the effect of music on postoperative pain in a population of women who have had abdominal surgery?"
5. *Critically read* these studies to determine their scientific merit.
   Use the critique guidelines contained in the course syllabus.
6. *Write a 5 to 8 page, typed, double-spaced paper* that includes the following:
   (a) a narrative statement of the clinical nursing problem;
   (b) the burning clinical question in PICO format;
   (c) identification of studies reviewed;
   (d) summary of the evidence base (as per sample);
   (e) strengths and limitations of the evidence base;
   (f) how these limitations affect the readiness of the new intervention for use in clinical practice; and
   (g) a conclusion that addresses the state of the art on your topic.

(continued)

Box 5.1 (continued)

Teacher Evaluation Criteria

1. The clinical nursing problem is identified and is stated according to PICO (Population, Intervention, Comparison, Outcome) criteria.
   10%
2. The summary is succinct, yet includes sufficient information about the studies for the reader to determine their overall validity.
   30%
3. Strengths and limitations are accurately identified and related to application of findings in practice. (This section reflects the writer's knowledge of the research process and critiquing ability.)
   30%
4. The paper concludes with the writer's opinion about whether or not the findings are ready to be implemented in practice. Sufficient rationale is clearly presented in relation to the overall strengths and limitations of the research base.
   10%
5. The paper reflects clarity of thought, logical progression of ideas, and is grammatically correct.
   10%
6. The paper adheres to APA Guidelines.
   10%

REFERENCE

Garrelts, L., & Melnyk, B. M. (2001). Pacifier usage and acute otitis media in infants and young children. *Pediatric Nursing, 27,* 516–519.

Appendix A

Pacifier Usage and Acute Otitis Media in Infants and Young Children

Laurie Garrelts
Bernadette Mazurek Melnyk

Acute otitis media (AOM) is a commonly encountered pediatric illness that affects approximately 70% of children by 3 years of age, with one third experiencing more than three episodes (Pichichero & Cohen, 1997). AOM is the most frequent diagnosis for office visits in children under the age of 15 years and is the primary reason that children receive antibiotics (Andrews, 2001). The estimated cost of treatment for AOM in the United States is 8 billion dollars annually (Fitzgerald, 1999). If not properly treated, AOM can lead to hearing loss, middle ear disorders, and delayed speech development (Petersen-Smith, 2000). Simultaneously, overly aggressive treatment with antibiotics has led to increased antibiotic resistance in children (Fitzgerald, 1999).

Illness prevention through anticipatory guidance is an important element of pediatric primary health care. Therefore, clinicians should become familiar with the risk factors for AOM so that parents can be educated about prevention strategies. Studies have indicated that several variables increase the risk for AOM, including: (a) bottle feeding infants, (b) feeding infants in the supine position, (c) passive smoke exposure, (d) attendance at group child daycare, and most recently, (e) pacifier usage (Fitzgerald, 1999).

Pacifier use is a common practice, as it is estimated that approximately 75–85% of all children in western countries use or have used a pacifier (Victora, Behague, Barros, Olinto, & Weiderpass,

1997). Use of a pacifier is typically thought of as a comforting and harmless habit, with only a temporary effect on dentition and occlusion. However, this habit may not be as risk-free as once thought, as some researchers contend there is a relationship between otitis media (OM) and pacifier use in children (Niemela, Pihakari, Pokka, Uhari, & Uhari, 2000).

Clinical Question
Is there a relationship between pacifier usage and AOM in infants and young children?

Search for the Evidence
The search for evidence began by accessing the Medline database and entering the key words "otitis media" and "pacifier." These key words were combined using the term "and" and the search was limited to humans, the English language, and the years 1995 through 2001. Only four of the 10 articles located were studies that addressed pacifier usage and OM. Three articles were selected to be included as evidence in this report; the fourth article was excluded because it was an older publication that analyzed several risk factors for AOM.

The Evidence
Study #1. The purpose of the first study by Niemela and colleagues (2000) was to evaluate the association between pacifier use and the occurrence of AOM through an intervention that educated parents on restricting pacifier use in their infants and young children. This study was a randomized, controlled, prospective clinical trial that was conducted at 14 well-baby clinics in Oulu, Finland between December 1996 and February 1997. The clinics were paired according to their size and the area they served, after which one clinic from each pair was randomly assigned to either the experimental or control group.

A total of 484 healthy children less than 18 months old were included in this study. There were no statistically significant differences between the experimental and control group children at baseline on variables such as age, gender, daycare, history of AOM, adenoidectomy, tympanostomy, pacifier use, parental smoking, atopic eczema, and breastfeeding.

The educational intervention used in the study by Niemela and colleagues (2000) was delivered by clinic nurses and consisted of providing parents with verbal and written information about the adverse effects of pacifiers, including an increased

Laurie Garrelts, BSN, RN, is a Pediatric Nurse Practitioner/ Care of Children and Families Graduate Student, University of Rochester School of Nursing, Rochester, NY; and Staff Nurse, Neonatal Intensive Care Unit and Pediatric Emergency Department, Children's Hospital, University of Rochester Medical Center, Rochester, NY.

Bernadette Mazurek Melnyk, PhD, RN-CS, PNP, is Associate Dean for Research and Director, Center for Research & Evidence-Based Practice and Pediatric Nurse Practitioner Program, University of Rochester School of Nursing, Rochester, NY.

The *Evidence-Based Practice* section focuses on the search for and critique of the "best evidence" to answer challenging clinical questions so that the highest quality, up-to-date care can be provided to children and their families. To submit questions or obtain author guidelines, contact Bernadette Mazurek Melnyk, PhD, RN-CS, PNP; Section Editor; University of Rochester School of Nursing; 601 Elmwood Avenue; Box SON; Rochester, NY 14642; (716) 275-8903; bernadette_melnyk@urmc.rochester.edu risk for AOM, oral candidiasis, dental caries, and malocclusion. Nurses in the experimental clinics informed the parents that the need for sucking during the first 6 months is often great and reflexive, therefore, pacifiers may be used as often as necessary during this time period. However, parents were advised to limit pacifier usage after 6 months and discontinue its use after 10 months of age (Niemela et al., 2000). The parents who attended the control clinics received standard care, which did not include counseling or educational materials about pacifier usage.

Parents at both clinics were instructed to document the occurrence of AOM on a daily symptom sheet that they mailed to the clinic on a monthly basis. During this time period, if a child was evaluated by a physician for an illness, the parents also were instructed to have their physician write the child's diagnosis and medication prescribed on the daily symptom sheet. In addition, parents recorded the dates that pacifier usage by the child changed (e.g., a change from using a pacifier continuously to use only while falling asleep). The effect of the intervention on pacifier use was evaluated by calculating the time for which children over 6 months old used a pacifier continuously, only when falling asleep, or not at all during the monitoring period (Niemela et al., 2000).

Glossary of Terms

Randomized, controlled, prospective trial: A true experiment in which subjects are randomly assigned to either the experimental or control group and the outcomes are studied over time.

Independent variable: The variable that is thought to cause or influence a change in the dependent or outcome variable.

Dependent variable: The outcome variable.

Convenience sample: A sample that is obtained by convenience (i.e., the most readily available subjects to participate in the study).

Relative risk ratio: the probability of contracting the illness.

Confidence intervals: The range of values in which a population parameter lies.

$p = .01$: The probability that the study results are due to chance is 1 in 100.

$p < .05$: The probability that the study results are due to chance is less than 5 in 100.

External validity: The extent to which the results of a study can be generalized from the sample to the population.

Interrater reliability: The extent to which two raters assign the same ratings for a variable that is being measured.

Follow-up data collection was successful in 91% of the children who were enrolled in the study. Reasons for attrition were that five families

moved away geographically, and 45 families did not return the symptom sheets. The time frame in which monitoring of data occurred ranged from 1 to 6 months with a mean of 4.6 months.

Findings indicated that at the end of the study 68% of the children in the intervention group and 66.5% of the children in the control group were still using a pacifier. However, time spent using a pacifier continuously was significantly reduced for children in the intervention group. For intervention group children who were 6 to 10 months of age, they spent 35% of their monitoring time using pacifiers continuously compared to 48% in the control group (Niemela et al., 2000).

Study findings also indicated that the occurrence of AOM was 29% less in the group that received the intervention compared to the control group. In addition, the occurrence of AOM was 33% higher in the group of children who continuously used the pacifier when compared to those children that only used the pacifier when falling asleep or not at all. Based on their findings, Niemela and colleagues concluded that health care providers should encourage parents to terminate pacifier usage in infants after 10 months of age. The rationale provided was that an infant's physiologic need to suck is greatest in the first 6 months of life, and the incidence of AOM prior to 10 months is low (Niemela et al., 2000).

Study #2. Niemela, Uhari, and Mottonen (1995) used a prospective, correlational, longitudinal design to investigate the relationship between the independent variable of pacifier use and the dependent variable of AOM over a 15-month period of time. The convenience sample consisted of 845 White children attending a daycare center full-time in Oulu, Finland between March 1991 and June 1992. The ages of the children ranged from 0.25 to 7.24 years, with a mean age of 3.29 years and a mean monitoring time of 10 months, with a range of 1 to 15 months.

Parents of the children were asked to record daily signs and symptoms of infectious disease in their children on monthly symptom sheets. Visits to their primary care provider, along with the child's diagnosis, medications, and number of days absent from daycare also were to be recorded on the symptom sheets. In the last month of the study, parents were asked to complete a questionnaire addressing their child's use of a pacifier at the start of the study, number of months in which the pacifier was used during the monitoring period, number of adenoidectomies and tympanostomies, duration of breastfeeding, parental smoking practices, and social class of the parents. The authors did not indicate how many hours per day that a child needed to suck on a pacifier in order for them to consider the child a "pacifier user." The authors defined the dependent variable as more than three episodes of AOM during the monitoring period and controlled statistically for age and other possible confounding variables (i.e., parental smoking) in their analyses. Relative risk ratios and 95%

confidence intervals were used to determine if children who used pacifiers had a statistically significant higher occurrence of AOM than nonpacifier users.

Findings indicated that more than three episodes of AOM occurred in 29.5% of children younger than 2 years of age using pacifiers compared to 20.6% of children who were not using pacifiers (relative risk of 1.6). In children 2 to 3 years of age, the incidence of AOM was 30.6% in pacifier users and 13.2% in nonpacifier users (relative risk of 2.9), which was statistically significant ($p = .01$). In addition, the use of a pacifier led to a statistically significant increase in the annual rate of AOM in children less than 2 years old and in children 2–3 years of age (Niemela et al., 1995).

Niemela and colleagues (1995) concluded that their study supports the theory that the use of a pacifier is a risk factor for AOM, especially for recurrent attacks. These authors also suggested that pacifier usage should be restricted to the first 10 months of life, when the need for sucking is the greatest and AOM is uncommon. The authors did address some study limitations, such as the lack of consistent diagnostic criteria between physicians and the fact that all children attended a daycare center, where infection rates are high due to the close contact between many children. They stated that pacifier use may not be such a potent risk for children that do not attend daycare centers (Niemela et al., 1995).

Study #3. Jackson and Mourino (1999) also sought to examine the relationship between pacifier use in 200 children, ages 12 months of age or younger, and the incidence of OM. Since the authors used the general term of OM, it is unknown whether OM was used to indicate only AOM or both AOM and OM with effusion. The study was conducted at a pediatric practice that was part of a university medical center in Virginia. The mean age of the children in the study who had been diagnosed with at least one episode of OM was 8.3 months. Seventy-five percent of the sample was African American, 22% White, 2% Hispanic, and 0.5% Asian. Seventy-six percent of the parents were reported as having a low education level.

The authors reviewed the children's past medical records and recorded the number of episodes of OM experienced by each child. The diagnosis of OM was made by practitioners that employed similar criteria via physical exam coordinated with reports of signs and symptoms. In addition, parents or guardians completed a questionnaire that elicited data regarding pacifier habits, length of time the pacifier was used per day, daycare utilization, breastfeeding practices, bottle feeding, parental smoking, thumb sucking, and parental educational level. The authors defined a "pacifier user" as a child who sucked on a pacifier for more than 5 hours a day. The parent questionnaire and definition of pacifier use was based upon informa-

tion gleaned from previous pilot studies (Jackson & Mourino, 1999). Findings indicated that the prevalence of OM in pacifier users (36%) was larger than the prevalence of OM in nonpacifier users (23%) ($p < .05$). This association remained significant after controlling for other confounding variables (e.g., parental smoking). Children who used a pacifier were twice as likely to develop OM. There were no associations between OM and gender, race, breastfeeding, parental smoking, and parent education level. Based on their study's findings, the authors concluded that there is an increased risk for OM in children who use pacifiers versus those who do not. As a result of their findings, Jackson and Mourino (1999) suggest that parents should be encouraged to discontinue the use of pacifiers with their infants before 10 months of age.

Critique of the Evidence

A strength of all three of the studies reviewed was that they had large sample sizes, which provided sufficient power to detect statistically significant results (Brown, 1999). However, the samples used in the studies were not randomly selected. In addition, the first two studies were conducted with exclusively White children in Finland, and the third study's sample was predominately comprised of African American children whose parents had a low level of education. Therefore, external validity of these studies is weak, and caution must be used in generalizing the results of these studies to other populations, such as those comprised of varied ethnicity and social classes (Brown, 1999).

Each study provided a detailed methodology section with a concise description of their research design. Although there is a paucity of research pertaining to this topic, Jackson and Mourino (1999) provided background information and a thorough literature review.

The first study by Niemela and colleagues (2000) was a randomized, prospective, controlled clinical trial, the strongest design for testing cause and effect relationships (Polit & Hungler, 1999). Although the investigators were not able to use true random assignment, they used cluster randomization to allocate the well-baby clinics to study groups in order to decrease the probability of contamination between the intervention and standard care groups. Because the second and third studies used correlational designs, findings only support that there is a relationship between pacifier usage and OM, not that pacifier usage causes OM.

A strength of the first two studies also is that both employed prospective designs, which are generally stronger than a retrospective design, as used by Jackson and Mourino (1999) (Polit & Hungler, 1999). Since the third study used a retrospective chart review, the authors were unable to determine if the pacifier habit had occurred before, concurrently, or after the first episode of OM (Jackson & Mourino, 1999). All three studies relied upon pa-

58

rental completion of symptom sheets or questionnaires for their data collection. As a result, parent self-report may have resulted in "response bias," as subjects may have distorted their answers to provide more favorable responses, which may have led to inaccurate study results (Polit & Hungler, 1999). In addition, parent reporting of symptoms may not be a valid strategy for documenting the incidence of AOM, which is a major limitation of the first two studies. All three studies reviewed also relied heavily upon parental memory of infant pacifier-sucking patterns, which may not be accurate. However, only Jackson and Mourino (1999) recognized this issue as an inherent limitation of their study.

Jackson and Mourino (1999) were the only researchers who attempted to develop some form of interrater reliability in their study in that they developed a predefined set of criteria for OM on which physicians were to base their diagnosis. These researchers also used pilot studies to test their questionnaires. No information is provided regarding the validity or reliability of the data collection methods used in either the Niemela et al. (2000) or Niemela et al. (1995) studies. However, a strength of all three studies is that each used appropriate statistical measures to analyze their data.

Future studies should use random samples that are heterogeneous and representative of the population at large so that results may be generalized. In addition, more valid and reliable methods for documenting episodes of AOM should be used in future research on this topic.

Implications for Practice

OM is a common pediatric illness that can have significant complications, such as hearing loss and speech delay. Therefore, it is critical for pediatric nurses and other pediatric health care providers to have knowledge regarding factors that may increase risk for AOM in children. Based on the studies reviewed, evidence is accumulating to indicate that there is a relationship between substantial pacifier usage (i.e., continuous usage or usage more than 5 hours per day) and AOM in infants and young children. Therefore, it is important to assess the extent to which parents use pacifiers with their infants at routine well-child care visits early in infancy and to educate parents regarding the potential for increased risk of AOM with substantial pacifier usage, especially after 6 to 10 months of age.

Simultaneously, parents need to be educated about the mechanism by which pacifier usage may contribute to AOM. Specifically, sucking on a pacifier lifts the soft palate in the mouth causing the contraction of the tensor veli palatine muscle. Contraction of this muscle results in the Eustachian tube becoming actively patent and provides an ideal medium for bacteria and viruses from the nasopharynx to be swept into the middle ear (Jackson & Mourino, 1999). In addition, sucking on a pacifier increases the amount of saliva in the mouth, which is an excellent medium for microorganisms. Thumbsucking, on the other hand, has not been shown to produce this same pathophysiological mechanism, and studies have not supported its relationship to AOM (Niemela et al., 1995).

If parents are using pacifiers with their young infants continuously or with their infants who are older than 10 months of age, they should not be made to feel guilty about this practice. Instead, sensitive interventions that support these parents in gradually weaning their children from the pacifier are needed. Nurse practitioners and nurses are in an ideal position to routinely incorporate assessment and appropriate anticipatory guidance related to pacifier usage with parents of young infants. Early intervention is important in that it could prevent costly physical, psychological, and financial negative outcomes associated with OM in children.

References

Andrews, J.S. (2001). Otitis media and otitis externa. In R.A. Hoekelman (Ed.), *Primary pediatric care* (pp. 1702–1706). St. Louis: Mosby.

Brown, S.J. (1999). *Knowledge for health care practice: A guide to using research evidence.* Toronto: W.B. Saunders.

Fitzgerald, M.A. (1999). Acute otitis media in an era of drug resistance: Implications for NP practice. *The Nurse Practitioner, 24*(10), 10–14.

Jackson, J.M., & Mourino, A.P. (1999). Pacifier use and otitis media in infants twelve months of age or younger. *Pediatric Dentistry, 21,* 256–260.

Niemela, M., Pihakari, O., Pokka, T., Uhari, M., & Uhari, M. (2000). Pacifier as a risk factor for acute otitis media: A randomized, controlled trial of parental counseling. *Pediatrics, 106,* 483–488.

Niemela, M., Uhari, M., & Mottonen, M. (1995). A pacifier increases the risk of recurrent acute otitis media in children in daycare centers. *Pediatrics, 96,* 884–888.

Petersen-Smith, A.M. (2000). Ear disorders. In C.E. Burns, M.A. Brady, A.M. Dunn, & N.B. Starr (Eds.), *Pediatric primary care: A handbook for nurse practitioners* (2nd ed.) (pp. 783–806). Philadelphia: W.B. Saunders Co.

Pichichero, M., & Cohen, R. (1997). Shortened course of antibiotic therapy for acute otitis media, sinusitis and tonsillopharyngitis. *Pediatric Infectious Disease, 16,* 680–695.

Polit, D.F., & Hungler, B.P. (1999). *Nursing research: Principles and methods* (6th ed.). New York: Lippincott.

Victora, C.G., Behague, D.P., Barros, F.C., Olinto, M.T., & Weiderpass, E. (1997). Pacifier use and short breast-feeding duration: Cause, consequence, or coincidence? *Pediatrics, 99,* 445–453.

Chapter 6

Teaching Meta-Synthesis: Summarizing Qualitative Research

Teresa L. Panniers

As knowledge increases, wonder deepens.

—Charles Morgan

Traditionally, the EBP movement has focused primarily on quantitative evidence, that is, meta-analyses of a clinical problem in medicine, nursing, and health care. Miller and Crabtree (2000) describe the randomized control trial (RCT) as having high internal validity but having almost no information about context. They also describe the quantitative RCT as being "heard from one voice" and in exclusion of "the cacophonous music of patients, clinicians, insurance companies, lawyers, government regulatory bodies, consumer interest groups, community agencies, office staff, corporate interests, and family turmoil" (p. 613). Although meta-analytic studies go a long way to synthesizing information for decision making by both health care providers and patients, missing is the rich information, which is also important to health care decision making, that is provided by studies conducted in the qualitative domain of research. Qualitative evidence offers nurses access to a rich source of information, generally provided from the *insider's view* to assist in health care decision-making processes. We need answers to all types of clinical questions, those that need quantitative evidence to provide answers and those that need qualitative or contextual evidence to provide answers. The kind of question one asks determines the appropriate evidence to answer the question, whether it is quantitative or qualitative.

In the last two decades, health care practitioners have increasingly recognized the importance of examining the experiences of life from the *insider's view* (Paterson, Thorne, Canam, & Jillings, 2001). This qualitative research uses in-depth, open-ended interviews with individuals who volunteer to tell an investigator about their experiences and to inform practitioners about their health care needs. Although qualitative researchers have conducted studies on a plethora of phenomena, there remains a need to synthesize these findings in a coherent manner so that we can better understand the implications of this knowledge for health care practice (Paterson et al., 2001).

Although there is a rich history of high quality primary qualitative research studies available to inform nursing practice, the availability of studies on clinical topics that have been summarized in a systematic way is relatively new. Sandelowski, Docherty, and Emden (1997) state that in order for qualitative findings to have an impact on health care policy, the qualitative primary studies will need to be interpreted in a larger context and presented in a way that makes the information usable for health care practice. One means of accomplishing this effort is through the use of a technique called qualitative meta-synthesis.

QUALITATIVE META-SYNTHESIS TO GUIDE PRACTICE

As noted, qualitative meta-syntheses are a relatively new entry to the scientific literature available to nurses. Even the term *qualitative meta-synthesis* is not used consistently in the literature. *Qualitative meta-synthesis* has been used to describe the method of summarizing qualitative findings so that they may be viewed in a larger interpretive context and presented in an accessible and usable form for practicing nurses (Sandelowski et al., 1997). The most comprehensive view of the synthesis of qualitative research studies is described by Paterson and colleagues (2001) as meta-study, "a research approach involving analysis of the theory, methods, and findings of qualitative research and the synthesis of these insights into new ways of thinking about phenomena" (p. 1). They use the term meta-synthesis, but in a more narrow sense, as the synthesis phase that follows the analysis of the findings, methods, and theory of qualitative research reports and that result in the generation of new and more complete understandings of the phenomenon under study. In this chapter, the term qualitative meta-synthesis is used to describe the process of analyzing primary qualitative research studies and synthesizing findings to provide a comprehensive, new understanding of how individuals experience illness and perceive their health care needs.

LOCATING QUALITATIVE META-SYNTHESES IN THE SCIENTIFIC LITERATURE

When considering methods of teaching students to become informed consumers of the evidence from qualitative research, a search of the scientific databases seems a good place to start for obtaining information. To demonstrate this process, I searched MEDLINE (1996 to November Week 3, 2004) and CINAHL (1982 to December Week 2, 2004) using the keywords *qualitative* and *meta-synthesis*; this search revealed 18 and 20 citations, respectively. The majority of the studies located were actual meta-syntheses, with a few articles devoted to didactic information related to conducting a qualitative meta-synthesis or related to understanding the state of the art in the area of qualitative meta-synthesis. Examples of topics covered in the retrieved sources include HIV-positive women (Sandelowski & Barroso, 2003b), nonvocal ventilated patients (Carroll, 2004b), and patients experiencing breast cancer (Arman & Rehnsfeldt, 2003). This simple, uncomplicated search strategy is but one type of search, yet the resultant number of studies found by this search highlights how relatively new qualitative meta-syntheses are in the scientific literature.

TEACHING STUDENTS TO BE INFORMED CONSUMERS OF QUALITATIVE META-SYNTHESES

Getting Started

Once a qualitative meta-synthesis related to a specific health care problem (such as maternal HIV infection [Sandelowski & Barroso, 2003b]) has been identified, students can begin to critique the value of the information provided in the meta-synthesis. To assist students in this critique, I use a list of questions, adapted from the work of Paterson and colleagues (2001), to help them evaluate the value of the qualitative meta-synthesis. Questions such as the appropriateness of the research question posed by the researcher to guide the meta-synthesis are included. Also, students should ask how effective the search strategy for primary studies was and how well the inclusion and exclusion criteria were chosen and adhered to by the author of the qualitative meta-analysis. Students should evaluate how well the researcher critically appraised the strengths and limitations of the primary studies included in the meta-synthesis and whether or not the researcher has strived to uncover the significant assumptions made about the phenomenon being studied in each of the primary studies. Finally, students should evaluate whether or not the researcher searched for alternative explanations for conflicting findings from the primary studies and discern whether or not the researcher interpreted the findings from each of the primary studies to provide new meaning for interpreting knowledge. Specific questions that can be used for this learning activity are listed in Box 6.1. The learning activity is generally useful for a homework assignment and can be used in class for reporting results of the assignment or for a group class assignment.

Examples of Evaluating Qualitative Meta-Syntheses

Now that a structure for evaluating qualitative meta-syntheses has been described, students can use the following examples to gain an understanding of the process of evaluating the value of qualitative meta-syntheses. One example of a qualitative meta-synthesis that is of high quality is the meta-synthesis conducted by Paterson, Thorne, and Dewis (1998) to advance the understanding of the lived experience of diabetes in published research and theses. The authors used an organizing framework by Curtin and Lubkin (1990) that provides a well-developed conceptualization of the experience of chronic illness. Paterson, Thorne, and Dewis used the method of meta-ethnography (Noblit & Hare, 1988) to analyze findings from 43 research reports identified by searching six computerized databases and the Canadian Nurses Association library for published and unpublished dissertations. The time frame covered was the years 1980 through 1996. The researchers described Noblit and Hare's method of meta-ethnography as consisting of six overlapping and sometime parallel phases: (1) deciding what is relevant; (2) reading selected research reports; (3) determining how studies are related; (4) translating the studies into one another; (5) synthesizing these translations; and (6) writing the synthesis. The researchers demonstrated their strategy for determining the trustworthiness of their findings by undertaking several activities. Initially, one researcher analyzed each study and then other members of the team reviewed the analysis. Then all the researchers met to identify differences in their analyses and to arrive at consensual agreement. If some of the

Box 6.1
Questions to Ask When Reviewing Qualitative Meta-Syntheses

1. How well was the research question guiding the meta-synthesis formulated?

2. Has the researcher used an effective method to select the primary research for the meta-synthesis?

   a. Has the researcher chosen inclusion and exclusion criteria for screening adequately primary studies?

   b. Has the researcher reviewed the databases and other sources of data adequately?

   c. Has the researcher used sound decisions for including a primary study or excluding a primary study in the meta-synthesis?

3. Has the researcher critically appraised the strengths and limitations of the primary studies included in the meta-synthesis?

4. Has the researcher strived to uncover the significant assumptions made about the phenomenon being studied in the primary study?

5. Has the researcher searched for alternative explanations for conflicting findings from the primary studies?

6. Has the researcher interpreted the findings to provide new meaning for interpreting knowledge?

Adapted from B. L. Paterson, S. L. Thorne, C. Canam, & C. Jillings, 2001.

cases presented in a primary study resulted in findings that were not consistent with what was found by the researchers who conducted the qualitative meta-synthesis, the researchers sought alternative explanations for their conclusions.

As a result of this exhaustive set of activities, Paterson et al. (1998) described the emergence of a unifying metaphor for understanding patients' experiences with diabetes. Specifically, the researchers identified the metaphor of *balance* to explain individuals' experiences with diabetes in their lives. The authors provided a table with the particular expressions of the metaphor, and for each expression the authors identified the associated source of primary study. Examples of expressions of the metaphor *balance* included "accepting oneself as a person with diabetes" and "maintaining a positive self-concept," "learning to manage the diabetes," and "not ill but having the disease" (p. 58). The authors included a detailed analysis of each of the expressions accompanied by the citation for the original source. For example, regarding "learning how to manage diabetes," the authors describe the findings of five authors of primary studies as the necessity of having basic knowledge about diabetes before a person can learn to manage the disease appropriately; and from authors of four primary studies that individuals with diabetes generally choose to experiment with diet before they adjust medication because dietary experiments are thought to have less drastic consequences than those involving medication (p. 59).

Not only did Paterson and colleagues (1998) analyze the primary findings to describe a unifying metaphor and the accompanying expressions of the metaphor, they also interpreted findings to provide new meaning for interpreting knowledge, as shown by their recognition that research that focused on using *balance* instead of *control* as a metaphor can facilitate new interpretations and understandings of behavior the individuals express, and as a result, can move health care practitioners away from describing diabetic individuals as "noncompliant" (p. 60). Finally, Paterson and colleagues, through their synthesis of these primary studies, found new meaning related to how health care professionals can interact with diabetic individuals to provide direction and support. They also interpreted findings from the primary studies to discern that the decision to assume control of diabetes is dynamic and can change with variations in life events and the disease itself (p. 61). The researchers further recognized some limitations of their qualitative meta-synthesis. They noted that qualitative research pertaining to diabetes had almost exclusively been conducted with well-educated female Caucasians who have insulin-dependent diabetes mellitus and who lived with an ally; as a result, the researchers identified a need to study people with a different demographic profile. They also found that the decision to control diabetes is not yet well understood and requires further study.

Students could be assigned this article for reading and then they could discuss the article in class. Table 6.1 shows an example of information in this and other articles that are summarized using the questions one should ask when reviewing a qualitative meta-synthesis.

A second example is the meta-synthesis by Carroll (2004a), with commentaries from Thorne (2004) and Paterson (2004). These publications appear in their entirety in Appendix A of this chapter. Carroll's meta-synthesis related to communication in nonvocal ventilated patients, not only providing the reader with data from the actual meta-synthesis, but also demonstrating an example of the dialogue among researchers

TABLE 6.1 Sample Meta-Syntheses and Authors' Responses to Critical Questions

	Paterson, Thorne, & Dewis (1998)	Carroll (2004)	Sandelowski & Barroso (2003b)
Research question guides the meta-synthesis	Authors wanted to advance the understanding of the lived experience of diabetes in published research and theses.	Author wanted to gain an understanding of the experiences of nonvocal ventilated patients experiences with communication.	State that few studies have been specifically directed toward examining motherhood in the context of maternal chronic illness, in this case HIV infection.
Effective method used to select the primary research	Searched six computerized databases and the Canadian Nurses Association library for published and unpublished dissertations. Time Frame: 1980 through 1996.	Searched a wide variety of databases using pertinent keywords, e.g., mechanical ventilator, mechanical ventilation etc. Qualitative studies focused on the communication experience while being mechanically ventilated or the general experience of being mechanically ventilated. Informants were hospitalized adults who were ventilated for a short period.	Very detailed; presents methods in separate publications (e.g., Sandelowski, Docherty, & Emden, 1997; Sandelowski & Barroso, 2003a)
Critical appraisal is made of the strengths and limitations of the primary studies	Meta-ethnography used—an interpretive approach requiring a researcher to compare and analyze textual reports, creating new interpretations in the process. Requires inductive analysis of data generated in the text of research studies	Data, methods, and theoretical frameworks of the original studies were critically analyzed. Each article read twice and line-by-line analysis conducted. Metaphors uncovered and translated from study to study to preserve holistic findings.	Suggests that qualitative findings, even those not rigorously synthesized, can be summarized and the meta-summary provides information and can form the basis for meta-synthesis
Significant assumptions uncovered about the phenomenon being studied in the primary study	Balance emerged as the predominant metaphor of the lived experience of diabetes. Particular expressions of the metaphor *balance* were provided accompanied by the associated source of primary study.	Patients who are ventilated experience an interruption of normal communication resulting in not being well understood. Understanding these patients' perceptions of communication needs is necessary for nurses to provide quality care.	Mothering work; paradoxical mother-child & illness outcomes; contrary decisions & contradictory outcomes; emergence of concept of "virtual motherhood"

(continued)

TABLE 6.1 *(continued)*

	Paterson, Thorne, & Dewis (1998)	Carroll (2004)	Sandelowski & Barroso (2003b)
Alternative explanations sought for conflicting findings in the primary studies	*Balance* was not viewed as a universal goal—some persons experienced rigidity in the workplace that affected their ability to maintain *balance*. Other researchers suggested that "maintaining balance" was dynamic and could be revised based on life events.	The incorporation of studies with varying methods was seen as a plausible source for conflicting findings, but the researcher noted the paucity of studies of nonvocal ventilated patients so viewed the study as providing the ability to address the strengths and weaknesses of each method.	Not really applicable since authors strived to be inclusive of all findings and used meta-summary, including data extraction, data abstraction, and calculation of frequency effect size to formulate a set of findings derived from all reports. Meta-summary results were used to conduct the meta-synthesis.
Findings interpreted to determine alternative explanations for conflicting findings from the primary studies	Authors recognized that the research was conducted almost exclusively on well-educated female Caucasians who have support. They stress the need for studying men, those living alone, and those with non-insulin dependent diabetes.	The commentaries and dialogue among the author of the present meta-synthesis and by other researchers practiced in meta-syntheses provided rich information on alternative explanations for interpreting findings from the present meta-synthesis.	Relates to the technique used. Researchers suggest that the meta-synthesis is at least 3 times removed from the original research. Suggest that the meta-synthesis can be viewed as a unique encounter between 2 readers—the researchers and the texts (in this case, 56 reports)

that is useful for assisting nurses in understanding phenomena in health care. Carroll's study (2004a) is presented and followed by two thoughtful responses by leading proponents of meta-synthesis of qualitative research, which are in turn followed by Carroll's (2004b) response to these comments from the other researchers. This discourse provides an example of the dynamic nature of qualitative meta-synthesis and how this dialogue can expand our understanding of qualitative research.

Carroll (2004a) conducted an extensive literature search using a wide variety of databases. The author used several keywords, including *mechanical ventilator, mechanical ventilation, ventilator, ventilation, respirator, communication, qualitative, and experience,* to search the databases. Regarding inclusion criteria, Carroll chose qualitative studies about the communication experience or the general experience for individuals while they are being mechanically ventilated. In all the studies chosen, patients were adults who were ventilated while hospitalized. The ventilation period was generally short. Studies focused on patient perceptions rather than nurses' perceptions of communication. Studies focusing on patients who were on a ventilator for extended periods of time were excluded because the length of time needed to conduct this type of study would have resulted in a different communication experience from patients who were on ventilation for a short period. Studies focusing on detailing the experience of being therapeutically paralyzed were excluded because patients in these studies were unable to communicate in any form. The final sample used for the meta-synthesis were 12 studies published between 1982 and 2000 with a total of 111 participants and sample sizes ranging from 1 to 30. Nine articles explored participants' general reactions to ventilation and included information on communication, and three articles focused on the patients' experiences specific to communication while being mechanically ventilated.

Carroll (2004a) critically analyzed the data, methods, and theoretical frameworks in each of the primary studies and detected and synthesized common threads across study participants' individual experiences. She discovered from the meta-synthesis that nonvocal ventilated patients experience an interruption of normal communication and perceive themselves as not being well understood. Characteristics of communication experienced by these patients included not being understood (inequality of communication, misunderstandings, and altered perceptions); loss of control (unmet needs, dependency, and dehumanization); and negative emotions. In addition, Carroll uncovered the idea that understanding nonvocal, mechanically ventilated patients' perspective of being understood is necessary for nurses to provide quality care to this population. These patients desired that nurses provide individualized care and a caring presence.

As mentioned earlier, following the meta-synthesis by Carroll (2004a), Thorne (2004) and Paterson (2004) provide commentaries. Thorne discusses the intent of meta-synthesis and stresses the need for authors to contribute new information not possible by conducting a traditional critical review the existing literature. Thorne states further that when a researcher conducts a meta-synthesis, the critical reflection undertaken results in findings of a higher order than can be found in the available research. She suggests that Carroll's (2004a) strategy for interpreting the findings should be made more explicit. In her commentary, Paterson noted the important contribution made by Carroll (2004a) in providing interesting insights about the communication experiences of ventilated patients; however, Paterson did comment on some methodological issues that may have affected the conclusions drawn. For example, she questions whether descriptive studies should be included because this type of qualitative study does not fit well with the intentions of a meta-synthesis. Paterson (2004) further states that Carroll provides "limited discussion of the influence of theoretical frame in researchers' analysis of data" (p. 108).

Carroll's (2004b) response to both commentators acknowledges a thought-provoking perspective. She offers further insight into her methodological plan by suggesting that inclusion of a combination of "atheoretical and theoretical primary reports provided a mix of broad structure and complete free flow of ideas" (p. 110). She stresses that there are few primary reports about the communication experiences of nonvocal patients available as of yet. She notes that researchers should thoroughly document all aspects of their research in the primary reports to increase the quality of the reports used for a meta-synthesis. The dialogue among these three authors provides insights into some of the issues surrounding meta-synthesis, demonstrates collegiality among qualitative researchers, and shows the interest of publishers in providing a forum for scholarly discourse. This particular article can be used as a reading assignment followed by a classroom exercise, wherein students discuss the original meta-synthesis and follow it by critiquing the merit of the commentaries. Students can also refer to Box 6.1 to view pertinent information from the Carroll (2004a) article using the questions one should ask when reviewing qualitative meta-syntheses.

A third example concerns the work of Sandelowski and Barroso (2003b), who conducted a qualitative meta-synthesis of primary research reports pertaining to HIV-positive mothers and their experiences with mothering. The rationale for studying motherhood in the context of HIV infection is based on the authors' recognition that few studies have been conducted on this population in order to gain insight into maternal experiences of those who experience chronic illness, and more specifically, those who are HIV-positive. The researchers conducted a thorough search of studies of U.S. women living with HIV infection from 1991 to 2002, with 114 reports obtained from the initial search, with 56 reports containing motherhood findings.

Sandelowski and Barroso (2003b) demonstrate how methods are used to summarize statements derived from primary studies related to women who are HIV-positive and how these summarizations can enlighten providers about individuals' experiences of motherhood in the context of HIV. The authors refer to this process as *meta-summary*. In an earlier methods paper, Sandelowski and Barroso (2003a) demonstrated how they were able to summarize the findings from qualitative research in the form of discrete statements that may not have been synthesized in the traditional, rigorous manner usually seen in qualitative research, but that nonetheless provided important information for guiding clinical practice. The authors developed a method for abstracting statements from studies, using a guide they have produced and a method of calculating frequencies of the appearance of these statements, to determine the themes prevalent in the overall group of primary studies (2003a). They refer to this technique as a meta-summary of findings.

Using meta-summary, Sandelowski and Barroso (2003b) note that the most relevant findings about motherhood in the context of HIV infection include issues such as struggling with decisions about disclosing their HIV status to their children, worrying about what would happen to their children as their disease worsened, and worrying about the negative impact of maternal HIV on their children, including negative reactions from other people. In a positive sense, children are viewed as a source of strength for mothers with HIV infection. The authors provide a complete list of the summarized findings related to motherhood in the context of HIV infection (p. 473).

Following the meta-summary of statements, Sandelowski and Barroso (2003b) apply meta-synthesis techniques for conceptual renderings and translation and synthesis of segments of these findings (p. 472). Results show that there exist phenomena described as mothering work in the context of HIV infection, mothering troubles in the form of paradoxes in mothering, and a distinctive kind of maternal practice—*virtual motherhood*—that allows mothers to have oversight of their children rather than demanding direct physical contact with them (p. 476). In addition to these general findings, the authors provide much more detailed information about women's experiences with mothering in the context of HIV from the meta-synthesis.

Sandelowski and colleagues (1997) and Sandelowski and Barroso (2003a) have devoted much effort to the methodologies used to produce qualitative meta-syntheses and have also provided substantive information from meta-syntheses about health-related issues (Sandelowski & Barroso, 2003a, 2003b). These scholarly papers can be used to teach students about qualitative methods and to demonstrate how these qualitative methods, when applied to a focal area of study, can produce information to guide nursing practice. Examples of information from these works, summarized using the set of questions for evaluating qualitative meta-syntheses, can be found in Box 6.1.

CONCLUSIONS

Teaching students to use the best in qualitative evidence to guide clinical decision-making may seem like a formidable task for educators; however, having this new and growing resource in the form of qualitative meta-syntheses provides educators with a new instrument for teaching students. Using synthesized information about patients' experiences from the patients' own view can be applied to real-life settings to improve the quality of patient, family, and community care. In addition, as recipients of information provided by qualitative meta-syntheses, we come to appreciate the diligent work of researchers who strive to increase our understanding of complex phenomena and assist us in educating students to provide care that now includes not only evidence from quantitative studies but also from the rich information that originates in the qualitative realm of research.

REFERENCES

Arman, M., & Rehnsfeldt, A. (2003). The hidden suffering among breast cancer patients: A qualitative meta-synthesis. *Qualitative Health Research, 13,* 510–527.

Carroll, S. M. (2004a). Nonvocal ventilated patients' perceptions of being understood. *Western Journal of Nursing Research, 26,* 85–103.

Carroll, S. M. (2004b). [Response by Carroll]. *Western Journal of Nursing Research, 26,* 110–112.

Curtin, M., & Lubkin, I. (1990). What is chronicity? In I. Lubkin (Ed.), *Chronic illness: Impact and interventions* (2nd ed., pp. 2–20). Boston: Jones & Bartlett.

Miller, W. L., & Crabtree, B. F. (2000). Clinical research. In K. Denzin & Y. S. Lincoln (Eds.), *Handbook of qualitative research* (2nd ed., pp. 607–631). Thousand Oaks, CA: Sage.

Noblit, G. W., & Hare, R. D. (1988). *Meta-ethnography: Synthesizing qualitative studies.* Newbury Park, CA: Sage.

Paterson, B. (2004). [Commentary by Paterson]. *Western Journal of Nursing Research, 26,* 107–109.

Paterson, B. L., Thorne, S. L., Canam, C., & Jillings, C. (2001). *Meta-study of qualitative health research: A practical guide to meta-analysis and meta-synthesis.* Thousand Oaks, CA: Sage.

Paterson, B. L., Thorne, S., & Dewis, M. (1998). Adapting to and managing diabetes. *Image: Journal of Nursing Scholarship, 30*(1), 57–62.

Sandelowski, M., & Barroso, J. (2003a). Creating meta-summaries of qualitative findings. *Nursing Research, 52,* 226–233.

Sandelowski, M., & Barroso, J. (2003b). Motherhood in the context of maternal HIV infection. *Research in Nursing & Health, 26,* 470–482.

Sandelowski, M., Docherty, S., & Emden, C. (1997). Qualitative metasynthesis: Issues and techniques. *Research in Nursing and Health, 20,* 365–371.

Thorne, S. (2004). [Commentary by Thorne]. *Western Journal of Nursing Research, 26,* 104–106.

APPENDIX A

Western Journal of Nursing Research, 2004, 26(1), 85-103

Nonvocal Ventilated Patients' Perceptions of Being Understood

Stacey M. Carroll

This metasynthesis presents an enlarged interpretation and understanding of nonvocal mechanically ventilated patients' experiences with communication. Peplau's interpersonal relations theory provided the theoretical framework for the metasynthesis. The final sample included 12 qualitative studies, for a total of 111 participants. The data, methods, and theoretical frameworks were critically interpreted. Common threads detected across study participants' individual experiences were synthesized to form a greater understanding of nonvocal ventilated patients' perceptions of being understood. Five overarching themes were divided into two groups. The first group of themes was categorized as the characteristics of nonvocal ventilated patients' communication experiences. Nonvocal individuals were often not understood, which resulted in loss of control and negative emotional responses. The second group of themes was categorized as the kind of nursing care desired by nonvocal patients in order to be understood. Nonvocal patients wanted nursing care that was delivered in an individualized, caring manner. This facilitated positive interpersonal relations between the patient and the nurse. Findings are discussed in relation to the current state of knowledge on this topic.

Keywords: *nonvocal; ventilated; communication; metasynthesis*

Patients who are mechanically ventilated are often nonvocal. As a result, the normal communication process is altered, and these individuals usually are not well understood by others. Because there are increasing numbers of patients on ventilators (Douglas et al., 1997), these communication issues are of paramount importance. Misunderstandings can adversely affect the nursing care these patients receive. Patients have demonstrated high recall rates of the ventilator experience, including communication while ventilated (Bergbom-Engberg, Hallenberg, Wickstrom, & Haljamae, 1988; Green, 1996). Understanding nonvocal mechanically ventilated patients' perspectives of being understood is necessary for nurses to provide quality care to this population. This could potentially reduce patients' frustration by enabling their needs to be met more appropriately.

Stacey M. Carroll, A.P.R.N., B.C., Ph.D. Candidate, Boston College School of Nursing.

DOI: 10.1177/0193945903259462

IMPORTANCE OF COMMUNICATION

Communication is a way for patients to have their physical, social, psychological, and spiritual needs met (Ashworth, 1987). Communication difficulties experienced by nonvocal ventilated patients frequently have resulted in negative emotions for patients and for the nurses caring for them (Fowler, 1997; Happ, 2001; Menzel, 1998; Pennock, Crawshaw, Maher, Price, & Kaplan, 1994; Riggio, Singer, Hartman, & Sneider, 1982; Russell, 1999). Confusion, such as Intensive Care Unit (ICU) psychosis, can become worse if the communication process is not effective (Ashworth, 1987; Granberg, Bergbom-Engberg, & Lundberg, 1996; MacKellaig, 1987). When the patient is not understood, the communication process becomes one sided, and feedback from the patient is limited.

Effective communication is part of quality nursing practice (Hemsley et al., 2001). Augmentative and alternative communication (AAC) strategies such as lipreading, communication boards, writing, hand gestures, and computers or electronic devices have been used for this population (Albarran, 1991; Helfrich-Miller, 1999) with varying levels of success. These supplementary strategies are slower than using and interpreting regular speech (Jones, 1986) and can therefore be time-consuming to utilize (Borsig & Steinacker, 1982; Hemsley et al., 2001). Successful communication may contribute to the recoveries of patients who are ventilator dependent (Wojnicki-Johansson, 2001), whereas unsuccessful communication may hinder their recoveries (Russell, 1999).

PURPOSE AND THEORETICAL FRAMEWORK

Numerous qualitative studies have been conducted to explore mechanically ventilated patients' experiences of communication, but a review of the literature revealed no published metasynthesis on this topic. The present metasynthesis was designed to answer the following research question: What characterizes nonvocal ventilated patients' perceptions of being understood across qualitative studies? The goal was to provide an enlarged interpretation and understanding (Beck, 2001; Paterson, Thorne, Canam, & Jillings, 2001) and to build cumulative knowledge (Estabrooks, Field, & Morse, 1994; Thorne & Paterson, 1998) of the communication experiences in this population.

February 2004, Vol. 26, No. 1 87

Peplau's (1992) interpersonal relations theory provided the overarching theoretical framework for this metasynthesis. This theory stresses the importance of reciprocal communication so mutual understanding by the patient and the nurse can occur (Forchuk, 1994; Peplau, 1992). Communication difficulties, such as those encountered when patients are nonvocal, can hinder interpersonal relationships between the patient and the nurse.

SAMPLE

Appropriate studies for inclusion were identified through an extensive literature search. Multiple computer databases were used, including CINAHL, Medline, Sociofile, Psychlit, and Dissertation Abstracts. Keywords entered included mechanical ventilator, mechanical ventilation, ventilator, ventilation, respirator, communication, qualitative, and experience. The qualitative studies chosen for inclusion were studies that were about the communication experience while mechanically ventilated or about the general experience of being mechanically ventilated. The latter group of studies identified and described communication as a relevant characterization of the ventilator experience, so the content was substantive and pertinent to this metasynthesis. In all the studies chosen, the participants were adults who were ventilated while hospitalized. The ventilation period generally was short term.

Studies that focused on the nurses' perceptions of the communication process, rather than patients' perceptions, were excluded. Studies that addressed the experience of individuals who were on ventilators but living in the community were also excluded, because the length of time that had elapsed was likely to have changed the communication experience. In addition, the environment and social support networks of those living in the community can be vastly different from the hospital environment, potentially affecting the communication and coping processes. Studies detailing the experience of being therapeutically paralyzed were excluded because such patients are unable to communicate in any form.

The final sample for this metasynthesis yielded 12 studies published between 1982 and 2000. The total number of participants was 111, with sample sizes of individual studies ranging from 1 to 30. Nine of the articles explored the participants' general reactions to ventilation and included information on communication, and three of the articles focused on the specific experience of communication while ventilated. Seven of the studies took place in the United States. The remaining five studies were conducted in other countries (two in Canada, one each in Iceland, the United Kingdom, and Israel). The majority of the studies used descriptive explorative or descriptive phenomenologic methodologies. The four narratives were descriptive in nature. One study used grounded theory methodology. Only one study utilized a theoretical framework. Almost all the participants had been extubated and were therefore vocal at the time of the interviews or while writing the narratives. As a result, their accounts were primarily retrospective. The disciplines represented by the studies were nursing, medicine, and sociology. Characteristics of the included studies are detailed in Table 1.

METHOD AND DATA ANALYSIS

For this metasynthesis, the data, methods, and theoretical frameworks of the original studies were analyzed and subsequently synthesized (Paterson, 2001; Paterson et al., 2001; Thorne & Paterson, 1998). Each article was read at least twice to reveal the overall themes expressed, and then a line-by-line analysis was conducted to delineate metaphors from the data. More than 50 metaphors were initially identified in the 12 articles. These metaphors were translated from study to study, with the aim of keeping them consistent from one account to another to preserve the holistic interpretation of the research findings (Noblit & Hare, 1988). The metaphors were grouped into categories of overarching metaphors until all themes represented in the original studies were included and appropriately classified.

The data were analyzed in light of the included studies' methods and theoretical frameworks. The included studies were predominantly descriptive and atheoretical. These factors limited the ability to formulate very complex depictions of the experience. The included studies also did not highlight information pertaining to system-level implications, as they focused on individual experiences. This limited the ability to explore how the environment might have altered the experience. The common threads detected across the study participants' individual experiences, however, were synthesized to form a greater understanding of nonvocal ventilated patients' perceptions of being understood. Detailed memos were documented to constitute an audit trail.

February 2004, Vol. 26, No. 1   **89**

TABLE 1: Studies Included in Sample for Metasynthesis

Citation	Sample	Purpose/ Research Question	Method
Fitch (1989)	N = 30. Canada. 2 ICUs. 23 women, 7 men. Ages 17 to 80 years. Intubated 17 to 144 hours. Interviewed after extubation.	Determine the patients' perceptions regarding the inability to speak while receiving mechanically assisted ventilator therapy	Exploratory, descriptive
Frace (1982)	N = 3. United States. 2 women, 1 man. Intubated 2 to 10 days. Interviewed after extubation.	Determine psychological stresses faced by patients on mechanical ventilators, how they cope, and how nursing personnel can assist these patients in facing stresses	Exploratory, descriptive
Gries & Fernsler (1988)	N = 9. 2 small U.S. hospitals. 5 men, 4 women. Ages 35 to 81. Interviewed 1 to 7 days after extubation.	Elicit patients' perceptions of the mechanical ventilation experience from the time of awareness of intubation until extubation	Exploratory, descriptive
Hafsteindottir (1996)	N = 8. Iceland. 2 ICUs. Intubated for at least 3 days. Interviewed after extubation.	How do respirator-treated patients experience communication?	Descriptive phenomenology
Jablonski (1994)	N = 12. United States. 5 men, 7 women. Ages 27 to 73. Interviews done after discharge, 2 to 108 months after ventilation.	Collect and analyze primary recollections of patients who were dependent on mechanical ventilation	Descriptive phenomenology
Johnson & Sexton (1990)	N = 14. United States. 3 still receiving nighttime ventilation, others extubated within 1 to 6 months.	Identify those factors that were recalled as distressing by individuals who have been mechanically ventilated	Exploratory, descriptive

(continued)

90   *Western Journal of Nursing Research*

TABLE 1   (continued)

Citation	Sample	Purpose/ Research Question	Method
Logan & Jenny (1997)	N = 20. Canada. 11 women, 9 men. Ages 19 to 83. Ventilated 5 to 214 days. Interviewed 6 to 13 days after ICU.	Describe patients' subjective experiences of mechanical ventilation and weaning and to extend an evolving nursing theory of weaning	Grounded theory
Parker (1984)	N = 1. United Kingdom. Male. Written after extubation.	Provide personal experience of ventilation and suggestions on avoiding communication breakdowns	Narrative
Rier (2000)	N = 1. Israel. Male. Spent 15 days on ventilator. Now extubated.	Notebooks the author used to communicate with staff were used to reconstruct his ventilator experiences	Narrative
Schumann (1999)	N = 11. United States. Interviewed after extubation.	Describe intensive care patients' experience of mechanical ventilation	Descriptive phenomenology
Urden (1997)	N = 1. United States. Female.	Comments patient made on a patient satisfaction survey used to remind critical care nurses of importance of communication, compassion, and patience	Narrative
Viner (1985)	N = 1. United States. Male. Had spent 31 days on ventilator. Now extubated.	Author sought to make physicians mindful of impact of patients' individual personality and background on coping	Narrative

FINDINGS

The reciprocal translations of the data metaphors in the present metasynthesis resulted in five overarching themes with subcategories (Table 2). These interrelated themes were categorized in two groups: the characteris-

February 2004, Vol. 26, No. 1   91

TABLE 2: Nonvocal Mechanically Ventilated Patients' Perceptions of Being Understood

Characteristics of Communication	Nursing Care Desired
Not being understood	Individualized care
Inequality of communication	Caring presence
Misunderstandings	
Altered perceptions	
Loss of control	
Unmet needs	
Dependency	
Dehumanization	
Negative emotions	

tics of nonvocal patients' communication experience and the kind of nursing care nonvocal patients wanted to receive to be understood.

Characteristics of the Nonvocal Communication Experience

The nonvocal communication experience was characterized by participants' not being understood. As a result, participants experienced a loss of control as well as negative emotions.

Not Being Understood

Nonvocal ventilated patients reported that they often were not understood because the communication process was unequal. This caused misunderstandings and altered perceptions.

Inequality of communication. In unimpaired communication, there theoretically is the capacity for an equal exchange of information between two or more people. The communication process became one of inequality when a patient was mechanically ventilated and nonvocal. This inequality of communication led to nonvocal participants' not being understood. One participant stated, "I couldn't make them understand anything" (Gries & Fernsler, 1988, p. 56). The nurse typically held a position of power, even if unintentional, with respect to the communication process. For example, "[Health care providers] don't ask me, as a patient, how I really feel and how I can contribute to my own care, and that's very frustrating" (Jablonski, 1994, p. 201). Participants were limited to whatever supplemental communication methods health care providers offered.

Nurses had the ability to make the communication process as limited or as involved as they wished. Nurses tended to limit their messages to concrete, factual information such as, "We're going to give you a bath" (Jablonski, 1994, p. 198). Participants wanted to hear more detailed information. Even if an attempt was made to involve the patient, at times the nurse still could not understand the patient, and thus changed the dynamics of the communication process. Mechanically ventilated patients often simplified their messages to make themselves more easily understood. This further increased the inequality of communication. Messages patients were trying to convey, even in their simplified version, often were not received in totality.

Misunderstandings. Participants misunderstood staff actions and were unable to clarify their erroneous interpretations, contributing to their feelings of disorientation. Patients who were nonvocal often did not know why they were unable to speak. In addition, participants had difficulty comprehending medical jargon and were unable to clarify this, leading to potential misunderstandings.

In addition to participants' misunderstanding others, health care providers sometimes misunderstood what nonvocal individuals were trying to say. One patient was receiving a tracheostomy under local anesthetic and felt that his heart was going to explode. He said, "You cannot speak—you mouth 'Heart, heart' moronically. 'Everything's fine, just relax,' smiles a disinterested surgeon. My perceptions were totally different" (Parker, 1984, p. 37). This participant's specific concern was misunderstood by the staff. Gestures, which participants used as attempts to communicate, were sometimes mistakenly attributed to anxiety.

Altered perceptions. When the nonvocal patient was not understood, the potential for altered perceptions increased. Altered perceptions ranged from disorientation to psychosis. Disorientation was common; one participant stated: "It took me a whole week to figure out where I was" (Logan & Jenny, 1997, p. 143). The strange environments contributed to participants' losing track of time or having other altered thought processes. One patient stated, "I couldn't distinguish the human from the spiritual world" (Urden, 1997, p. 104). Such disorientation sometimes progressed to paranoia as evidenced by a participant who stated, "At times I was frankly psychotic" (Viner, 1985, p. 9).

February 2004, Vol. 26, No. 1   **93**

Loss of Control

When patients were not adequately understood, they reported a loss of control over their situation. Loss of control was characterized by having unmet needs, feelings of dependency, and being dehumanized.

Unmet needs. When participants were not understood, their needs were often not met. A nurse was unable to understand one participant's statements about his severe arm pain (Johnson & Sexton, 1990). Incontinence resulted when participants were unable to convey that they needed to void (Jablonski, 1994). The need for spiritual connection was sometimes unmet because of impaired communication (Schumann, 1999). A nonvocal patient was unable to tell the nurse that she was afraid she would never get off the ventilator and thus did not receive the reassurance she needed (Frace, 1982). Another participant similarly stated: "What I really wanted was for [the nurse] to reassure me and acknowledge my fears" (Urden, 1997, p. 104). Some participants' needs were unmet because time or fatigue impeded communication efforts:

"My eyes would not focus to write" (Fitch, 1989, p. 16).

"[Writing] didn't work out, because I was so terribly weak. I felt terrible about it. Just realizing that I could not even communicate with a pen" (Hafsteindottir, 1996, p. 264).

"[The nurse] never gave me time to finish my questions when I tried to write them" (Urden, 1997, p. 104).

Inconsistency of nursing staff contributed to unmet needs. One participant asserted, "It is a form of neglect to leave the patient to be cared for by a colleague who does not know the system" (Parker, 1984, p. 39). Another explained, "Every time I'd get a new nurse, I'd have to try to tell her all over again how to turn me so the [chest] tubes didn't hurt" (Johnson & Sexton, 1990, p. 55).

Dependency. Dependency occurred because the patient was not able to communicate control over his or her own care. "It [being on the ventilator] was a strange feeling, like you're not in control of your own body," said one participant (Logan & Jenny, 1997, p. 145). The inability to be understood created a situation of great dependency. One participant explained, "My condition rendered me fully dependent on my doctors and nurses, with little physical or mental strength with which to challenge them" (Rier, 2000, p. 72). Others stated, "[There was a] basic frustration inherent in not being in control of one's destiny" (Viner, 1985, p. 8) and "Life has changed totally, it is no longer mine" (Parker, 1984, p. 37).

Dehumanization. When patients perceived that nurses were focusing more on the machine than on the person attached to the machine, they felt dehumanized (Logan & Jenny, 1997; Urden, 1997). One participant stressed, "We must always keep our perspective, and not get lost in the maelstrom of our technology" (Viner, 1985, p. 13). This perspective was not always remembered, however:

> "[Some nurses] forget the personal side and forget that you are a person too" (Logan & Jenny, 1997, p. 145).

> "They don't care, they don't give a hoot or anything, as long as that thing [the ventilator] keeps [going] up or down, or does its own thing. As long as the body is there, the machine is there" (Jablonski, 1994, p. 201).

> "[The nurse] looked afraid and repulsed, never making eye contact with me, and didn't come past the front of the bed unless she had to" (Urden, 1997, p. 104).

Such dehumanization made participants feel like "a stranger from another planet" (Logan & Jenny, 1997, p. 145) and feel that they were being treated like "live corpses" (Jablonski, 1994, p. 192). Patients were denied involvement in their own care and were treated as passive objects.

Dehumanization can encompass outright neglect. Participants perceived that it was easier for health care staff to ignore them because they were nonvocal. For example, one participant stated, "[The staff was] totally indifferent to my facial protests" (Parker, 1984, p. 39). Another participant stated, "They could understand me when I said, 'bedpan.' They would come running. Anything else I was trying to say, they couldn't understand" (Jablonski, 1994, p. 198). Participants sometimes felt that staff purposely denied them information or ignored them.

Negative Emotions

Every study in this metasynthesis sample included information about the negative emotions ventilated patients experienced with respect to communication. The most prominent emotion expressed was frustration. Other emotions included fear, anger, agony, distress, anxiety, stress, and panic. Comments demonstrating negative emotions included the following:

> "It seems like a nightmare at times" (Logan & Jenny, 1997, p. 142).

"It was so terrible. I couldn't talk and I couldn't ask what was wrong with me" (Johnson & Sexton, 1990, p. 56).

"I was always apprehensive or frightened" (Parker, 1984, p. 37).

Participants reported futility when their communication efforts were useless. Futility occurred when there was a buildup of negative emotions from not being understood. It was closely related to the negative emotion of frustration because the goal of successfully conveying a message was not met. Statements such as "I was left screaming, but silently" (Urden, 1997, p. 104) and "I felt that I was crying out, but no one could hear anything" (Hafsteindottir, 1996, p. 266) indicated that patients wanted to convey information but were unsuccessful in doing so. Such futility further increased negative emotions.

If patients' attempts to communicate were futile, they often gave up, became resigned, or became passive and apathetic. As one participant stated, "It sometimes happened that I just gave up, because I became so tired, trying to explain what I meant" (Hafsteindottir, 1996, p. 266).

Nursing Care Desired by Nonvocal Ventilated Patients

Nonvocal ventilated patients wanted nursing care that was delivered in an individualized and caring manner. This type of care helped them to be more easily understood, or mitigated the negative effects of not being understood. This facilitated positive interpersonal relations between the patient and the nurse.

Individualized Care

When nurses used an individualized, holistic approach to the care of nonvocal mechanically ventilated patients, the communication process was more effective. If participants were understood, they generally experienced fewer negative emotions. One participant stated that when she was able to express herself, "It would calm you down, and everything would just be a whole lot better" (Logan & Jenny, 1997, p. 144).

Participants were reassured when nurses anticipated their needs and provided information. Participants stated a need to "understand what was going on" (Logan & Jenny, 1997, p. 143). Participants' fears were allayed when they were given explanations of what was happening. Because some participants reported that they did not know why they were unable to speak, it would have been helpful if the nurse had explained this to them. Provision of information reduced altered perceptions by orienting participants to reality. One participant appreciated selective disclosure by staff when he was critically ill: "I was for the first time in my adult life content mainly to leave the details to the medical staff" (Rier, 2000, p. 73). When he was recovering, however, this changed and he stated, "[I] preferred to know all the details of my treatment" (Rier, 2000, p. 82).

Consistent staff facilitated continuity of care and, thus, effective communication. Nurses who knew patients well provided more individualized care and made more accurate assessments. As one participant stated, "I was saved from a fair degree of oxygen starvation only by the entry of my beloved night sister, who knew immediately from the look in my eyes that all was not well" (Parker, 1984, p. 39).

AAC methods that were identified by participants as being helpful included writing, gestures, letter boards, mouthing words, and questions asked by the nurses. Because these AAC methods each had benefits and drawbacks in different situations, an individualized and creative approach was necessary to discover which method worked for each patient (Fitch, 1989; Hafsteindottir, 1996; Schumann, 1999). For example, one participant reported that he found it easy to communicate with a deaf person who was an expert lipreader (Viner, 1985). A combination of methods was often needed to facilitate communication, and the patient needed to be involved in the identification of appropriate communication methods. When participants were intubated for longer periods of time, coping skills were more developed and the repertoire of appropriate supplemental methods increased.

Being understood decreased feelings of dependency. When communication was facilitated, participants felt that they had more control over their care. The ability to speak, which occurred when patients were removed from the ventilator, also greatly increased patients' perceptions of being in control. Some participants judged the success of their communication efforts by whether their needs were met. Schumann (1999) found that patients who were connected to spiritual resources had greater energy to communicate with staff. A holistic individualized approach would allow for assessment of each patient's spirituality.

Caring Presence

Participants expressed appreciation when nurses provided them with support. When nurses had a caring presence, this conveyed patience and facilitated communication. A participant stated, "Not only did the staff

February 2004, Vol. 26, No. 1 **97**

engage quite actively in sentimental work, but I consider this to have been crucial in my recovery" (Rier, 2000, p. 78). Staff patience was important, especially when using supplemental methods of communication that could be time-consuming.

Presence and caring of the nurse were important qualities, especially if the patient was not truly able to be understood. A participant in one study said, "Just be there!" when asked how nurses could help patients (Logan & Jenny, 1997, p. 144). Other participants added the following:

> "It is very important to have someone you care for and trust by your side. People need to understand that one has very much need for that" (Hafsteindottir, 1996, p. 265).

> "There was always . . . [a nurse] by my side . . . of course, it wasn't like having my mum. But it was the second best [smiles]" (Hafsteindottir, 1996, p. 266).

A participant stated, "It is time to pause and remember that there is a living, thinking, feeling, and frightened human body on the other end of that machine" (Viner, 1985, p. 3). Some nurses did this successfully:

> "[The nurse] would humor me and talk to me about her children; it made me feel human" (Logan & Jenny, 1997, p. 145).

> "Both doctors and (especially) nurses took great pains to preserve my 'personhood'" (Rier, 2000, p. 78).

Having a supportive relationship with the nurse enhanced the communication experience: "I developed a close bond and quite sophisticated rapport with these nurses," (Parker, 1984, p. 37). Nonvocal ventilated patients had heightened perceptions and "everyone who enters his day assumes a magnified role" (Viner, 1985, p. 6). Participants acutely perceived whether the nurse cared or not, and this affected the trust placed in that nurse. As one participant stated, "It is the nurse...who is the single most important person in the critically ill patient's life. In turn, the single most important attribute of the nurse is *whether she cares*" (Viner, 1985, p. 6).

DISCUSSION

The results suggest that communication is a significant concern in this population, as negative outcomes resulted when nonvocal ventilated individuals were not understood. Nurses were found to be in an ideal position to facilitate nonvocal patients' abilities to communicate. Interpersonal relations between the patient and the nurse were affected when reciprocal communication was not effectively utilized. Communication difficulties were expressed even when the studies did not focus solely on the communication experience. For example, Schumann (1999) focused on ventilated individuals' general perceptions of mechanical ventilation and spirituality, but communication issues emerged as a significant component of the participants' experiences.

Peplau (1999) stressed the importance of reciprocal communication so misinterpretation can be avoided. The present metasynthesis suggests that nonvocal patients who could not be understood were not equal partners in the communication process. Feedback, which has been identified as an integral part of the communication process (Simonds, 1995), was often not able to be provided by nonvocal patients. Feedback is especially important in health care where complex information replete with medical jargon is provided to patients. Without feedback, clarification often could not occur, and misunderstandings resulted.

Communication difficulties may worsen ICU psychosis (Ashworth, 1987; Black, Deeny, & McKenna, 1997; Granberg et al., 1996), an experience of confusion that can include hallucinations and delusions. If nurses could understand ventilated patients, more accurate assessments of confusion could be made. This would facilitate appropriate reality orientation and mitigate the effects of these altered perceptions. If the nurse misunderstands what the patient is trying to convey, this can lead to unnecessary and potentially harmful interventions. Sedatives may be used when a patient is gesturing (de Toledo, 1980; Hansen-Flaschen, 1994), but sedatives can further suppress respiratory drive (Manthous, Schmidt, & Hall, 1998). The patient who is gesturing may simply be trying to convey a message. The patient may also misunderstand the nurse, resulting in negative emotions and confusion for the patient. If patients are understood, their autonomy would likely increase, and they would be more active participants in their own health care. This could decrease feelings of dependency and dehuman-zation.

The results show that nonvocal ventilated individuals have unmet needs. This is consistent with the findings of Happ (2000), who noted that patients' preferences were often unclear or unknown. Fowler (1997) reported that the messages intubated patients most often wanted to communicate were pain and discomfort, inability to breathe, and intense emotional feelings. Meeting these patient needs is a basic nursing responsibility but one that is difficult to accomplish when communication is ineffective. Chang (1997) found that

February 2004, Vol. 26, No. 1   **99**

hospitalized patients perceived better nursing care quality if their needs were met by the nurses. If patients' varied needs are not met because of communication difficulties, their healing and coping processes could be adversely affected. For nurses to make accurate assessments, they need to be able to understand nonvocal patients. Appropriate assessments could reduce the possibility of altered perceptions, misunderstandings, dependency, and dehumanization.

A cycle of negative emotions and futility ensued when mechanically ventilated patients were not understood. This is not surprising, as communication impairments in this population have been linked to many negative emotions including powerlessness, withdrawal, frustration, aloneness, anger, and fear (e.g., Belitz, 1983; Happ, 2000; Riggio et al., 1982). Patients' responses to their illnesses are an essential component of Peplau's interpersonal relations theory (Haber, 2000), and communication is necessary to assess these responses. When nurses cannot understand nonvocal patients, emotional responses of the patients may go unrecognized.

When an individualized approach to the communication needs of the patient was used, this was likely to facilitate the patient's being understood. This is consistent with existing literature, which has demonstrated that an individualized approach leads to determination of appropriate AAC methods so those methods can be documented to ensure continuity of care (Connolly & Shekleton, 1991; Ecklund, 1999). Patients with critical illness generally have demonstrated a strong need to know throughout their illnesses (Hupcey & Zimmerman, 2000). When nurses anticipated a patient's need for information, the patient did not have to expend as much energy trying to express those needs. Happ (2000) found that when nurses successfully interpreted what voiceless patients were trying to say, the patients had more control over their care. She stressed that continuity and presence were necessary for effective interpretation to occur. These factors help the nurse to know the patient and thus provide more effective care. "Knowing the patient" has been documented as being critical to skilled clinical judgment (Tanner, Benner, Chesla, & Gordon, 1993) and as a necessary antecedent to individualized care for the patient (Jenny & Logan, 1992; Radwin, 1995). The caring aspects of nursing can ameliorate the technologically defining environment that often surrounds patients who are mechanically ventilated (Cooper, 1993).

Most of the studies examined in the present metasynthesis used descriptive methodologies and no theoretical framework. Participants' accounts were also primarily retrospective, as the interviews generally occured after extubation. These factors may account for the basic similarities in findings across the studies. Nonvocal ventilated patients described their experiences in a fairly similar manner when given open-ended questions or when writing narratives. This relative homogeneity persisted despite improvements in ventilator technology and AAC methods over the years.

Greater depth of the meaning of nonvocal communication experiences was obtained when the experiences were examined in a broader context. For example, Logan and Jenny (1997) used grounded theory and found that difficulty communicating contributed to the "work" involved in ventilator weaning. Their findings contributed to a theory about ventilator weaning. Gries and Fernsler (1988) examined participants' responses within Neuman's model of nursing, and they identified communication problems as a major interpersonal stressor that can lead to disequilibrium in ventilated individuals. Neuman's model can then be utilized by nurses to better understand the relation of communication to ventilated patients' well-being. Schumann (1999), although using a descriptive approach, explored nonvocal ventilated participants' responses in light of spirituality. The connection between spirituality, communication, and the patient's overall experience was established.

A potential limitation of the present metasynthesis is the incorporation of studies with varying methods. Such blending of methods has been criticized because of the inherent differences among the methods (Jensen & Allen, 1996). There are not a sufficient number of qualitative studies on this topic, however, to focus solely on studies utilizing one method for the purposes of a metasynthesis. Incorporating various methods can address the strengths and weaknesses of each method. An attempt was made to stay faithful to the data in the included studies, but the original data from the studies were not used. This metasynthesis was, therefore, derived from other authors' interpretations of the data.

The present metasynthesis identifies the negative consequences to patients when they are not understood, and it highlights the critical role nurses play in facilitating communication in this population. Patients deserve to have their suffering eased, their comfort promoted, their healing facilitated, and their quality of life improved. These goals are difficult to accomplish when communication is impaired. By enhancing communication and providing appropriate information, nurses can ensure that patients are understood and reassured. This facilitates positive interpersonal relations between those who are nonvocal and mechanically ventilated and the nurses caring for them.

February 2004, Vol. 26, No. 1 **101**

NOTES

1. The author gratefully acknowledges the assistance and encouragement of Margaret Kearney, Ph.D., RNC, and Ellen Mahoney, DNS, RNCS, on this manuscript.

REFERENCES

Albarran, J. W. (1991). A review of communication with intubated patients and those with tracheostomies within an intensive care environment. *Intensive Care Nursing, 7*, 179-186.

Ashworth, P. (1987). The needs of the critically ill patient. *Intensive Care Nursing, 3*, 182-190.

Beck, C. (2001, April). *Metasynthesis: Implications for nursing practice.* Paper presented at the Eastern Nursing Research Society, Atlantic City, NJ.

Belitz, J. (1983). Minimizing the psychological complications of patients who require mechanical ventilation. *Critical Care Nurse, 3*, 42-46.

Bergbom-Engberg, I., Hallenberg, B., Wickstrom, I., & Haljamae, H. (1988). A retrospective study of patients' recall of respirator treatment (1): Study design and basic findings. *Intensive Care Nursing, 4*, 56-61.

Black, P., Deeny, P., & McKenna, H. (1997). Sensoristrain: An exploration of nursing interventions in the context of the Neuman systems theory. *Intensive and Critical Care Nursing, 13*, 249-258.

Borsig, A., & Steinacker, I. (1982). Communication with the patient in the intensive care unit. *Nursing Times*, S2-S11.

Chang, K. (1997). Dimensions and indicators of patients' perceived nursing care quality in the hospital setting. *Journal of Nursing Care Quality, 11*, 26-37.

Connolly, M. A., & Shekleton, M. E. (1991). Communicating with ventilator dependent patients. *Dimensions of Critical Care Nursing, 10*, 115-122.

Cooper, M. C. (1993). The intersection of technology and care in the ICU. *Advances in Nursing Science, 15*, 23-32.

de Toledo, L. W. (1980). Caring for the patient instead of the ventilator. *RN, 43*, 21-23, 103, 105.

Douglas, S. L., Daly, B. J., Brennan, P. L., Harris, S., Nochomovitz, M., & Dyer, M. A. (1997). Outcomes of long-term ventilator patients: A descriptive study. *American Journal of Critical Care, 6*, 99-105.

Ecklund, M. M. (1999). Successful outcomes for the ventilator-dependent patient. *Critical Care Nursing Clinics of North America, 11*, 249-260.

Estabrooks, C. A., Field, P. A., & Morse, J. M. (1994). Aggregating qualitative findings: An approach to theory development. *Qualitative Health Research, 4*, 503-511.

Fitch, M. (1989). The patient's reaction to ventilation. *Canadian Critical Care Nursing Journal, 6*, 13-16.

Forchuk, C. (1994). Peplau's theory-based practice and research. *Nursing Science Quarterly, 7*, 110-112.

Fowler, S. B. (1997). Impaired verbal communication during short-term oral intubation. *Nursing Diagnosis, 8*, 93-98.

Frace, R. M. (1982). Mechanical ventilation: The patient's viewpoint. *Today's OR Nurse, 11*, 16-21.

Granberg, A., Bergbom-Engberg, I., & Lundberg, D. (1996). Intensive care syndrome: A literature review. *Intensive and Critical Care Nursing, 12*, 173-182.

Green, A. (1996). An exploratory study of patients' memory recall of their stay in adult intensive therapy unit. *Intensive and Critical Care Nursing, 12,* 131-137.

Gries, M. L., & Fernsler, J. (1988). Patient perceptions of the mechanical ventilation experience. *Focus on Critical Care, 15,* 52-59.

Haber, J. (2000). Hildegard E. Peplau: The psychiatric nursing legacy of a legend. *Journal of the American Psychiatric Nurses Association, 6,* 56-62.

Hafsteindottir, T. B. (1996). Patient's experiences of communication during the respirator treatment period. *Intensive and Critical Care Nursing, 12,* 261-271.

Hansen-Flaschen, J. (1994). Improving patient tolerance of mechanical ventilation: Challenges ahead. *Critical Care Clinics, 10,* 659-671.

Happ, M. B. (2000). Interpretation of nonvocal behavior and the meaning of voicelessness in critical care. *Social Science and Medicine, 50,* 1247-1255.

Happ, M. B. (2001). Communicating with mechanically ventilated patients: State of the science. *AACN Clinical Issues, 12,* 247-258.

Helfrich-Miller, K. R. (1999). A life of language. *Advance for Providers of Post-Acute Care,* 47-48.

Hemsley, B., Sigafoos, J., Balandin, S., Forbes, R., Taylor, C., Green, V. A., et al. (2001). Nursing the patient with severe communication impairment. *Journal of Advanced Nursing, 35,* 827-835.

Hupcey, J. E., & Zimmerman, H. E. (2000). The need to know: Experiences of critically ill patients. *American Journal of Critical Care, 9,* 192-198.

Jablonski, R. S. (1994). The experience of being mechanically ventilated. *Qualitative Health Research, 4,* 186-207.

Jenny, J., & Logan, J. (1992). Knowing the patient: One aspect of clinical knowledge. *Image: Journal of Nursing Scholarship, 24,* 254-258.

Jensen, L. A., & Allen, M. N. (1996). Meta-synthesis of qualitative findings. *Qualitative Health Research, 6,* 553-560.

Johnson, M. M., & Sexton, D. L. (1990). Distress during mechanical ventilation: Patients' perceptions. *Critical Care Nurse, 10,* 48-57.

Jones, E. (1986). Communication aids for the critically ill. *Care of the Critically Ill, 2,* 117-122.

Logan, J., & Jenny, J. (1997). Qualitative analysis of patients' work during mechanical ventilation and weaning. *Heart and Lung, 26,* 140-147.

MacKellaig, J. M. (1987). A study of the psychological effects of intensive care with particular emphasis on patients in isolation. *Intensive Care Nursing, 2,* 176-185.

Manthous, C. A., Schmidt, G. A., & Hall, J. B. (1998). Liberation from mechanical ventilation: A decade of progress. *Chest, 114,* 886-901.

Menzel, L. K. (1998). Factors related to the emotional responses of intubated patients to being unable to speak. *Heart and Lung, 27,* 245-251.

Noblit, G. W., & Hare, R. D. (1988). *Meta-ethnography: Synthesizing qualitative studies.* Newbury Park, CA: Sage.

Parker, H. (1984). Communication breakdown. *Nursing Mirror, 158,* 37-39.

Paterson, B. L. (2001). The shifting perspectives model of chronic illness. *Image: Journal of Nursing Scholarship, 33,* 21-26.

Paterson, B. L., Thorne, S. E., Canam, C., & Jillings, C. (2001). *Meta-study of qualitative health research: A practical guide to meta-analysis and meta-synthesis.* Thousand Oaks, CA: Sage.

Pennock, B. E., Crawshaw, L., Maher, T., Price, T., & Kaplan, P. D. (1994). Distressful events in the ICU as perceived by patients recovering from coronary artery bypass surgery. *Heart and Lung, 23,* 323-327.

Peplau, H. E. (1992). Interpersonal relations: A theoretical framework for application in nursing practice. *Nursing Science Quarterly, 5,* 13-18.

Peplau, H. E. (1999). Psychotherapeutic strategies. *Perspectives in Psychiatric Care, 35,* 14-19.

Radwin, L. (1995). Knowing the patient: A process model for individualized interventions. *Nursing Research, 44,* 364-370.

Rier, D. A. (2000). The missing voice of the critically ill: A medical sociologist's first-person account. *Sociology of Health and Illness, 22,* 68-93.

Riggio, R. E., Singer, R. D., Hartman, K., & Sneider, R. (1982). Psychological issues in the care of critically ill respirator patients: Differential perceptions of patients, relatives, and staff. *Psychological Reports, 51,* 363-369.

Russell, S. (1999). An exploratory study of patients' perceptions, memories and experiences of an intensive care unit. *Journal of Advanced Nursing, 29,* 783-791.

Schumann, R. R. (1999). *Intensive care patients' perceptions of the experience of mechanical ventilation: A dissertation.* Unpublished doctoral dissertation, Texas Woman's University.

Simonds, S. K. (1995). Communication theory and the search for effective feedback. *Journal of Human Hypertension, 9,* 5-10.

Tanner, C. A., Benner, P., Chesla, C., & Gordon, D. R. (1993). The phenomenology of knowing the patient. *Image: Journal of Nursing Scholarship, 25,* 273-280.

Thorne, S., & Paterson, B. (1998). Shifting images of chronic illness. *Image: Journal of Nursing Scholarship, 30,* 173-178.

Urden, L. D. (1997). Endnote: From the patient's eyes. *Critical Care Nurse, 17,* 104.

Viner, E. D. (1985). Life at the other end of the endotracheal tube: A physician's personal view of critical illness. *Progress in Critical Care Medicine, 2,* 3-13.

Wojnicki-Johansson, G. (2001). Communication between nurse and patient during ventilator treatment: Patient reports and RN evaluations. *Intensive and Critical Care Nursing, 17,* 29-39.

Western Journal of Nursing Research, 2004, 26(1), 104-106

Commentary by Thorne

A meta-synthesis represents an opportunity to critically interpret the body of qualitative literature that has accumulated in a field, to rigorously interpret the conclusions that are possible because of it, and to add something new to our understanding that would not have been possible based on a mere critical review of the existing literature. This meta-synthesis makes a valiant attempt to build on what is known about health care communication under compromised circumstances and add an original dimension to the evolving discourse on "voice." It focuses our attention on those who are mechanically ventilated, or explicitly "voiceless." With the chilling reminder that such patients characteristically recall their experiences after the fact, this meta-synthesis attempts to link the discoveries that have been made using qualitative approaches to enhance our understanding of this profoundly vulnerable state in which some patients find themselves.

The foundations for the meta-synthesis begin effectively, with accessible and reasoned explanations for the inclusion criteria and logic trail that guides the study. As the analysis unfolds, however, we begin to glimpse the struggle that meta-synthesis can become in this genre and the distinctions between primary, secondary, and meta-analytic logic become somewhat obscured. When a researcher engages in meta-synthesis, he or she is making a claim about a different or higher order conclusion that can be generated from the available research. Thus, meta-synthesis inherently invites critical reflection on what exists in the scholarly literature and why it exists, and the claims made based on a meta-synthesis study similarly invite an ongoing dialogue. In this instance, I take up that invitation to wrestle with some of the apparent assumptions that have been made and with the conclusions that are drawn because of them.

First, the author assumes that the atheoretical nature of the primary studies limits the potential of the meta-synthesis to formulate complex depictions of the phenomenon. This is a claim with which I would take issue and counter with the suggestion that the absence of a theoretically driven set of studies might also represent a distinct advantage toward this end. Too often, the theoretical entanglement of qualitative investigations in the applied health sciences makes it difficult to discern that which is original scholarship within the conceptual structure of the research report (Sandelowski, 1993; Thorne, Joachim, Paterson, & Canam, 2002). Because of this, atheoretical

DOI: 10.1177/0193945903259463

February 2004, Vol. 26, No. 1   **105**

research may yield a more pure form of inductive reasoning about a phenomenon that becomes possible based simply on engagement with the data.

Second, although the meta-synthesis report consists mainly of similarities in findings across the studies, the author proposes that its credibility might have been limited by the variation in methodological approaches. In my view, the discussion starts to become interesting when it attempts to provide us with a brief glimpse of findings that did not conform to the common themes reported here. However, in the absence of an explicit critical analysis, it becomes difficult to discern what sense the author makes of why certain aspects of the research are similar and why the variations might have occurred. Although some might argue that methodological variation limits the credibility of a meta-synthesis (Jensen & Allen, 1996), I would propose that methodological diversity enhances the possibility of finding alternatives to the common themes we might ordinarily assume to obtain a complex and multifaceted portrait of the phenomenon. When methods are overly similar, we may more often revert to aggregation rather than actual synthesis of new conceptualizations.

Third, the complications inherent in representation in meta-synthesis become apparent in the reporting style, in which individual data examples from participants in primary studies rather than the interpretive claims made by the authors of the primary conclusions become the reference point for new findings. In the absence of explanations for the interpretive strategy, we are left with claims about aggregations of common themes. On this basis, some of the conclusions and recommendations seem less critically derived than we might anticipate, and their legitimacy as conclusions of this kind of research comes into question. We are told, for example, that inconsistency of nursing staff contributes to the unmet needs of this population but have no access to the kinds of interpretive claims from the body of original work from which this conclusion might have been drawn. Could it be that the primary studies were dominated by the research agenda of one particular academic discipline? Do persons who recall their mechanically ventilated experiences actually spontaneously report experiences related to inconsistency of nursing staff? Or, as we might imagine, is it more likely that they would tell us that certain nurses are better at communicating with them than others, in which case consistency might be relevant only if one had access to the better communicators? One wonders whether the primary researchers might have been so captured by the frustrating vulnerability of the circumstance they were studying that they may have grasped at the kind of recommendation that would seem most acceptable to the profession.

The attraction of meta-synthesis is that it offers to take us beyond a critical review of existing qualitative research and into a new domain of understanding. Ideally, therefore, it exposes new questions at least as often as it provides new answers. Yet we are left at the conclusion of this study with the disquieting feeling that the most relevant questions may still lie beyond reach. Perhaps meta-synthesis is best understood as a "work in progress." In that context, this article invites us into the initial phase of a journey into the complex world of "voicelessness" so that we can reflect on our aspirations when we attempt to provide it voice as qualitative researchers. We look forward to the insights and inspirations that such a journey might yield in the fullness of time.

REFERENCES

Jensen, L. A., & Allen, M. N. (1996). Meta-synthesis of qualitative findings. *Qualitative Health Research, 6*, 553-560.

Sandelowski, M. (1993). Theory unmasked: The uses and guises of theory in qualitative research. *Research in Nursing and Health, 16*, 213-218.

Thorne, S., Joachim, G., Paterson, B., & Canam, C. (2002). Influence of the research frame on qualitatively derived health science knowledge. *International Journal of Qualitative Methods, 1*(1). Available from www.ualberta.ca/~ijqm/

Sally Thorne
University of British Columbia,
School of Nursing

Western Journal of Nursing Research, 2004, 26(1), 107-109

Commentary by Paterson

The author of the article "Nonvocal Ventilated Patients' Perceptions of Being Understood" is quite right that we need to be able to synthesize bodies of qualitative research to determine what we know and where we should go in the field of research that is our phenomenon of interest. The topic of the communication experience of ventilated patients is timely and important. The fact that this topic is one that is often overlooked was emphasized by the few studies that have been conducted in this area over the last 2 decades. The article raises some interesting insights about the communication experience of ventilated patients and about research within this particular field of study.

Reading participants' quotes and the author's discussion of the implications of the research findings for practitioners moved me. I was reminded about the challenge that nonvocal patients, not only those who are ventilated, present to nurses who rely largely on verbal interchange as communication. I recalled a patient who had a talking computer because her amylotrophic lateral sclerosis (ALS) had resulted in her not being able to talk. She took a great deal of time to type out sentences, using a blowing technique, on her computer. In my impatience, I sometimes finished sentences for her. She responded by changing her message. For example, when she wrote: "I wish my doctor would . . . ", I interjected: "tell you that you can go home." She would then type: "No. I wish my doctor would visit me more." She taught me that her need to communicate was being compromised because of my hurry to get on with the tasks of the day. She taught me to be more patient.

There are some methodological ambiguities in the study. My interpretation of meta-synthesis differs from that of the author. I believe that the article represents the meta-analysis component of meta-synthesis. Meta-analysis can make valuable contributions to our understanding of the research within a particular field. For example, we conducted a meta-analysis of qualitative experience in the area of diabetes and were able to identify the somewhat paradoxical metaphors of balance and control as central in researchers' conceptualization of the diabetes experience (Paterson, Thorne, & Dewis, 1998). A synthesis of this research extended the analytic component to include the influences of research methodology and theoretical frames, as well as sociocultural and historical contexts, in researchers' interpretations of their research findings. The synthesis resulted in a new model of chronic

DOI: 10.1177/0193945903259464

108   *Western Journal of Nursing Research*

illness. I would encourage those interested in the method to read writing by Sandelowski and Barrosso (2002a, 2002b) or Thorne, Joachim, Paterson, and Canam (2002) about the complexities of meta-synthesis and some ways to address these.

The author clearly identifies some of the central debates surrounding meta-synthesis, such as the decision to include studies representing a variety of research approaches or to include only those studies in which one approach was used. I agree that the decision to select studies with various research approaches is justifiable. However, I am concerned that as meta-synthesis as an interpretive method is a construction of what researchers have constructed in their research reports; it does not fit with either the intentions or the research frame of descriptive research approaches, such as descriptive phenomenology. The role of the researchers' selection of research method was not discussed in the article. The author states: "Greater depth of the meaning of nonvocal communication experiences was obtained when the experiences were examined in a broader context" and gives as an example a grounded theory study by Logan and Jenny (1997) in which the work of ventilation was described. The fact that grounded theory is an interpretive method in which the phenomenon under study is assumed to be a social process (i.e., ventilation involves the exchange of meaning interpretation) is not discussed. Likewise, there is limited discussion of the influence of theoretical frame in researchers' analysis of data. The author indicates that Gries and Fernsler (1988) confirmed the use of Neuman's model of nursing in their research but did not discuss how the selection of Neuman's model of nursing as a theoretical framework may have shaped how the researchers studied communication (i.e., interviews rather than participant observation) and interpreted their research findings.

There are a number of other features of the primary research reports selected for the meta-synthesis that are striking and worthy of further analysis, particularly in regard to sample selection. For example, there is a variation in the time since extubation among participants, ranging from 17 hr to 108 months. It would be interesting for the author to investigate how the story of the ventilated experience differs over time. For example, after 108 months, do people recall only the horrific and startlingly aspects of the experience or do they minimize the trauma of the experience because the passage of time has resulted in their mediating the emotional outcomes? Another interesting finding would be to compare the data associated with people who had been ventilated for lengthy periods (e.g., 214 days as in Logan & Jenny, 1997) with those who had been ventilated for short periods. Is it possible that one develops means of communication over time and with experience as a ventilated patient?

In conclusion, the research is an excellent reminder that just because people cannot talk, it does not mean they do not have needs for communication. It also emphasizes the need for nurses' sensitivity to the experience of ventilated patients.

REFERENCES

Gries, M. L., & Fernsler, J. (1988). Patient perceptions of the mechanical ventilation experience. *Focus on Critical Care, 15*, 52-59.

Logan, J., & Jenny, J. (1997). Qualitative analysis of patients' work during mechanical ventilation and weaning. *Heart and Lung, 26*, 140-147.

Paterson, B., Thorne, S., & Dewis, M. (1998). Adapting to and managing diabetes. *Image: Journal of Nursing Scholarship, 30*(1), 57-62

Sandelowski, M., & Barroso, J. (2002a). Finding the findings in qualitative studies. *Journal of Nursing Scholarship, 34*(3), 213-219.

Sandelowski, M. & Barroso, J. (2002b). Reading qualitative studies. *International Journal of Qualitative Methods, 1*(1). Available from http://www.ualberta.ca/~ijqm/

Thorne, S., Joachim, G., Paterson, B., & Canam, C. (2002). Influence of the research frame on qualitatively derived health science knowledge. *International Journal of Qualitative Methods, 1*(1). Available from http://www.ualberta.ca/ijqm/

Barbara Paterson
University of British Columbia,
School of Nursing

Western Journal of Nursing Research, 2004, 26(1), 110-112

Response by Carroll

These thorough commentaries offer thought-provoking perspectives that are helpful in furthering the interpretation of the nonvocal experience through the process of meta-synthesis. I concur with the commentators' suggestion that this meta-synthesis is an initial step in a research area that surely requires further exploration. The commentators touched on the many controversial issues that have arisen as meta-synthesis, a relatively young method of research, continues to be developed.

Although both commentators support methodological diversity within the primary studies, one commentator raises the concern of whether descriptive approaches should be part of an interpretive meta-synthesis. As addressed in the article, there were a limited number of studies on this topic; so the decision was made to include primary studies with varying methodologies despite some authors' criticisms of blending methods (e.g., Jensen & Allen, 1996). Because of the limited selection, a great number of the primary studies of this meta-synthesis were descriptive. As a result, basic similarities across studies were found. The descriptive studies, however, also were helpful in corroborating interpretive findings. Although it likely would be unadvisable to use solely descriptive studies to compose a meta-synthesis sample because of the interpretive nature of the meta-synthesis process, a combination of methodologies may lead to a fuller understanding of the phenomenon. I agree that if a large group of primary studies is accessible, limiting purely descriptive studies and including more interpretive studies would highlight variances and the reasons for those variances.

One commentator proposed that using atheoretical primary studies would lead to more pure inductive reasoning. Studies with some structure, via a theoretical framework, actually provided greater detail about the themes and their linkages in this meta-synthesis. The studies with no theoretical framework, perhaps surprisingly, contributed to more similarities in the findings than did those with a theoretical framework. Because qualitative studies about the experience of being nonvocal while ventilated had not been synthesized previously, a combination of atheoretical and theoretical primary reports provided a mix of broad structure and complete free flow of ideas. The central inductive nature of the meta-synthesis process was not compromised by including studies with a theoretical base.

DOI: 10.1177/0193945903259465

February 2004, Vol. 26, No. 1   **111**

Through reciprocal translation, which Noblit and Hare (1988) described as a form of synthesis, the connections among various interpretive claims as well as potential causes and effects were made clearer in this meta-synthesis. Inconsistent nursing staff, for example, was seen as a cause of unmet needs of nonvocal persons who therefore experienced a loss of control. These linkages were borne out in descriptive and interpretive primary studies within this meta-synthesis. The interpretation of synthesized themes was portrayed partly by selecting quotations from primary study data that most effectively demonstrated the essence of the particular theme. For example, one participant spoke of not being in control of his destiny. Although this comment is an individual data example, it illustrates the broader interpretive claim of loss of control; a richer depiction of the experience was portrayed. The quotations used in a meta-synthesis can be likened to exemplars, which Benner (1994) described as conveying aspects of a thematic analysis.

One of the challenges of undertaking meta-synthesis is the reliance on the primary researchers' interpretations (Paterson, Thorne, Canam, & Jillings, 2001). Many of the primary studies did not describe variations in their themes based on respondent characteristics. For example, some studies had respondents with wide ranges of intubation times but did not specify whether certain themes applied to those with longer versus shorter intubation times. This points to the importance of thorough primary research reports when determining a sample for a meta-synthesis. As more research is generated about the nonvocal experience, there will be a wider pool of primary studies from which to select thus enhancing the ability to explain variations.

As more meta-syntheses are conducted, clearer guidelines likely will be developed regarding the difficult issues raised by the commentators. If there were a larger pool of accessible primary studies, I would select studies with mostly interpretive methodologies and fewer studies with purely descriptive methodologies so that variances would be more prominent and explainable. I would continue to select primary studies with theoretical and atheoretical bases, as both offer unique perspectives. I look forward to observing the evolution of meta-synthesis as a research method, because it offers a wonderful potential to broaden our understanding of many complex issues in nursing. In addition, continuing research in the area of nonvocal communication issues will enable nurses to better understand the experience and ultimately enhance care for this population.

REFERENCES

Benner, P. (1994). The tradition and skill of interpretive phenomenology in studying health, illness, and caring practices. In P. Benner (Ed.), *Interpretive phenomenology: Embodiment, caring, and ethics in health and illness* (pp. 99-127). Thousand Oaks, CA: Sage.

Jensen, L. A., & Allen, M. N. (1996). Meta-synthesis of qualitative findings. *Qualitative Health Research, 6,* 553-560.

Noblit, G. W., & Hare, R. D. (1988). *Meta-ethnography: Synthesizing qualitative studies.* Newbury Park, CA: Sage.

Paterson, B. L., Thorne, S. E., Canam, C., & Jillings, C. (2001). *Meta-study of qualitative health research: A practical guide to meta-analysis and meta-synthesis.* Thousand Oaks, CA: Sage.

Chapter 7

Teaching Meta-Analysis: Summarizing Quantitative Research

Michael J. Barnes and Rona F. Levin

> To understand God's thoughts we must study statistics, for these
> are the measure of His purpose.
>
> —Florence Nightingale

Meta-analysis is a quantitative technique used to summarize research.
Participants of a meta-analysis are the actual studies that are summarized.
Like many other quantitatively oriented topics, meta-analysis is difficult
to understand, and thus difficult to teach. Our experience has shown us
that the first principle of teaching meta-analysis is to tailor the presentation to the audience. That is, if the audience is quantitatively savvy, then
the presentation could be mathematically oriented and full of quantitative
theory, formulas, and calculations. Otherwise, as is usually the case with
nursing students or clinicians, the presentation is best prepared in a
way that is engaging and conceptually oriented with little in the way of
mathematical formulae. This chapter contains the content we share with
students about meta-analysis in simple terms. It also includes some of

the strategies we use to make the content interesting, understandable, and, yes, even fun.

HISTORICAL SIGNIFICANCE

The beginning use of quantitative techniques for summarizing studies dates back to the early eighteenth century, when mathematician Roger Cotes attempted to combine the findings of different astronomers (Shadish, Cook, & Campbell, 2002). He combined computed weighted averages (to be discussed later in the chapter) of the measurements that astronomers were calculating. Later, in 1904, Sir Karl Pearson combined the results of six studies regarding a newly developed inoculation of typhoid fever. Other early historical accounts exist of such summaries (Cooper & Hedges, 1994; Dickerson, Higgins, & Meinert, 1990; Hunter & Schmidt, 1990; Shadish & Haddock, 1994). Widespread use of meta-analysis did not occur until 1976. As the story goes, Gene V. Glass was the first to detail a general method for accumulating effect sizes over studies from any literature, coining the term *meta-analysis* to describe the method.

Including the impetus behind the "first" meta-analysis makes the reason for such an approach to research come alive, especially if is presented in a humorous way. Thus the first author (Barnes) has told the following story to students. In his work, Glass was attempting to determine the effectiveness of psychotherapy. Glass's interest was instigated by claims made by Hans Eysenck (1978), who beginning in 1952 stated that psychotherapy had no "real" positive effects. In fact, it is rumored that he called psychotherapy a "bunch of hogwash." In addition to creating an intense debate in the academic field of clinical psychology that lasted decades, Eysenck created quite a clamor amidst practicing clinicians, posing a threat to their very livelihood. In the academic realm, and with the aid of practicing clinicians, more than 370 studies were conducted by the mid 1970s in response to Eysenck's edict. Unfortunately, due to the contradictory results of these studies, no qualitative summary of the research could provide conclusive evidence to either support or refute Eysenck's claims.

To attempt to bring some resolve to this issue (not to mention some possible relief to panicking clinicians), Glass and his colleague Mary Lee Smith embarked on a summary of these studies. In contrast to qualitatively summarizing the 375 studies that addressed the effects of psychotherapy, they standardized and averaged the findings of this huge body of work. Results were published in their classic paper (Smith & Glass, 1976). They concluded that indeed psychotherapy was effective, marking the occasion of the first systematic modern attempt at quantitatively combining the results of many studies. (It is important to note that Eysenck, never one to accept the results of just "one" study as conclusive evidence, held firm to his notion, calling this meta-analysis "mega-silliness" [Eysenck, 1978]. It seems he missed the boat, disregarding the fact that this one study encompassed 375 *single empirical* studies. "Despite the criticisms of Eysenck and other scholars, meta-analysis is now widely accepted as a method of summarizing the results of empirical studies within the behavioral, social, and health sciences" [Lipsey & Wilson, 2000, p. 1].)

THE BASIS OF META-ANALYSIS

In our teaching we move from the history of meta-analysis to a presentation and discussion of its basic principle: the use of a common metric over studies. The essential motivation of Glass and his colleagues was the use of the effect size as the common metric. A common metric is needed because different studies rarely use identical ways to measure outcome variables, even if the individual studies address similar questions and invoke similar outcome constructs. Providing examples of the concept of using a common metric is an essential strategy for facilitating students' understanding. One example we use has to do with a hypothetical meta-analysis of depression. Studies investigating depression might have used different measures of depression; that is, one study of psychotherapy for depression might have used the Beck Depression Inventory, whereas another may have used the MMPI Depression scale. By utilizing different measures, the studies have operationalized depression differently. The measures have different metrics with different means and standard deviations, so averaging the scores across studies without converting them into a common metric would yield nonsensical results. Meta-analysis converts each study's outcomes to a common effect-size metric, so that different measurements of outcomes wind up having the means and standard deviations that have a common meaning and can thus be averaged across studies.

THE PROCESS OF META-ANALYSIS

The conduct of a meta-analysis, like any other form of research, must go through stages. These include, but are not limited to, problem formulation, review of literature, coding of studies, data collection (computing of effect sizes) and interpretation, data analysis, and evaluation. Last, a review of a study's limitations (examining possible threats to its validity) is done. As always, research should end with a public presentation of results. A presentation of the stages of a meta-analysis follows.

Problem Formulation

All reviews necessitate preliminary thoughtfulness about the problem to be addressed. The topic of reviews can be very broad, as a study that assesses the overall effect of psychotherapy (Smith, Glass, & Miller, 1980), or very narrow, such as a study that assesses whether the paradoxical interventions in psychotherapy improved outcomes (Shoham-Salomon & Rosenthal, 1987). As with any study, it is essential to develop a clear research question for a meta-analysis. This question provides direction for developing criteria that are used to determine which studies to include in the meta-analysis. The independent variables or treatments should be clear, as well as the dependent variables or outcomes of the meta-analysis. Also, whether or not the meta-analyst is trying to determine relationships of causality or correlation between the independent variable (i.e., treatment) and the dependent variable (outcome) are of primary importance and should be established at the start.

Review of the Literature

Persons conducting meta-analyses then need to conduct a literature search to find studies relevant to the problem. Studies should be located from a variety of sources. Published studies can be located from computerized databases, by inspecting reference lists of previous reviews, by scanning tables of contents of recent journals, and by identifying registers of past and ongoing clinical trials.

Although it may seem somewhat counterintuitive, both published and unpublished studies should be obtained. Because criteria for publication usually involve evidence of significant findings, studies that report nonsignificant findings are often not accepted for publication. Meta-analyses, however, are to be *all inclusive*; therefore, the inclusion of studies with nonsignificant results are needed to give a more objective and balanced picture of all research that bears upon the topic of interest. Unpublished studies are often hard to find. These may include unpublished dissertations and master's theses, final reports of grants and contracts, convention papers, technical reports, and even papers that were rejected for publication (the latter being those typically relegated to a file drawer). Failure to include studies that report "nonsignificant" findings results in what is referred to as the "file drawer problem." Also important is the identification and connection with any and all scholars who are interested in the research question. Therefore, personal contact with authors who have published in the area of interest is encouraged. These authors are usually aware of others of lesser-known reputations and who may have conducted unpublished works. Often, these individuals are involved in works in progress.

Regardless of the source of the work, studies must meet substantive criteria. They must address the question of interest and be relevant to the treatments, units, settings, measures, and times outlined in the guiding formulated problem.

Coding of Studies

Meta-analyses use a common coding scheme to quantify study characteristics and results. Individual codes should, first and foremost, reflect the researcher's hypothesis. For example, the hypothesis might be that a clean technique for urinary catheterization is as effective as a sterile technique in controlling urinary tract infection (UTI) in a population of homebound elderly clients. Codes for each important study characteristic should be developed. Codes often include the following:

- Characteristics of the study report: This includes such things as the date the study was published and the form of the publication.

- The participants: This would include the presenting problem and gender composition of the studies, as well as other demographic variables of importance to the studies comprising the domain of the study. Any exclusionary criteria restricting the scope of studies used should also be included.

- The intervention: This includes the type of intervention and dosage. Also to be noted is who provides the intervention and the setting where it is provided.

- The intervention process: This would involve the use of a manual to increase intervention fidelity. Intervention fidelity involves the use of a protocol to ensure that the intervention is operationalized in detail and applied similarly across studies.

- The methodology of the study: Elements conforming to this area include the sample size, method of assignment to conditions, and attrition, as well as kinds of measures employed. For example, experimental studies of treatment for depression using treatment versus control group comparisons generally will not be combined with observational (i.e., nonexperimental) studies in which level of depression was correlated with the level of service received by a group of patients in the same meta-analysis. Rather, all studies would be either of an experimental nature or of a nonexperimental nature.

Often a coding protocol is used to facilitate this process. One teaching strategy we have used when presenting this content is to circulate a coding form used for an actual meta-analysis.

Data Collection

Computation of Effect Sizes

A discussion of data collection is the most quantitatively oriented part of the presentation. As such, students might have tremendous difficulty following this part of the material. Therefore, we attempt to simplify this part of the presentation by minimizing the mathematical details and formulas we include. Rather, we offer a few effect size indices and emphasize under what circumstances they are used (see Table 7.1). A narrative of how we present this material follows.

As noted above, meta-analysis is done using a common metric, namely, effect size. For every statistical analysis there is an effect size. For example, when a study employs a correlational analysis, the correlation coefficient is informative of the effect size. When employing a *t* test, Cohen's *d* (a derivative of standardized and unstandardized mean differences; see below) is the pertinent index of effect size.

Effect size statistics embody information about both the direction and the magnitude of quantitative research findings. Which effect size statistic is appropriate depends on the nature of the research findings, the statistical forms in which they are reported, and the hypotheses being tested by the meta-analysis. As noted above, commonly used effect size indices, and the context in which they are used, are presented in Table 7.1.

Ideal Values for Effect Sizes

At this juncture, a comment or two should be made regarding the computation of effect sizes. Complex formulas are unnecessary; however, it is important to note the "ideal" values associated with the aforementioned

TABLE 7.1 Commonly Used Effect Size Indices and Indications for Their Use

Effect Size Index	When Used
1. Standardized Mean Difference	Experiment (or nonexperiment) when all dependent variables are measured on a continuous scale; studies use different measures/scales.
2. Unstandardized Mean Difference	Experiment (or nonexperiment) when all dependent variables are measured on a continuous scale; studies use the same measures/scales.
3. Correlation Coefficient	Nonexperiment when all dependent (criterion) variables are measured either on a continuous or a noncontinuous scale. Studies can use either the same or different measures/scales.
4. The Odds Ratio	Compares two groups in terms of the relative odds of a status of an event (e.g., death, illness, successful outcome, receipt of treatment, gender, exposure to a toxin). The dependent variables are inherently dichotomous.
5. Relative Risks Ratios	The risk ratio is a ratio of two conditional probabilities. This is sometimes confused with the odds ratio. The risk ratio is also used when the data are dichotomous. The relative risk ratios often represent the probability of failure in the treatment condition to the probability of failure in the control outcome.

Note: The latter two indices often are used in medical and nursing research.

effect sizes, that is, those values that are representative of a positive outcome.

The Standardized and Unstandardized Mean Difference

The mean difference (both standardized and unstandardized) is typically used in experimental studies contrasting treatment and nontreatment conditions. As noted above, means are standardized when the measures used in studies differ, for example, different measures of depression. When the same measures were utilized, unstandardized means are employed. The (1) standardized and (2) unstandardized mean difference (across studies) reflects the advantage (or disadvantage) of the treatment mean over that of the control group.

1. Standardized Mean $_{\text{Treatment}}$ – Standardized Mean $_{\text{Control}}$
2. Unstandardized Mean $_{\text{Treatment}}$ – Unstandardized Mean $_{\text{Control}}$

When either of the above indices is greater than zero, a positive treatment effect is noted. Conversely, when either of the differences is less than zero, the control condition results in a more favorable outcome than the treatment. When the effectiveness of the treatment condition is equal to that of the control condition, the mean difference in either case is zero.

The Correlation Coefficient (r)

When summarizing results of nonexperiments, especially correlational research, correlations are typically employed. A positive correlation co-efficient (across studies) is representative of a positive relationship be-tween treatment and outcome. Therefore, the ideal value associated with the correlation coefficient is positive or greater than zero. When the effectiveness of the treatment condition is equal to that of the control condition, the correlation coefficient is equal to zero.

Odds Ratio

The odds ratio is an effect size statistic that compares two groups in terms of the relative odds of a status of an event (e.g., death, illness, successful outcome, receipt of treatment, gender, or exposure to a toxin). The dependent variables are inherently dichotomous (e.g., good outcome or bad outcome).To understand the odds ratio, it is worth clarifying the meaning of *odds*. The odds of an event are defined as **odds of an event or outcome** $= p/1 - p$, where p is the probability of an event or outcome. A hypothetical example is used to clarify this concept.

For example, let's assume the **probability** of a successful outcome of treatment is .25, then the **odds** of that outcome is .33 or 1/3, that is, .25/1 − .25. Thus the *odds* of a successful outcome, given treatment, are 1 to 3 (one success in three failures). Contrast that with the *probability* of that successful outcome which is 1 in 4, that is, one success in four cases. In this same study, suppose that, for the control group the *probability* of a successful outcome is .20. The *odds* of a successful outcome, given no treatment (i.e., control condition), is then .25 or 1/4, that is, .20/1 − .20.

From the odds of success for the treatment and control groups, we can calculate the odds ratio, which is the ratio of those two odds, that is, .33/.25 or 1.33. Therefore, for these data the odds of a successful outcome are 1.33 times greater for the treatment group than for the control group.

It is easy to determine, therefore, that the ideal value associated with the odds ratio is a value greater than 1. When the odds ratio is greater than 1, it means that the ratio of succeeding exceeds that of failing, or a positive outcome. In other words, it is desirable that the odds of success (the numerator) be greater than the odds of failure (the denominator). Therefore, we want a very large fraction here (i.e., a fraction greater than 1). Note that if the odds of the treatment condition were identical to that of the control condition, then the overall odds ratio would be equal to 1.

Relative Risk Ratio

The relative risk ratio or index is just the opposite of the odds ratio. This index relates to the probability of risk (or lack of success) to that of success. Therefore, the ideal value of this index is less than 1. In other words, we want the probability of failure (the numerator) to be less than the probability of success (the denominator). Therefore, we want a very small fraction here, one that is less than 1. An example is employed to clarify this construct.

Suppose the risk of women who use a known antiseptic catheter made from silver oxide is compared to women who use a standard catheter regarding their asymptomatic bacteriuria. The data indicated that of 451 women who used a known antiseptic catheter made from silver oxide, 56 of them exhibited asymptomatic bacteriuria. Therefore, their risk ratio was .124 (56/451). Across the same studies, data also indicated that of the 285 women who used a standard catheter, 56 of them exhibited asymptomatic bacteriuria. Therefore, their risk ratio was .196 (56/285).

A comparison of the two risk ratios was revealed. The ratio of the treatment (i.e., use of the silver oxide catheter) to the standard catheter is .63 (.124/.196). Therefore, the risk associated with the treatment condition is less than that associated with the standard condition, because the ratio is less than 1. If the risk associated the treatment condition was greater than that associated with the standard condition, this ratio would be greater than 1. If the risk ratios of the treatment condition were identical to that of the standard condition, the overall risk ratio would be equal to 1.

Data Interpretation: Point Estimates and Confidence Interval Estimates of Effect Sizes

Point Estimation of Effect Size

Next, it is important to emphasize that any effect size statistic is like any other inferential statistic; that is, it is only a guess of a population parameter. For example, a mean of a sample, when computed, is only a guess of the population mean. As such, it has a degree of error associated with using it, because we are only using a fraction of the elements of the population in deriving it. So if we were to calculate the mean of a sample and the answer was 35, we would say that our best guess of the population mean is 35. But realize that it probably is slightly different from 35. This guess is what is referred to as "point estimation."

After arriving at the value of the effect size, it is important to gauge the strength (e.g., strong, weak, or moderate) of the effect size estimate. Guidelines exist for determining the strength of effect sizes. For example, in the case of the standardized and unstandardized mean difference, divide the mean difference by the standard error associated with the mean difference, which results in an index referred to as Cohen's d. The difference is a standardized index of strength of the effect of the treatment (if positive) or control (if it is negative) condition. The guidelines and parameters of d are as follows:

If d is less than .50, the strength of the effect is considered weak.

If d is .50 but less than .80, the strength of the effect is considered moderate.

If d is greater than .80, the strength of the effect is considered strong.

As stated above, guidelines exist for all effect size indices.

Using Confidence Intervals to Estimate Effect Size

In addition to making estimates with the use of a point estimator, we usually make estimates through the use of a confidence interval. In other words, we estimate with the use of an interval or range of values. In the case mentioned above, we would estimate the population mean with an interval. So, although we might say that our best guess of the population mean is 35, we would say that it is probably somewhere between 20 and 50. This estimation is done with a level of confidence, usually 95%, reflecting our confidence in obtaining a value in this range if we were to conduct this study over and over again. Putting it all together, we would say that our best point estimate of the population mean is 35; however, we are 95% confident that it is between 20 and 50.

Effect sizes are conceptualized the same way. Point estimates and confidence intervals of effect sizes are regularly computed in the course of a meta-analysis and appear on the computerized output during analysis. The idea is to understand the meaningfulness of these numbers. For example, if we were looking at a difference between means (treatment minus control), and we obtain a positive point estimate value for effect size, we would say that the effect size, because it is positive, suggests that there is a benefit of receiving treatment. If we look at the 95% confidence interval limits and see two positive values, we are confident that there is a consistent positive effect of treatment. If, however, the lower limit is negative and the upper limit is positive, there is no consistency in the benefit of treatment. Far worse, if both of the limits are negative, it is reflective of a consistent negative effect of treatment (i.e., a benefit to no treatment).

The same reasoning applies in the cases of all of the effect sizes. Therefore, one would want (1) two positive confidence limits for the confidence intervals of each of the following indices: the unstandardized mean difference, the standardized mean difference, and the correlation coefficient; (2) two confidence limits greater than 1 for the odds ratio; and (3) two confidence limits less than 1 for the relative risk ratio.

Many computerized programs are equipped with graphs of confidence intervals. This graphic display is of the utmost importance to clarify these concepts for novice students and researchers. For example, in Figure 7.1, which of the relative risk ratios are indicative of a positive outcome? If you answered number 2, you made the right call.

Data Analysis and Evaluation

Although topics such as the following are important to the person conducting meta-analyses, only casual mention need be given to students.

> *Data Analysis: Combining Effect Sizes.* Meta-analyses involve combining effect sizes over relevant studies. They require a researcher to arrive at an overall effect size for a given outcome across studies. Once effect sizes are obtained for separate primary studies, a mean or average across studies is calculated.

Outcome	Values for Risk Ratios (RR) (Point Estimation)	Values for 95% Confidence Intervals of Risk Ratios (Interval Estimation)	Charted Intervals of Risk Ratios Midpoint
			1
1	1.37	1.15 to 1.59	X——X
2	.85	.78 to .92	X—X
3	1.05	.90 to 1.20	X——X

FIGURE 7.1 Point estimates and confidence interval estimates of relative risk ratios.

Data Analysis: Weighting Effect Sizes. Prior to averaging effect sizes across studies, effect sizes are usually weighted. The most common weighting schemes include weighting according to sample size, weighting according to the reliability and validity of the outcome measures, weighting according to the quality of the studies, and weighting through the use of the standard error associated with the effect size.

Data Evaluation (testing of homogeneity of effect sizes). This is a test of the stability of the effect size being utilized. Computer programs conduct this test for the meta-analyst. This testing is done to assess whether a set of effect sizes varies only as much as would be expected due to sampling error. In other words, it examines the part of the difference between the population effect size and the sample estimate of that effect size that is due to the fact that only a sample of observations from the population were observed or selected.

If the variability of the effect sizes seems reasonable, then the observed effect sizes are said to be homogenous. The effect sizes in this case are considered to be *reliable* and the procedure continues without any special considerations or manipulations. If homogeneity is rejected, it is determined that the distribution of effect sizes contains more variance than we would expect by chance. The effect sizes in this case are considered *unreliable.* Additional analyses would be required in this case. In-depth discussion of these topics will prove distracting and of minimal importance to the overall understanding of most audiences. Remember, most audiences will be consumers of research rather than researchers.

Pointing Out of Possible Threats to the Validity of Meta-Analysis

All research suffers from possible threats to validity. Experiments, which are known to have high internal validity, are also known to have threats to their external validity. On the other hand, nonexperiments, which are famous for their external validity, do not enjoy their high internal validity. For those who need a review, internal validity is the ability to assign outcome effects to the influence of the independent variable, and external validity is the ability to generalize findings. Threats to the validity of meta-analyses may be grouped into four categories (Shadish et al., 2002). Although we mention the four broad areas to students, we do not spend a great deal of time describing them in detail. These threats are as follows:

1. Threats to inferences about the existence of a relationship between treatment and outcome: These threats endanger the re-

searcher's ability to say that the independent variables or treatments are related to the dependent variables or outcomes. These types of threats are the results of any or all of the following: (a) restriction of range in the primary studies; (b) missing effect sizes in primary studies; (c) the unreliability of coding in meta-analysis, and selection bias.

2.   Threats to inferences about the causal relationship between treatment and outcomes: These threats compromise the ability of the researcher to claim that the independent variables or treatments under study are actually causing observed changes in the dependent variables or outcomes. These threats result from (a) failure to assign to primary treatment at random; (b) primary study attrition; or (c) moderator variable confounding.

3.   Threats to inference about the constructs represented in meta-analysis—validity threats that apply when generalizing to target constructs: These threats compromise the researcher's ability to declare that the constructs the researcher claims to study are in actuality what the researcher is studying and compromises the construct validity of the independent or dependent variables of the meta-analysis. These threats are possible when any of the following is present: (a) monomethod bias, (b) rater drift, (c) reactivity effect, (d) confounding constructs with levels of constructs, (e) confounding constructs with other constructs, or (f) misspecification of causal mediating relationship.

4.   Threats to inferences about external validity in meta-analyses—threats to inferences about how effect size is influenced by variation in persons, settings, times, outcomes and treatments: These threats jeopardize the researcher's ability to generalize findings of the meta-analysis to the population of studies. When these threats are present, no confidence can be given to the conclusion that there is a relationship between the independent and dependent variables under investigation across all situations. These threats result when any of the following are present in the primary studies: (a) sampling biases associated with the persons, settings, treatments, outcomes, and times entering a meta-analysis; (b) failure to test for heterogeneity in effect sizes; and (c) lack of statistical power for studying disaggregated groups.

Interpreting, Analyzing, and Presenting Meta-Analytic Data: The Use of a Sample Problem

As is the case with any complex topic, the use of a sample problem or study is instrumental in helping students relate the conceptual to the real.

Oftentimes, inexperience with new concepts and lack of confidence on the part of students result in their perception that the material is too abstract and impractical for their use. The meaningfulness of the technique is lost, and its understanding is compromised. Therefore, the use of a sample problem in the domain of the audience enhances the presentation. Moreover, it presents an opportunity to make concrete references to the abstract concepts presented above. Having them read the study prior to presentation is also beneficial.

Although we have used several meta-analyses published in nursing research journals as samples in the past, more recently we have begun to use meta-analyses from the Cochrane Library (specifically, Cochrane Reviews) as sample studies, particularly when we are conducting workshops for clinicians. We do this for a number of reasons:

1.   When teaching students how to find evidence on a clinical problem, we usually recommend accessing the Cochrane database first.

2.   All meta-analyses conducted by the Cochrane Collaboration must meet preset criteria.

3.   Studies tend to use a variety of treatment effectiveness measures, such as relative risk (RR) and odds ratios (OR) in addition to the traditional Cohen's d. Thus, students see the application of previously learned content on treatment effectiveness formulas and the difference between clinical and statistical significance.

4.   Cochrane reviews contain the type of table and graph contained in Figure 7.1. Once students see the results of studies (i.e., effect sizes and confidence intervals) in a picture, they seem to gain a quicker understanding of the meaning of the numbers.

5.   Cochrane reviews also contain a myriad of tables, which provide information that includes the characteristics of each study reviewed, criteria used to rate the quality of each study, and the rating given to each study in the meta-analysis. This is much more information about each individual study than is usually presented in a traditional journal article.

6.   Finally, a Cochrane review is often more difficult to read and interpret than a traditional article found in a journal, such as *Nursing Research*. Thus, if a student masters the reading and understanding of a Cochrane review, then the reading and critical appraisal of a meta-analysis in traditional format should be easier.

We also try to tailor the study we use in this learning activity to our audience. For example, when we conducted a workshop for nurses in the acute care setting, we used a meta-analysis entitled "Types of Urethral

Catheters for Management of Short-Term Voiding Problems in Hospitalised Adults" (Brosnahan, Jull, & Tracy, 2004). When conducting a workshop for community health nurses, we used a study entitled, "Interventions for Preventing Falls in Elderly People" (Gillespie, Gillespie, Robertson, Lamb, Cumming, & Rowe, 2004), which targeted elderly people in the community as one group of studies.

Box 7.1 contains the handout we use to review meta-analyses with students and clinicians. In the academic setting, Levin has used these questions to guide students in writing a required paper that critically examines a meta-analysis. Levin also uses the questions as criteria to evaluate the paper. Important to note, however, is that the authors always conduct a class in which instructor and students review a sample study before requiring students to critique a different study on their own.

As an example, when presenting to graduate nurses in an academic setting or to a group of nurses in the clinical setting, we have used a meta-analysis conducted by Brosnahan and colleagues (2004). The article summarizes a group of studies that address the effectiveness of types of urethral catheters for management of short-term voiding problems in hospitalized adults. The presentation of this meta-analysis included helping students to identify the following components of the study:

1. Independent and dependent (outcome) variables;
2. The nature of the study, that is, what type of studies were included in the meta-analysis (i.e., experimental, nonexperimental, both experimental and nonexperimental);
3. The effect size statistic utilized in the study (relative risk ratios);
4. The methodology employed by the author, including all topics included in the *Coding* section above;
5. Results, including the average relative risk ratios regarding each of the outcomes, as well as the confidence intervals of the effect sizes per outcome. A summary sheet is often used to aid in recording and summarizing results (see Table 7.2). Providing this type of table with an audience and having them complete it (fill it in) is another strategy we have found successful in helping students and clinicians understand the results of a meta-analysis;
6. Limitations of and threats to the validity of the meta-analysis are then explored;
7. Implications for practice.

Pedagogical Considerations

We have noted above several strategies we use to help students learn how to read, interpret, and critically appraise meta-analyses. These include

Box 7.1
Critical Appraisal of a Meta-Analysis

Purpose: To develop beginning skill in the critical appraisal of systematic reviews of the available evidence on a topic of clinical interest.

Definitions:
    "A systematic review . . . is a rigorous summary of all the research evidence that relates to a specific question; the question may be one of causation, diagnosis, or prognosis [of a clinical problem] but more frequently involves the effectiveness of an intervention [for a clinical problem]. Systematic reviews differ from unsystematic reviews in that they attempt to overcome possible biases . . . by following a rigorous methodology of search, research retrieval, appraisal of the retrieved research for relevance and validity (quality), data extraction, data synthesis, and interpretation" (Ciliska, Cullum, & Marks, 2001).
    A meta-analysis is "a statistical approach to synthesizing the results of a number of studies that produces a larger sample size and thus greater power to determine the true magnitude of an effect" (Johnston, 2005).

Questions for Critical Appraisal:

Validity of the Review

- What types of studies are included in the systematic review? How many of each type are included?

- Are the types of studies included appropriate for answering the question? Elaborate on the type of question that gave direction to the review, that is, one of harm or prognosis, or one of treatment effectiveness.

- Does the systematic review include a description of how the validity of individual studies was assessed? If yes, describe the method(s) of assessment.

- How did the results compare from study to study?

- Were individual patient data or aggregate data used in the analysis?

Box 7.1 (continued)

Significance of Results

- How large was the treatment effect?
- What method was used to ascertain the effect?
- How precise is the estimate of treatment effect?

Usability of Results

- Are my patients so different from those in the study that the results don't apply?
- Is the treatment feasible in my setting?
- Were all the clinically important outcomes (harms as well as benefits) considered in the review? Explain.
- What are my patients' values and preferences related to the desired outcomes of treatment as well as side effects that may arise?

making the whole topic of meta-analysis come alive by sharing how this statistical technique evolved and the little known humorous anecdotes related to its history. The use of humor when presenting any difficult or anxiety-provoking material helps students relax and thus assimilate this information more readily. Another essential strategy for learning is to share this topic with students in a conceptual rather than a mathematical discussion, for example, by talking about the meaning of an effect size as an indication of treatment effectiveness and showing how seemingly complex formulas are really quite simple. Eliminating jargon and mathematical terms and putting explanations in simple language goes a long way to eliminating the mystique surrounding meta-analysis, or any statistical topic for that matter. In addition, the plentiful use of clinical examples throughout the discussion of meta-analytic techniques and the interactive critique of a clinical study helps nursing students to see the value of meta-analysis for them as clinicians. Moreover, going through an actual meta-analysis step by step during a class demonstrates that students do not have to be math prodigies to read and understand this type of research.

TABLE 7.2 Summary of Findings

	Outcomes of the Meta-Analysis		
1. Number with Asymptomatic Bacteruria	Effect Size Index (Relative Risk—RR)	Confidence Interval of RR	Conclusion
Silver oxide versus standard			
Silver alloy versus standard (duration of treatment < 1 week)			
Silver alloy versus standard (duration of treatment > 1 week)			
2. Number with Asymptomatic Bacteruria— Subgroup Analysis for Silver Oxide Catheters			
All participants			
Women only			
Men only			
All participants received Systemic antibiotics			
All women received Systemic antibiotics			
All men received Systemic antibiotics			
3. Number with Asymptomatic Bacteruria—Urinary Infections	Effect Size Index (Relative Risk—RR)	Confidence Interval of RR	Conclusion
Silver alloy versus standard			
4. Number with Urethral Secretions	Effect Size Index (Relative Risk—RR)	Confidence Interval of RR	Conclusion
Silver oxide versus standard			

TABLE 7.2   *(continued)*

	Outcomes of the Meta-Analysis		
5. Number with Pain	Effect Size Index (Relative Risk—RR)	Confidence Interval of RR	Conclusion
Silver oxide versus standard			
6. Number with Asymptomatic Bacteruria	Effect Size Index (Relative Risk—RR)	Confidence Interval of RR	Conclusion
Antibiotic impregnated (minocycline + rifampicin) versus standard (silicone)			
7. Number with Asymptomatic Bacteruria	Effect Size Index (Relative Risk—RR)	Confidence Interval of RR	Conclusion
Silicone versus Latex			
8. Number with Asymptomatic Bacteruria (Urinary Tract Infection)	Effect Size Index (Relative Risk—RR)	Confidence Interval of RR	Conclusion
Hydron-coated latex versus plain latex			
Hydron-coated latex versus PVC balloon			
PVC balloon versus plain latex			
Hydrogel-coated versus silicone			
9. Number with Burning Sensation in Urethra	Effect Size Index (Relative Risk—RR)	Confidence Interval of RR	Conclusion
Silicon versus non-silicon			

(continued)

TABLE 7.2 *(continued)*

Outcomes of the Meta-Analysis			
10. Number with Urethritis	Effect Size Index (Relative Risk—RR)	Confidence Interval of RR	Conclusion
Silicon versus latex			
11. Urethral Reaction	Effect Size Index (Relative Risk—RR)	Confidence Interval of RR	Conclusion
Hydrogel-coated latex versus siliconized latex			
Full silicon versus hydrogel-coated latex			
Full silicon versus siliconized latex			

In addition, the constant use of illustrations and diagrams, such as the one in Figure 7.1, facilitates students' understanding of meta-analytic techniques. In fact, whenever possible several whiteboards or chalkboards are set up around the presentation area so that the first author can draw as he talks. Many who cannot conceptualize the meta-analytic techniques by listening or reading text are aided by a visual version of the concepts being taught.

Finally, we would like to comment on the ideal situation of having a nurse researcher and statistician teach this topic together. Such a partnership combines quantitative competence with clinical nursing knowledge, allowing us to cover all the bases. We are able to handle technical quantitative questions for those few who are so interested. More important, we are able to answer questions about the relevance and application of these studies to clinical practice. Answers to the latter questions address the meaningfulness and purpose of meta-analysis to the field of nursing and, one hopes, leave students believing in its usefulness for answering burning clinical questions and improving patient care.

REFERENCES

Brosnahan, J., Jull, A., & Tracy, C. (2004). Types of urethral catheters for management of short-term voiding problems in hospitalised adults. *The Coch-*

rane Database of Systematic Reviews. Issue 1, Art. No. CD004013.pub2. DOI:10.1002/1465552858.

Ciliska, D., Cullum, N., & Marks, S. (2001). Evaluation of systematic reviews of treatment or prevention interventions [Electronic version]. *Evidence-Based Nursing, 4,* 100–104.

Cooper, H., & Hedges, L. V. (Eds.). (1994). *The handbook of research synthesis.* New York: Russell Sage Foundation.

Dickerson, K., Higgins, K., & Meinert, C. L. (1990). Identification of meta-analysis: The need for standardized terminology. *Controlled Clinical Trials, 15,* 11–14.

Eysenck, H. J. (1978). An exercise in mega-silliness. *American Psychologist, 33,* 517.

Gillespie L. D., Gillespie, W. J., Robertson, M. C., Lamb, S. E., Cumming, R. G, & Rowe, B. H. (2003). Interventions for preventing falls in elderly people. *The Cochrane Database of Systematic Reviews,* Issue 4. Art. No.: CD000340. DOI: 10.1002/14651858.CD000340.

Hunter, J. E., & Schmidt, F. L. (1990). *Methods of meta-analysis: Correcting error and bias in research findings.* Newbury Park, CA: Sage.

Johnston, L. (2005). Critically appraising quantitative evidence. In B. M. Melnyk & E. Fineout-Overholt (Eds.), *Evidence-based practice: A guide to best practice.* Philadelphia: Lippincott Williams & Wilkins.

Lipsey, M. W., & Wilson, D. B. (2000). *Practical meta-analysis.* Thousand Oaks, CA: Sage.

Shadish, W. R., Cook, T. M., & Campbell, D. T. (2002). *Experimental and quasi-experimental designs for generalized casual inference.* Boston: Houghton Mifflin.

Shadish, W. R., & Haddock, C. K. (1994). Combining estimates of effect size. In H. M. Cooper & L. V. Hedges (Eds.), *The handbook of research synthesis* (pp. 26–281). New York: Russell Sage Foundation.

Shoham-Salomon, V., & Rosenthal, R. (1987). Paradoxical interventions: A meta-analysis. *Journal of Counseling and Clinical Psychology, 55,* 22–28.

Smith, M. L., & Glass, G. V. (1976). Meta-analysis of psychotherapy outcome studies. *American Psychologist, 32,* 752–760.

Smith, M. L., Glass, G. V., & Miller, T. I. (1980). *The benefits of psychotherapy.* Baltimore: Johns Hopkins University Press.

Chapter 8

Creating Clinical Protocols With an Apgar of 10

Ellen R. Rich and Jamesetta A. Newland

> Learning is something students do, NOT something done to students.
>
> —Alfie Kohn

Clinical protocols are key components of advanced nursing practice. Many states mandate that advanced practice nurses use clinical protocols in order to diagnose and treat client problems. In addition to being legally required, clinical protocols aid health care providers to give consistent, up-to-date care, help clarify the scope of nursing practice in a particular clinical setting, and allow clinicians to tailor their care to the population mix they serve. Even in states where they are not required, protocols can be excellent resources for the novice practitioner, and the processes of protocol creation and revision compel providers to examine their practices in light of the most current evidence. As they constitute a basic foundation of advanced nursing practice, clinical protocols must be reflective of the most current and best available evidence. This chapter is designed to help the instructor teach—or the advanced practice nurse (APN) to learn—the process of evidence-based clinical protocol development.

WHAT IS A PROTOCOL?

The first and most basic step in teaching and learning about protocol development is to ensure that the learner understands what constitutes a clinical protocol. Recommendations and guidelines are frequently found in the literature, and novices will often confuse these with protocols. If the learner has never used a clinical protocol in practice, he or she may not have a clear idea of what the final product looks like (see Box 8.1).

A recommendation is a suggestion or endorsement of something as "worthy of acceptance or trial" (Merriam-Webster, 1996, p. 976). Recommendations for a good restaurant or movie are commonly shared among individuals, denoting that they are worth a try. In health care, recommendations are frequently made by professional organizations for general topics, such as promotion of physical activity, smoking cessation, and healthy eating. Guidelines, on the other hand, are "official" recommendations, outlining a more proscribed approach to specific conditions. In an effort to standardize patient care management, there has been a movement toward the use of nationally recognized guidelines. The Agency for Healthcare Research and Quality, part of the U.S. Department of Health and Human Services, has created an online national guideline clearinghouse (www.guideline.gov) to provide access to a wide variety of current evidence-based guidelines. These tend to be disease-focused and address broad populations (Slutsky, 2005). They are extremely useful in the development of clinical protocols.

The dictionary definition for protocol is "a detailed plan of a scientific or medical experiment, treatment, or procedure" (Merriam-Webster, 1996, p. 939). A protocol may be even more specific than a guideline, as it is not only disease-focused, but also can be tailored to a specific population and practice situation. For example, national guidelines address the global management of asthma, but a protocol might outline the management of asthma by APNs practicing in an inner city clinic with

Box 8.1
Comparison of Terms

Recommendation	Do or do not do this*
Guideline	Include this* in 'doing'
Protocol	Do it this way

*"this" refers to an action by the provider

adolescents. Protocols outline what elements of the health history should be taken, what physical findings should be assessed, what diagnostic tests need to be performed, and what plan of care should be followed. Protocol content is discussed in a subsequent section. A sample protocol may be found in Box 8.2.

Assessing Need and Finding Focus

How would the APN determine the need for a specific clinical protocol? The following are examples of situations where a unique rather than standard clinical protocol is needed.

- Lack of currency of textbooks

- Constraints on providers inherent in a particular health care setting or with a particular population

- A condition that is not thoroughly addressed in existing protocols

- Failure of existing protocols to address a specific population

- Cultural remedies that are not taken into account with standardized protocols

- To blend different national guidelines from various sources (e.g., National Heart, Lung, and Blood Institute [NHLBI], American Heart Association, and American Academy of Family Practice

In addition, an APN who develops a protocol must select a focus. The first step in determining what specific protocols need to be developed is to look carefully at patient characteristics. Local governments or past practice statistics can provide information relating to demographics, such as age, gender, and ethnicity. The local health department can identify morbidity and mortality information and epidemiologic trends. Computerized medical management systems can track frequently seen diagnoses. Advanced practice nurses can identify presenting problems that seem to require frequent MD consultation; these could be more easily handled by using a well-structured protocol.

Other elements to examine are the provider mix and level of autonomy in the practice. A practice where there are many physicians and few APNs, with easy accessibility to consultation, may not require extensive protocol creation. Alternatively, when there are no physicians on site or consultation is not easily available, APNs, especially if they are novices, might require a number of well-written protocols.

Box 8.2
Chlamydia in Women

Definition: Chlamydia is a common sexually transmitted infection caused by small intracellular, membrane-bound organisms. They may infect the cervix, urethra, Bartholin's glands, uterus, tubes and peritoneum. As the infection ascends the female reproductive tract, it causes pelvic inflammatory disease (PID), resulting in infertility, ectopic pregnancy, and chronic abdominal pain.

Subjective: Age (less than 25 is a risk factor).

Sexual history: Risk factors include multiple partners, new partner within last 2 months, not using a barrier method of contraception consistently, history of STDs, recent abortion, or partner with suspected or known chlamydia.

Dysuria, lower abdominal pain, abnormal bleeding.

Vaginal discharge, if present, may be scant.

80% of women with chlamydia have no symptoms.

Routine screening during annual examinations is recommended for those at risk.

Objective: Mucopurulent cervicitis—may have positive "swab test" (swab inserted into os has purulent material on it when removed)

Cervical erythema (redness may be patchy), friable cervix

Cervical, uterine, or adnexal tenderness.

Labs: Chlamydia Microtrak, culture, or genprobe

Gonorrhea culture or genprobe

Wet mount of vaginal smear to R/O coexistent vaginitis—many WBC's seen

Negative urine culture (with dysuria as a complaint).

Inflammation on Pap

RPR approximately 12 weeks after exposure

Box 8.2 (continued)

Differential: Gonorrhea, trichomoniasis, candidiasis, bacterial vaginosis, ureaplasma

Assessment: Chlamydia cervicitis or contact

*Consult/
Refer:*   Severe PID

Plan: May treat based upon clinical assessment or history of contact in absence of a positive test.

Treatment: 1. Doxycycline 100 mg po bid × 7 days   OR

2. Azithromycin 1 gm po in a single dose   OR

3. Ofloxacin 300 mg po bid × 7 days

If tetracyclines are contraindicated or patient is on OCPs or pregnant, may use:

4. E.E.S. 800 mg po qid × 7 days   OR

5. Amoxicillin 500 mg pot id × 7 days

If patient has PID, follow protocol for gonorrhea as well as chlamydia and use dual therapy.

*Patient
Education:*   1. Avoid coitus until treatment for both partners is complete and partners are asymptomatic.

2. Use condoms and spermicide to avoid transmission of STD.

3. Patient to notify all partners so they can be treated at UHC.

4. Provide counseling support or arrange appropriate referral, if needed.

Follow-up: 1. Return if symptomatology persists or for routine Pap and pelvic if needed.

2. Repeat testing for cure is optional if patient was treated with doxycycline or azithromycin.

May consider retest if treated with EES. If done, it must be delayed until at least 3 weeks after treatment.

Source: J. A. Newland & M. L. Huppuch (Eds.). (1998). *Clinical protocols manual* (3rd ed.). Rev. 2004. Pleasantville, NY: Pace University.

Determining Depth and Breadth

In addition to assessing areas of need for, and focus of, protocol development, the APN needs to determine the appropriate depth and breadth of protocols to be written. Determining the correct depth of information requires finding a balance between a protocol replete with information and one that is concise and quickly readable. After gathering extensive information about a topic, it is tempting to incorporate a good deal of it into a protocol. Does every possible symptom of a certain disease need to appear in the subjective section, or only those that are most commonly observed? The answer depends on who will be using the protocol and the frequency with which the condition is seen. In settings where students commonly see patients, or where there are many APNs, including novices, it is better to err on the side of more than less depth of information. The same is true for conditions that are less commonly seen in a particular practice. Providers who are less familiar with certain conditions may be more comfortable with a protocol that contains more detailed information. When a particular condition is frequently seen, or when providers are more experienced, protocols can be less detailed.

The breadth of a clinical protocol refers to how prescriptive it is for the provider. A narrowly focused protocol details the plan of care very exactly. Typically, specific medications are mentioned, with few alternative options. The need to perform certain diagnostic tests is clearly dictated by the protocol. Many find this "cookbook" approach comforting and safe. Others feel that narrow protocols are too restrictive, deprive the practitioner of the ability to make decisions, and remove the art from practice. The more specific the protocol is, the larger the task becomes of reevaluating the evidence for revision. For example, a protocol that provides the option to use any statin medication for a patient with hyperlipidemia would be less sensitive to revision than one that limits treatment to one particular brand name. New evidence about that one particular drug would require prompt revision of the narrower protocol.

Broader protocols allow for more autonomy when making decisions, and often suit situations where there are higher levels of provider expertise. Choice and flexibility are common; creating greater opportunity to tailor the plan of care to a variety of patients. Less prescriptive protocols may be threatening to the novice practitioner and may offer less support in the case of a legal challenge (Newland & Rich, 1996).

Gathering Information

Gathering essential information, based on current evidence, is perhaps the most important step in protocol development. For areas where evidence is conflicting, scarce, or not compelling, expert consultation may be sought. For example, when writing a protocol for Lyme disease at a time when little was known about that entity, an entomologist specializing in that illness was consulted. Supportive materials, such as patient information pamphlets, may be helpful to use as handouts or in the development of supplemental patient education tools.

THE GUTS

First, the topic of the protocol must be selected. Most protocol foci are disease-based, ruling out other conditions that may present in a manner similar to the illness in question. An alternate approach, however, and one that may be well suited to the novice practitioner, is symptom-based. This approach is suitable when a broad range of diagnoses are possible for a particular complaint. Examples are chest pain, syncope, and abdominal pain. Symptom-based protocols can direct the workup of more complex problems. There then can be additional protocols specific to the particular diagnoses included in the symptom-based protocol. Additionally, protocols may be developed to address different genders. For example, because of the location of the female reproductive organs, there is a wider range of differential diagnoses for a woman presenting with abdominal pain than for a man with the same complaint. Finally, a protocol may not be related to an illness state, but may be for health maintenance or promotion activities. Examples include protocols for providing particular immunizations, well-child visits at various ages, smoking cessation care, and management of Pap smear results.

Clinical protocols are generally organized in a problem-oriented medical record format, using categories based on subjective data, objective data, assessment (diagnosis and differential diagnoses), and last, plan of care. This facilitates an organized method of data gathering and interpretation, well aligned with the format of a patient visit, with history-taking followed by the physical examination, any on-site laboratory tests, and documentation.

Subjective

The subjective section of the protocol should include presenting patient complaints associated with the protocol topic. For example, if the protocol is for infectious mononucleosis, subjective complaints would include symptoms such as fatigue, sore throat, and fullness or pain in the area of the cervical lymph nodes. Generally, the more typical complaints are represented, unless the approach is to be more detailed (see the section on Depth and Breadth). Presenting symptoms may be listed in a format consistent with the seven parameters of symptom analysis: location, quality, severity, timing, setting, aggravating/alleviating factors, and associated manifestations (including pertinent negatives). This helps remind the APN to address the presenting complaint in a comprehensive manner. It is also extremely important to include symptoms of complications associated with the disease in question, to alert the provider to situations that might require emergency intervention or immediate referral. These are considered "not-to-miss" indicators, and are especially important for novice providers and for risk management. In the above example, a complaint of inability to swallow solids or liquids would likely necessitate intravenous hydration or possible hospital admission. Serious consequences could arise if a provider sent home without standard treatment a patient who had that complaint. The protocol author may choose to highlight (bold or italic print, for example) those complaints that would signal the need for consultation with or referral to a physician, or for emergency care.

Objective

The objective section should list signs that would point to the diagnosis that is the subject of the protocol. The author may choose to list signs in order of commonality, yet should not eliminate atypical but diagnostic findings. For example, a less common presenting sign of mononucleosis is periorbital edema. If a patient with a sore throat and vague symptoms of fatigue also presents with periorbital edema, the diagnosis of infectious mononucleosis would be far more likely. The protocol could also function as an educational tool when a provider who did not know about this particular presenting sign becomes newly informed. This section is also the place to include differences in presentation based on characteristics of a particular target population. For example, if a large number of a practice's patients are African American, the manifestation of a particular rash or color change in dark-skinned individuals should be included. Again, not-to-miss signs should be clearly highlighted.

The objective section should also include diagnostic tests when the results are available at the time of the visit, prior to making the diagnosis. Results of these tests would contribute to the diagnostic process. Again, this is site specific, and depends on the type of equipment and testing available. Examples of diagnostic tests that could be readily available include rapid streptococcal A tests, electrocardiograms, and urine microscopy.

Assessment

The assessment section necessarily includes the condition that is the topic of the protocol, but should also list differential diagnoses—other conditions that may present in a way that is similar to the illness in question. Depending on the topic of the protocol, there may be few or many differential diagnoses. For example, there are many more differential diagnoses that should appear in a protocol for tension headache than there would be for one dealing with ankle injury. The assessment section presents another opportunity to indicate not-to-miss conditions that would necessitate referral or consultation. When highlighting these red flag areas, the author can be quite specific, noting whether a problem should prompt consultation, referral, or emergency care, and also noting how quickly the action should occur.

Plan

The plan section provides a road map for the provider's actions. A thorough protocol includes the following elements within the plan section: orders for further diagnostic testing, if needed; the treatment plan; patient education; referral, if any; and follow-up instructions. Health maintenance or promotion issues should also be included. For example, the plan section for a protocol on asthma could address smoking cessation and annual influenza immunization.

The treatment plan should include not only medications, but also other therapeutic measures, for example, warm soaks, rest, or stretching exercises. If current evidence supports their use, suggested nutritional supplements, herbal products, and complementary modalities should be included. Patients' cultural values should also be considered and addressed as needed. Patient education should be specific, so that all providers give consistent information. It can be helpful to refer to specific patient education materials when in-depth information must be imparted.

Referral and follow-up instructions are critical, helping to assure continuity of care and as a legal mandate. The provider is obliged to track the status of referrals that are made, particularly if the consequences of a missed referral are dire. Clearly written follow-up instructions within a protocol guide the practitioner and help ensure that patients are told when to return. A protocol for hypercholesterolemia would outline timing and frequency of follow-up visits. If a return visit for a particular complaint is not required, the patient should be informed when their next health maintenance visit is due. Most important, clinical protocols should spell out what signs or symptoms of potential complications should prompt patients to return sooner or seek emergency care. These warning signs may include adverse effects of prescribed treatments.

References

Clinical protocols that are evidence-based are incomplete without a section that includes references. These should be current and reflect research and clinical expertise. A reference list might also include additional sources the clinician may consult when greater depth of information is needed.

UPDATING AND TROUBLESHOOTING

Even though writing a clinical protocol requires significant time and effort, the work does not end after the protocol is completed. There are always novel evidence, fresh guidelines, new treatments, and even medications that may be removed from the market. Clinical protocols should be systematically reviewed and revised on an annual basis. Some may require no changes whereas others will need extensive alteration. A helpful strategy is to keep an electronic or paper folder for each protocol, and file new information over the year as it becomes available. Then when updating is due, critical information is easy to locate. Radical changes based on new evidence may require that protocols be revised before the scheduled time, particularly when something included in the protocol is found to be hazardous or when a new beneficial therapy becomes available for use.

Troubleshooting is a less frequent necessity when a protocol has been carefully crafted. Once a protocol is in use, however, unforeseen problems may become evident. Perhaps a particular medication is too costly for most of the patients and a less expensive substitute would be as efficacious. Providers using the protocol should be urged to evaluate continuously its practicality, utility, advantages, and disadvantages, and provide constructive feedback to the author or coordinator.

CREATIVE ASSIGNMENTS FOR PROTOCOL DEVELOPMENT

There are a variety of student assignments that may be used to teach the process of evidence-based clinical protocol development. Group work is often preferred; as that modality promotes idea generation and exchange. Examples of learning activities are listed below.

1.   To promote conceptualization of what a protocol actually is, the instructor may provide the students written materials on a specific topic with which to create a protocol: fact sheets, current recommendations, guidelines, and an established protocol on the topic. Ask students to use these references to develop a rudimentary protocol. For example, to design a protocol for the diagnosis and management of genital chlamydia infection, the instructor provides students (a) a fact sheet on chlamydia (Centers for Disease Control, 2003)); (b) the U.S. Preventive Services Task Force's (USPSTF) *Recommendations and Rationale: Screening for Chlamydial Infection* (Berg & USPSTF, 2001); and (c) a commentary on the USPSTF document (Newland, 2002). After students have attempted to construct a protocol, they then are shown two protocols (Newland & Huppuch, 1998; Running & Berndt, 2003) for comparison. (Note: Or find similar resources for another topic.)

2.   Another exercise asks students to take an existing protocol and tailor it to various population groups. These groups can be based on gender, age, or ethnicity.

3.   A "protocol scavenger hunt" assignment directs groups of students to collect evidence-based material to construct a new protocol. Students may be assigned to search for (and evaluate) competing guidelines for the protocol as a whole, or the protocol may be divided into four parts (subjective, objective, assessment, and plan), with each student looking for literature related to one of the four parts.

4.   Ask students to compare protocols that have different foci. They would examine samples of disease-based, symptom-based, and health maintenance protocols. Questions to consider are: How are the structures of these similar or different? What types of evidence are used in the various cases? How are the sources similar or different? Who wrote the protocol?

CONCLUSIONS

By using the information included in this chapter, students will hopefully be able to develop protocols with an Apgar of 10. Nurses learn during basic training that the Apgar score is an accurate indicator of the immediate condition and chances for survival of an infant at birth. A higher score indicates a more favorable outcome. By approaching the development of a clinical protocol from an evidence-based perspective, you can create a protocol with an Apgar of 10. Allot 2 points for each of the five sections: subjective, objective, assessment, plan, and references. If your score is less than 10 initially, work to achieve and maintain a 10. The ultimate benefactors of a protocol with an Apgar of 10 are patients.

REFERENCES

Berg, A. O., & U.S. Preventive Services Task Force. (2001). Screening for chlamydia infection: Recommendations and rationale. *American Journal of Preventive Medicine, 20*(Suppl.3), 90–93. Retrieved April 29, 2004, from http://www.ahrq.gov.clinic/uspstfix.htm

Centers for Disease Control and Prevention. (2002). Sexually transmitted diseases treatment guidelines 2002. *Morbidity and Mortality Weekly Report, 51*(No. RR-6), 32–36.

Centers for Disease Control and Prevention. (2003). *Chlamydia.* Retrieved April 29, 2004, from http://www.cdc.gov/std.Chlamydia/STDFact-Chlamydia.htm

Merriam-Webster's collegiate dictionary (10th ed.). (1993). Springfield, MA: Merriam-Webster.

Newland, J. A. (2002). Commentary on screening for chlamydial infection: Recommendations and rationale. *American Journal of Nursing, 102*(10), 93.

Newland, J. A., & Huppuch, M. L. (Eds.). (1998). *Clinical protocols manual* (3rd ed.). Pleasantville, NY: Pace University.

Newland, J. A., & Rich, E. (1996). Nurse-managed primary care center. *Nursing Clinics of North America, 31,* 471–486.

Running, A. F., & Berndt, A. E. (Eds.). (2003). Chlamydial infection. In *Management guidelines for nurse practitioners in family practice* (pp. 678–680). Philadelphia: Davis.

Slutsky, J. (2005). Using evidence-based practice guidelines: Tools for improving practice. In B. M. Melnyk & E. Fineout-Overholt, *Evidence-based practice in nursing and healthcare: A guide to best practice* (pp. 221–236). Philadelphia: Lippincott Williams & Wilkins.

Torkko, K. C., Gershman, K., Crane, C. A., Hamman, R., & Baron, A. (2000). Testing for chlamydia and sexual history taking in adolescent females: Results from a statewide survey of Colorado primary care providers. *Pediatrics, 106*(3), E32.

Uphold, C. R., & Graham, M. V. (2003). *Clinical guidelines in family practice* (4th ed.). Gainesville, FL: Barmarrae Books.

Weiner, H. R. (1999). Chlamydia infection: The hidden epidemic. *Emergency Medicine, 31*(11), 88–91.

Chapter 9

How to Assess Clinical Protocols for an Evidence Base

Rona F. Levin and Lillie M. Shortridge-Baggett

> Education is what remains when we have forgotten all that we
> have been taught.
> —Lord Halifax

Practice protocols are used by clinicians to provide effective health care and ensure consistency among providers. Thus, we believe that developing skills to appraise critically the validity of protocols is a necessary outcome for nursing programs at both graduate and undergraduate levels. To accomplish these outcomes we have devised learning exercises that we use in both undergraduate and graduate nursing research courses to teach students to conduct assessments of the protocols they use in their nursing practices so that their practices can be evidence-based.

We use the term *protocol* here to refer to any written documentation of standards that has been developed to guide the practice of nursing in specific health care situations. These documents may be called policies, procedures, recommendations, guidelines, protocols, or decision guides. Although there are no consistent definitions of these terms, we have listed them by levels of increasing specificity for practice from policy to protocols to decision guides. In clinical situations that are very complex, decision guides, the highest level in protocol development, are used. These expert guides provide health care practitioners formulas for assessing clients and health care problems, making diagnoses based on findings of the assessment, and then designing a plan of care. Using decision guides helps practitioners tailor care to the individual patient (van Meijel, 2003). Decision guides also provide expected outcomes so that the effectiveness of interventions may be evaluated.

In chapter 8, Rich and Newland provided definitions for the different types of protocols available to the clinician. They also discuss steps to developing evidence-based protocols. In this chapter we present a guide for teaching students how to appraise protocols critically. The approach to teaching this critique in both undergraduate and graduate research courses is described.

Because nursing students at all educational levels need to approach practice with a critical eye and questioning mind, we use the learning activities in this chapter to teach undergraduate and graduate students why and how to assess the basis of practice protocols. An ideal place to introduce such a topic is the nursing research course, especially if it is taught from an EBP perspective. Regardless of specialty, graduate students and program graduates who use protocols in their own practice need to ensure that they and those they mentor are engaged in best practice and participate in developing recommendations, guidelines, protocols, and decision guides.

The purposes of the assignments differ depending on level of student. With undergraduate students, the main objective is to facilitate students' awareness of different types of evidence (knowledge) upon which protocols are based, and the kind of evidence used in developing specific practice protocols. At the graduate level, the process recommended for assessing protocols includes a careful review of protocol development, a determination about the level of evidence on which it is based, and the outcomes related to its use. The research course that we teach at Pace University Lienhard School of Nursing emphasizes assessing the scientific evidence for the protocol rather than other sources of knowledge. There are several resources to assist in locating the protocols, evaluative criteria, and information needed in using the strategies with specific clients (Courtney, 2005; McSweeney, Spies, & Cann, 2001; Melnyk & Fineout-Overholt, 2005; Sackett, Straus, Richardson, Rosenberg, & Haynes, 2000; Titler, 2001). Regardless of the guidelines used, an effort is made to determine the type, strength, quality, and consistency of the evidence in assessing the validity of the protocol.

METHOD FOR TEACHING UNDERGRADUATE STUDENTS IDENTIFICATION OF THE BASIS OF NURSING PROTOCOLS

Purpose

This learning activity/assignment is intended to create an awareness of the various sources of human knowledge by providing students with an opportunity to question the research or evidence base of standard nursing interventions. The goals of this assignment are for students to (a) identify the bibliographical and other sources used in the development of a selected nursing technique or protocol; (b) determine whether the nursing technique or protocol was based on research or other types of evidence; and (c) suggest potential problems that may arise from using nursing techniques or protocols that are not based on valid evidence (Levin & Feldman, 2002).

Assignment

The learning activity described below is placed at the beginning of a nursing research course. Students are asked to work independently in their clinical practice sites to complete the assignment. You may ask them simply to take notes about their findings and share with classmates as a class exercise or to write a short paper describing their findings. In any case, they can use the following criteria as a guide to their presentation or paper:

- Describe the technique/protocol and the process of its development.

- Categorize the sources of knowledge used to develop the procedure/protocol that was identified by the interviewee (i.e., authority, tradition, experience, or scientific).

- State a conclusion about whether or not the protocol is evidence-based and identify the specific evidence you found to support it.

Learning Activity

Students are asked to select a nursing protocol/technique (such as urinary catheterization or intravenous maintenance) from a clinical agency's policy and procedure manual. They may obtain a copy of the selected protocol from an agency's nursing or nursing education office. Then students determine who wrote the protocol. This information may be obtained from an in-service educator or nursing administrator. Students request an interview with one or more individuals who are involved in developing practice protocols for the agency. The purpose of the interview is to determine the basis for the existing protocol. Suggested interview questions include the following:

- Can you explain how protocols are written in your agency?

- On what information was this specific protocol based?

- If references are not cited on the protocol, ask the following: "Are there any references that will give me a better understanding of the rationale for the practices included in the protocol?"

- If references are listed on the protocol ask, "Can you tell me the type of references these are?"

METHOD FOR TEACHING ASSESSMENT OF PROTOCOLS AT THE GRADUATE LEVEL

Purpose

Because the ability to assess practice protocols is so essential for the advanced practice nurse, we have included course content and an assignment related to this topic in the graduate research course we teach. The course was revised 2 years ago from a traditional research course to one with an EBP focus. The assignment and learning activity presented here were originally developed and introduced into the course by Levin and have been expanded upon by Shortridge-Baggett. This learning experience is designed to help graduate students develop beginning skill in determining the evidence base, and therefore the validity of practice protocols. An earlier version of the learning exercise described below was originally published in the *Instructor's Manual to Accompany Nursing Research: Methods, Critical Appraisal and Utilization* (Levin & Feldman, 2002). As described there, specific learning objectives for this exercise are to "1) create awareness of the types of knowledge used by health care providers to develop practice protocols; 2) develop an appreciation for evidenced-based practice protocols; and 3) apply EBP rating systems to the assessment of existing practice protocols" (pp. 20–27). We have since expanded and embellished upon the original version as described below.

Assignment

The assignment, entitled Assessing Practice Protocols, is placed at the end of the course because we view it as helping to synthesize and integrate the material previously learned. You may request students to hand in a formal paper addressing the items contained in Box 9.1, or ask students to present their findings orally in class. In either case the assignment may or may not be graded. We have used both approaches in different classes. When we do grade this assignment we use the criteria and weights shown in Box 9.2. Another consideration is to have students work independently or in small groups to complete this assignment. Again, we have done it both ways, and each approach has advantages and disadvantages. See section on Alternate Approaches for further discussion of this teaching/learning strategy.

Box 9.1
Directions for Preparation of Paper

Prepare a paper (approximately 4 to 6 pages) describing your experience, findings, and conclusions. Be sure to include the following:

- a brief description of the protocol you chose

- the title and credentials of the individual(s) you interviewed (no names, please)

- a summary of the information you obtained during the interview about how the protocol was developed

- the parameters of your literature search and a summary of what you found

- your conclusion about the types of knowledge upon which the protocol was based with supporting rationale

- a description of the rating scale you used to assess the protocol

- your assessment of the validity of the protocol

Append a copy of the protocol to your paper.

Box 9.2
Criteria for Evaluating the Paper

Criteria	Percentage of Grade
The description of the protocol is succinct, yet clearly identifies the specific practice it addresses.	5%
Appropriate information about the interviewee is provided.	5%
The information obtained during the interview is presented succinctly, yet is sufficient for the reader to make his/her own judgment about the sources of knowledge used for protocol development.	10%
There is an accurate conclusion about the sources of knowledge used to develop the protocol.	10%
A rationale to support the above conclusion is provided.	20%
An accurate description of the EBP rating scale is presented.	10%
An accurate conclusion is presented about the validity of the protocol.	20%
There is a logical flow of ideas.	5%
There is correct grammatical usage and accurate spelling.	5%
The paper is presented according to APA style.	10%

Learning Activities

The following are learning activities in which students engage and which we give to students in written form in order to complete this assignment.

1. Select a practice protocol from your employment or student clinical practice agency. (This protocol may be obtained from a policy and

procedure manual that guides your practice.)

2. Determine who wrote the protocol. (You may need to ask your supervisor or preceptor for this information if it is not apparent on the written protocol.)

3. Request an interview with one or more individuals who were involved in developing the protocol. Interview questions may include, but are not limited to the following:

    (a) Can you explain how protocols are developed in your agency?

    (b) On what specific information did you base this protocol?

    (c) Are there any references you can identify that would give me a better understanding of the rationale for the practices you included in the protocol?

    (d) What rating system was used to critique the protocol guidelines?

4. After the interview, categorize the sources of knowledge identified by the interviewee (e.g., authority, experience, research-based). Be specific.

5. Then, using one of the rating scales included in the chapter on EBP in the library reserve files, assess the protocol for its validity in application to practice.

6. After the interview, you may not have enough information on which to rate the protocol. If, for example, the interviewee has not provided you with sources from the literature, you will have to do a search to determine whether research exists to support the protocol you are assessing.

This does not have to be an exhaustive review, yet you should be able to determine whether there is valid research out there to support your rating.

DIFFERENT MODELS

Several different models have been used in courses during past semesters to teach assessment of protocols. As discussed above, one approach is to have students work independently or in small groups to complete the assignment. Both are effective in having students complete the assignment, but most students believe they gain greater depth when doing the evaluation as a group, especially if this provides access to current practice protocols and people in agencies where the protocols were developed. Students have commented that they can have more confidence in their assessment when a group critiqued the protocol. Therefore, the assignment has been done as a group activity for the past few semesters.

One way to conduct this learning exercise is for each student to share with the class the clinical problems of interest to them. Then, students with similar interests form groups and spend time agreeing on a topic on which their group will focus. Once this decision is made, they proceed with instructions for the assignment. The advantage of this approach is that students learn about the assessment of a large number of protocols on a wide range of topics. Issues might be similar across protocols, but the exposure to so many protocols increases comfort in doing the assessments.

Another model we have used in the course is for all students to select one clinical problem on which all the groups will focus. This approach provides depth in a specific area and the opportunity to critique many different protocols from a variety of sources on the same topic. Quality can vary greatly across these protocols, from ones that are well supported by evidence to others that have no documented support at all, with some totally outdated.

Another successful model we have used is having students begin to link assignments in the course. The same clinical problem may be used for a review of literature and critique of research studies; a critique of a systematic review, whether an integrative review or meta-analysis; and selection of a protocol to critique. This permits more in-depth understanding of a clinical topic and has led to changes in protocols in the students' health care agencies. Furthermore, the assignment has resulted in students' being published in a newsletter and manuscripts being written. See the description of some of these activities in the section on student outcomes below.

Permitting the use of a mixed approach in the class has been done, too. Some students are very interested in a specific topic and really want to learn more about any protocols that might be available on the area. Other students might want to work on the same topic. Therefore, a mixed approach is used. The most successful students have been the ones who linked all three assignments in the course.

Another model used in teaching assessment is for the class to select a specific clinical problem area and then have one group consider the individual factors, another group assess the family factors, and a third group review the community factors. This model was used in fall 2004 for one section of the course with excellent results and great satisfaction by students. In fact, students taking the course in spring 2005 have extended the search for additional protocols on the topic to review. Again, these students linked the three course assignments.

Graduate nursing students have selected a wide range of topics over the different semesters. Some of their questions have been background and others foreground. The topics have included health promotion, for example, smoking cessation programs; screening, for example, tuberculin skin testing; chronic illness management, for example, type 2 diabetes; and compliance or adherence with medications from individual, family, and community perspectives. The impact of the learning activity is that students select topics of interest to them, so the learning activity is very meaningful. Once the students have expressed their interests, the groups are formed. The groups work to refine the clinical question. At this stage, students share their clinical question with the entire class to see if there is interest in a similar question by other groups or by the entire class. The approach for conducting the search of evidence is similar for an individual group with one topic, two or more groups with a shared topic, or an entire class focusing on the same topic.

STUDENT OUTCOMES

As mentioned above, a wide range of outcomes have been achieved by students. The one of greatest interest to us is the ease with which students learned to complete the assignment regardless of the model used. They express how helpful it will be for them in their future roles to learn to appraise practice protocols critically.

The experience was very satisfying to all. There were a few unanticipated positive outcomes as well. For example, one group of students who linked their class assignments on different hand-washing techniques were able to change clinical practice in the hospital where two of them worked. These students were asked to write an article, which was subsequently published in a hospital newsletter. For one of the classes that focused on the same topic of tuberculin skin testing, a manuscript is being prepared for submission. Through their search and critique of the literature, so much new information was found with excellent guidelines that students want to share their findings so that their efforts will not need to be repeated by other nurses. They can take what they found and extend the work. In many instances students have been unable to locate a current protocol even in agencies in which the latest protocol was expected to be found. The students then searched for a protocol to assess, which is supported by the highest level of evidence. If appropriate, students may share the protocol with their agencies.

One of the most recent outcomes is that papers from one semester are being reviewed for possible extension by students in the next semester's class. The depth of the assessment and the number of protocols reviewed will provide excellent information on the clinical topic of the students' choice and the protocols reviewed.

SUMMARY AND RECOMMENDATIONS

Teaching nursing students how to develop and appraise practice protocols is necessary in order for them to be able to use protocols effectively to provide high quality, cost-effective care. Important learning outcomes for the students are to become critical appraisers of guides for practice, to realize that many are not evidence-based, and to recognize the level of specificity at which they are developed. Immediate learning outcomes for students have been excellent, and learning a systematic approach to assessment will be very beneficial for them throughout their careers.

In addition to learning the value of assessing protocols and an approach to assessment, students learned that nursing research is important to their practice. This is not simply a course they require to get a degree, but one that provides essential tools for their practice. Just as they would not give a medication, for example, without knowing how it works and the expected outcomes, they would not use a protocol without knowing its effectiveness. Having students say they need to have the nursing research course early in the curriculum, as well as later for more advanced research knowledge, may lead to introducing an additional course on research or integrating more in current courses on research and EBP.

REFERENCES

Courtney, M. (2005). *Evidence for nursing practice*. Sydney, Australia: Elsevier Churchill Livingstone.

Levin, R. F., & Feldman, H. R. (2002). *Instructor's resource manual to accompany nursing research: Methods, critical appraisal, and utilization* (5th ed.) [Electronic resource]. St. Louis, MO: Mosby.

McSweeney, M., Spies, M., & Cann, C. J. (2001). Finding and evaluating clinical practice guidelines. *Nurse Practitioner, 26*(9), 30–49.

van Meijel, B. (2003). *Relapse prevention in patients with schizophrenia: A nursing intervention study*. Utrecht, The Netherlands: Utrecht University.

Melnyk, B., & Fineout-Overholt, E. (2005). *Evidenced-based practice in nursing and healthcare*. Philadelphia: Lippincott Williams & Wilkins.

Sackett, D. L., Straus, S. E., Richardson, W. S., Rosenberg, W., & Haynes, R. B. (2000). *Evidence-based medicine: How to practice and teach EBM* (2nd ed.). London: Churchill Livingstone.

Titler, M. G. (2001). Use of research in practice. In G. Lo-Biondo-Wood & J. Haber (Eds.), *Nursing research* (5th ed., pp. 413–445). St. Louis, MO: Mosby.

Chapter 10

Evaluating Educational Outcomes: Measuring Success

Ellen Fineout-Overholt

Achievement is a we thing, not a me thing, always the product of many heads and hands.

—J. W. Atkinson

As the fifth critical step of the EBP process, evaluation of outcomes is integral to best practice. Therefore, it would be dissonant to teach EBP and not evaluate outcomes for learners, educators, and programs. Evaluation of EBP principles is imperative for clinician educators identifying criteria for evaluating a new nurse's performance and for academic instructors attempting to develop a "good" test item. In addition, evaluation of EBP education must span entire curricula. To relegate EBP to an orientation class or to one course in an academic program does the learner a disservice. All health care educational courses and programs need to integrate EBP into every offering and course. Subsequently, all courses must evaluate how well the learner learns, the educator educates, and the program conveys EBP principles.

Most traditional evaluation techniques focus on evaluation of knowledge retention. Although this type of evaluation is important, it is insufficient to provide educators with the full scope of how learners are integrating the knowledge we desire them to learn. This chapter addresses levels of evaluation, the infrastructure necessary to evaluate EBP principles, and practical methods for evaluating knowledge, skills, and application of EBP knowledge to practice.

In 1997, Kessenich, Guyant, and DiCenso strongly advocated for change in clinical nursing education. They espoused that tradition and ritual imbued current nursing curricula. Traditional education in healthcare academic and clinical settings is in need of careful evaluation to determine if clinicians are being prepared to practice based on the best available evidence. Outcome evaluation of EBP education must be a focus of health care education, and this must work in tandem with methods used to teach EBP. Traditional methods of evaluation focus primarily on assessing knowledge retention and therefore do not provide enough scope to evaluate integration and application of EBP principles into students' and clinicians' practices. Both educator and learner need to fully understand the scope of EBP, and then appropriate evaluation methods can be used. Kessenich and colleagues also stated, "The new paradigm for nursing education requires an emphasis on systematic observation and experience and a reliance on the research literature to substantiate nursing decisions" (p. 26). This new focus requires rethinking the usual evaluation methods common to nursing education. Educators must consider what methods are effective for evaluating how clinical decisions are made, with a particular emphasis on clinicians' integration of evidence *in combination with* their expertise and the family's and patient's values and preferences.

Cole and colleagues (2004) discussed the need for education to have an experiential aspect that includes reflection. Reflection, according to Sparks and colleagues (1991), is being aware of one's thoughts, feelings, beliefs, and behaviors and how these influence one's interpretation of health care situations. Benner and Leonard (2005) advocated that clinicians' clinical judgment incorporate knowing the patient and understanding the trajectory of the processes in which the patient is involved. These aspects of the evidence-based decision-making process are important to teach and important to evaluate; however, their evaluation is not likely to be encompassed in traditional educational outcome evaluation methods. That is why we are presenting a model for conceptualizing educational evaluation, identifying some of the resources needed to support evaluation of outcomes, and suggesting strategies and tools to do so.

LEVELS OF EVALUATION

There are many ways to conceptualize evaluation in education. Kirkpatrick (1994) identified four levels of evaluation: reaction, learning, transfer, and results. Each of Kirkpatrick's levels of evaluation builds upon the next. Often in continuing education, reaction is the only level of evaluation (e.g., were the participants satisfied, did they feel the program met their objectives). The learning level encompasses evaluating knowledge and skills and is often assessed via a test or observation of activity (e.g., learners may be asked to demonstrate a skill). Evaluation of the extent to which a learner integrates EBP principles is called transfer. Transfer of knowledge or skill is not readily evaluated in teaching EBP. Melnyk and colleagues (2004) found that those who had increased knowledge and beliefs in EBP were more likely to transfer their knowledge to others. In a Cochrane systematic review, however, Parkes and colleagues (2004) found a dearth of evidence aimed at evaluating the effectiveness of teaching EBP (i.e., how learners integrated EBP principles). In their review of 47 studies on teaching EBP, they found one randomized controlled trial (RCT) that met their criteria for evaluating the effectiveness of teaching critical appraisal of outcomes.

Upon evaluating the addition of EBP to an existing curriculum, Holloway, Nesbit, Bordley, and Noyes (2004) found that students felt there was too much EBP content. The conclusion of the authors was that of uncertainty about how and when faculty should introduce EBP into an existing curriculum. Without diffusely integrating the principles of EBP across the curriculum, whether in a clinical or academic course, learners may perceive a disconnect between the steps of EBP and their own practice, increasing the challenge of accurate evaluation. For learners to grasp the need for integrating EBP principles and to evaluate this transfer of information effectively, the culture must be imbued with EBP. Evaluation of Kirkpatrick's results demonstrates that principles of EBP are not only integrated but also applied. For learners of EBP, this level of evaluation would indicate that they have fully engaged the paradigm shift and now operate in a culture and mind-set underpinned by EBP principles. The challenges increase for educators to evaluate adequately at the transfer and results levels of evaluation.

Kirkpatrick's (1994) levels of evaluation focus primarily on the learner. For comprehensive information on how well EBP is being taught, the educator and program also need to be evaluated. Program and educator evaluations may influence each other. For example, the program may be well designed, but if the educator has difficulty in communicating principles to learners, the program evaluation may not reflect the excellence in design. For successful, accurate program evaluation, educators need to be skilled in EBP and other content areas that they are responsible to teach to learners. Educators need to be mentored to set their own evaluation goals and be encouraged to take time to self-reflect to determine if they are meeting them. Chapter 17 further elucidates the need for teaching practices that are evidence-based. Often it is helpful to ask self-evaluation questions to assist in determining factors that may influence educators' effectiveness (see Box 10.1). In addition, learner and program evaluation data can assist educators to know how well they are doing.

To determine the effectiveness of educational programs, goals first must be determined. Program goals should reflect the evaluation results expected of the learner. In addition, these goals would determine the outcomes to be evaluated. For example, if the program goal was to produce nurses who practiced based on evidence in conjunction with their clinical expertise and with data about patient values and preferences, then the outcomes to be measured could be (a) the extent to which clinicians' practices are based on the best available evidence; (b) the extent to which clinicians seek assistance in using the evidence as needed; and (c) the extent to which clinicians gather information about patient preferences and values.

Evaluating the process by which EBP is taught requires the program administrator to ensure that key stakeholders have been asked to provide their input into what the process should be, including the scope and purpose of the program (Bryant-Lukosius & DiCenso, 2004). For example, if the EBP teaching program is in the clinical setting, the educator may gather perspectives from those in administration, care providers, receivers of care, and other educators about what program outcomes need

Box 10.1
Questions for Evaluation of Educator Effectiveness

1. To what extent is the care that I deliver to my patients evidence-based?
2. How much do I believe that basing my care on the best evidence will lead to the highest quality outcomes for my clients and their families?
3. How much knowledge of the EBP process do I possess?
4. Do I have strong knowledge and skills related to EBP?
5. What is my personal commitment to EBP?
6. Do I model EBP in clinical settings?
7. Do I have adequate computer skills?
8. Do I have a relationship with librarians who have knowledge of EBP who can assist me with EBP?

to be to meet these key stakeholders' expectations. Their expectations may also assist in determining the content and methods chosen for the program. In addition, the perspectives of the program recipients, or participants, will provide the educator with a preliminary estimate of the proposed impact of the program; this impact will then need to be evaluated to determine if it was realized. Other outcomes will become evident through discussion with key stakeholders about what impact they think the EBP teaching program will have on the community or agency. Measurement of these outcomes will indicate the program's success to the educator, key stakeholders, and others. It is important to remember that measures of outcome, process, and impact must consider cultural, language, and gender differences (Bakken, 2002).

INFRASTRUCTURE TO SUPPORT EVALUATION

Congruence between the mission and philosophy of the organization and an EBP program's goals and objectives is imperative to evaluating these principles in teaching. It can be helpful to have a designated cadre of educators whose focus is primarily on evaluation strategies for learners, educators, and entire programs. Designated resources are necessary for educators to be able to collect data on their teaching effectiveness and learners' integration of taught content. Clear mechanisms need to be delineated in order for educators to know the procedure to collect data in the least biased manner. In addition, feedback loops must be evident for how those data will be returned to educators, who subsequently will use them to improve their courses or classes. Cultivating enthusiastic educators is essential for effective role models in EBP who set the stage for effective evaluation of EBP principles. Some of the resources necessary to evaluate teaching programs are computers and database software to house and analyze data about individualized programs, educator goals, and learner goals. In addition, ongoing educator development programs are necessary to provide the latest and best evidence in strategies for teaching EBP (Krugman, 2003). How faculty development is approached can make a difference in outcomes (Gruppen, Frohna, Anderson, & Lowe, 2003). For example, educators responded positively to a collaborative, cutting-edge program that fostered faculty development through mentorship (Pololi, Knight, Dennis, & Frankel, 2002). Part of mentorship needs to be assisting educators in turning data into program improvements. Specified mechanisms for data to be consistently returned to the educator contribute to a positive culture of using data for program and personal improvement.

PLANNING FOR EVALUATION

The first step is to plan for evaluation from the beginning. For example, before educators offer a program and then apply for continuing education credit, they must identify their objectives, the methods to meet them, and how they will evaluate whether the objectives are met. The methods of evaluation and accompanying successful criteria must be clearly identified. Educators must consider what assignments they will use to evaluate learners' knowledge, skill, and application of information presented in the EBP program. These assignments need to be clearly articulated for the learner. Learners do not need to use their energy trying to decipher what the successful criteria are for evaluating their learning. Rather, they need to be fully engaged in the EBP process and demonstrate their proficiency in it.

In planning for evaluation, budget considerations are important. It is also essential that all key stakeholders have buy-in to how evaluation methods will be used, and access to feedback data for the purpose of improving EBP education. An attitude of continuous improvement in educational courses and classes provides a context for data collection and interpretation (Beecroft, Kunsman, Taylor, Gevenis, & Guzek, 2004).

EDUCATOR EVALUATION

Most educators evaluate themselves on their own as well as by standardized criteria that are applied to all instructors. In addition, learner evaluations can provide important insight into how well the educator is communicating with this group. Generic evaluations that provide only a number to rate the educator against a set of standardized criteria are helpful, but are not specific enough to provide data for improving teaching skills. For this level of specificity the educator may have to request data from the learners in a nonstandardized way. Table 10.1 provides an example of the types of questions educators may ask learners to gather evaluation information to improve teaching. It is helpful to quantify data, if appropriate, and have a database set up for data entry. Qualitative information needs to be analyzed appropriately and can provide a rich perspective for educators about program process and outcome evaluation, as well as learner transfer and results evaluation.

Educators need to be cognizant of the impact their teaching style has on learners. What values educator place on the content they are teaching is reflected onto learners. Often the best way to evaluate an educator's impact is to ask learners about their perception of how educa-

TABLE 10.1   Informal Survey to Improve the Course

What should be changed to make the learning experience for this course better?					
What was the best part of course?					
Rate the required texts Mark an X in the appropriate box	Poor	OK	Not so bad	Pretty good	Excellent
TEXT 1					
TEXT 2					
Were there any articles especially helpful to the understanding of course content?					
How can the courses 1 and 2 be more seamless?					
Suggestions for improving teaching effectiveness?					
What were benefits of writing the EBP paper?					
How could the EBP paper be improved as a learning experience?					
What were the benefits of the Outcomes Management project?					
How could the Outcomes Management project be improved as a learning experience?					
Other comments about this course or the educator:					

tors value what they teach and their enthusiasm about the content (Glick, 2002). Other strategies for evaluating educators may include questioning the educator about self-generated goals, agency goals for programs, and key stakeholders' expectations. Also, evaluating how an educator creates a culture of data gathering for improving teaching and practice needs to be conducted. For other educators and learners to evaluate the teachers' enthusiasm for EBP and how it influenced evidence-based teaching or practice is helpful to understanding program and learner outcomes.

LEARNER EVALUATION

Each step of the EBP process needs to be evaluated (e.g., how a learner formulates the clinical question; does the question drive the search strategy and whether or not the search strategy is streamlined and focused). It also is important for educators to evaluate how learners gather evidence other than research. Evidence from the history and physical exam enter into the decision-making process and the accuracy and efficiency of gathering this evidence need to be evaluated (Munro, 2004). It is important to determine how well learners assess patients' preferences and what they value in life. Integration of evidence-based theories to inform practice also is essential to learners' evidence-based decision making. There is a paucity of information about how to evaluate these aspects of EBP. Because the primary focus of clinical education and academic EBP courses is on interpretation of research, the evaluation strategies tend to focus primarily on this aspect. Evaluation methods of a well-rounded EBP program should reflect all aspects of evidence-based clinical decision making.

Evaluation strategies may differ depending on the setting of the learner. For example, in the clinical setting an evidence-based performance improvement project can provide evaluation of transfer of knowledge and skills to a clinical situation. Learners can demonstrate their ability to apply the knowledge to a single problem involving performance or quality improvement. A successful outcomes management program can be used to determine if the learner has reached the results level of integration of knowledge and skill. This type of program focuses on continuous improvement of practice by monitoring specified outcome data and using those results for practice improvement.

In an academic setting, an EBP synthesis paper can assist in evaluating learners' integration of EBP principles. This kind of paper allows the learner to demonstrate skills gained in writing a clinical question, searching for best evidence, and critically appraising evidence for validity and applicability. Box 10.2 provides an example of criteria that could be used for an EBP synthesis paper. A project using evidence to generate an outcomes management plan for real-life clinical practice can assist in evaluating the application of evidence to practice. Essential to this evaluation method is application of the evidence in combination with the clinicians' expertise and families and patients' preferences and values. Box

Box 10.2
Criteria for EBP Synthesis Paper

10 pages maximum, excluding references and table

Part 1 (90 pts)

1. **Background and clinically meaningful question** are clear (5 points).

   Support "why ask" question; address each of the PICO components.

2. **Sources and search process** are clear (5 points).

   Databases, keywords, limits, combinations, number found (per database and final number included), inclusion/exclusion criteria (DO NOT LIMIT TO FULL TEXT).

3. **Critical appraisal of evidence, including appropriateness of statistics** is clear (10 points).

   Synthesize information from studies reviewed citing table. Clearly present details of reviewed studies (not background articles) in table with sufficient detail (no sentences, be succinct); address critical appraisal questions of what the results are, whether they are valid results (e.g., strengths and weaknesses of studies), and applicability to the question; identify statistics (NNT, OR, RRR, ARR, or more traditional tests); give details about them (in table); interpreted statistics in text.

4. **Conclusions (not findings) about evidence** are clear (10 points).

   Flows from evidence; true conclusions about evidence, not findings.

5. **Implications for practice based on the evidence** (from a population standpoint, not personal practice) are clear (10 points).

   Identify plan that flows from evidence; provide specific steps.

6. **Obstacles, facilitators and challenges to the plan** are clear (5 points).

   Name or address presence or lack of each; explain how to overcome the ones identified or how to use facilitators.

(continued)

Box 10.2 (continued)

7. **Outcomes for plan** are clear and measurable (10 points).
   Name outcomes for evaluation of plan, define how to measure and the time frame for measuring the outcomes, provide definite link to plan for addressing evidence.

8. **Contribution of theory to evidence** is clear (5 points).
   Briefly explain theory and apply theory to your plan.

9. **Description of evaluation of using the EBP process in writing the paper (*your reflection* on formulating the question to outcome evaluation)** is clear (5 points).

10. **Description of the benefit of the evidence to your personal practice** (albeit hypothetical) is clear and includes theoretical implications (15 points).
    Speak to your clinical expertise (including ability to interpret research reports) and the assessment data on patient preferences and values.

11. **Table** listing for each study included in the review: (a) author(s) and date of publication, (b) title, (c) conceptual framework, (d) study design, (e) major variables studied, (f) sample description, (g) measurement instruments for each variable, (h) data analysis used, (i) study findings, and (j) study strengths and weaknesses. (DO NOT include these kinds of details in the narrative portion of the paper. Instead refer the reader to the table.) (20 points)

Part 2 (10 pts.)

1. Argument is clearly made and logical (5 points).
   Paper builds on each section; connections are clear.

2. APA format is correct (5 points).
   Properly cite in text; properly cite reference list; attend to grammar and punctuation.

10.3 provides an example of criteria that could be used for an outcomes management project evaluation.

PROGRAM OR OFFERING EVALUATION

In an academic or clinical setting where a series of courses is required (e.g., a critical care orientation series), it is imperative that all courses reflect integration of EBP principles. Having only core courses providing learners with EBP content without application to other areas, particularly clinical courses, reinforces the disconnect that often exists between research and practice. Workshops on EBP can provide a starting point for clinicians where they can gain knowledge and skills; however, educators must provide further opportunities for clinicians to integrate their knowledge and skill within a clinical context. Establishing relevant links between EBP initiatives and patient outcomes is a starting point for evaluating clinical programs that teach EBP.

Gathering evidence from clinicians who are entering a clinical program about the use of EBP principles, and then upon graduating or completing that program, is important to program evaluation. Box 10.4 contains examples of questions for those who have completed EBP teaching programs. Evaluating integration and application of EBP principles is most important for these clinicians.

EVALUATION OF EBP MAY INFLUENCE CHANGES IN HEALTH CARE

Developing a program of evaluation for teaching EBP can sometimes seem daunting. Prioritizing what is important for learners to take away from clinical and academic programs can help educators know what is important to evaluate. Knowing, however, does not necessarily translate into gathering data, in the same way that knowing EBP principles does not necessarily equal best practice (Davis, O'Brien, Freemantle, Wolf, Mazmanian, & Taylor-Vaisey, 1999).

Making a difference in health care requires commitment from educators—those who prepare people to care for consumers—to have program outcomes as part of the educational plan. Best practice cannot be achieved without evidence. Outcome data are evidence for educators to be the best and to know that their "practice" of education is evidence-based. (Refer back to chapter 17 for an extended discussion of evidence-based teaching practices.)

Box 10.3
Assessment Criteria for Outcomes Management Project

Evidence base of project is clear (15 points). (Include evidence [external evidence] to support why you need to do this project, i.e., support that there is insufficient or no evidence to fully answer your clinical question; provide evidence that there is an existing problem—provide baseline data [internal evidence] to support that the problem does indeed exist; provide evidence of family/patient preferences and values and how they influence project; provide influence of collective group clinical expertise.)

Clinically meaningful question is clear (5 points). (Use PICO.)

Project outcomes are reasonable and clearly identified (5 points). (The outcomes flow from the question. All possible outcomes are considered and addressed to answer the question.)

Data collection methods (sources and process) are clear (5 points). (How approval is obtained, collection tool [submission with project is required], who is collecting data and from whom or what.)

Data analysis approach assists in answering the clinical question (5 points). (Did you use the right statistical test for the level of data you collected?)

Proposed presentation of data is clear (10 points). (Graphs are readable on slide/handout, anchors are identified. All data are presented to audience in written form, slide/handout. Data are **synthesized.** Do not provide raw data to audience. Raw data must be submitted with presentation packet for grading.)

Implications *for practice changes* based on the data and supporting evidence are clear (10 points). (What your data tell you that needs to be different in practice, particularly in light of the existing evidence [internal and external].)

Plan for change is clear (5 points). (Specific steps for change. Include theoretical framework for change)

Anticipated barriers, facilitators, and challenges *to plan* are clear (5 points). (These are specific to plan for change.)

(continued)

Box 10.3 (continued)

Outcomes for evaluation *of plan* are clear and measurable (including costs) (10 points).

Dissemination plan is clear and feasible (5 points). (What are you going to do with the information you gathered in your project?)

Lessons learned through the use of the EBP process are clear (2 points). (Evaluation of how the project changed based on what you learned while doing it, or what you would have done differently.)

PowerPoint presentation and supporting documents enhance presentation (6 points).
   Group work is evident in the presentation (2 points)
   Handouts were helpful to learning (1 point)
   Power Point presentation was creative (2 points)
   Completed presentation within time limit (1 point)

Overall argument is compelling and worthy of clinician change in practice (10 points).

Packet to be turned in for grading (2 points).
   Hard copy of slides in 4-on-a-page format
   Handout
   Data collection tool
   Raw data and summarized data

Box 10.4
Examples of Questions for Evaluating EBP Program Effectiveness

Closed Questions:

1. I am confident that critically appraising evidence is an important step in the EBP process.
2. I discussed evidence from a research study with a practice colleague at least three times weekly.
3. The content I learned in _____ (fill in the blank with the course/program of interest) has helped me to implement EBP principles.

Open Questions:

1. How has your confidence in critically appraising evidence increased since taking _____ (fill in the blank with the course/program of interest) program?
2. How does discussing evidence with colleagues influence your daily practice?
3. How did attending _____ (fill in the blank with the course/program of interest) program/course make a difference in how you practiced?

REFERENCES

Bakken, L. (2002). An evaluation plan to assess the process and outcomes of a learner-centered training program for clinical research. *Medical Teacher,* *24*(2), 162–168.

Beecroft, P., Kunsman, L., Taylor, S., Gevenis, E., & Guzek, F. (2004). Bridging the gap between school and workplace: Developing a new graduate. *Journal of Nursing Administration, 34*(8), 338–345.

Benner, P., & Leonard, V. (2005). Patient concerns, choices and clinical judgment in evidence-based practice. In B. M. Melnyk & E. Fineout-Overholt (Eds.), *Evidence-based practice in nursing and healthcare: A guide to best practice* (pp. 163–182). Philadelphia: Lippincott Williams & Wilkins.

Bryant-Lukosius, D., & DiCenso, A. (2004). A framework for the introduction and evaluation of advanced practice nursing roles. *Journal of Advanced Nursing, 48*(5), 530–540.

Cole, K., Barker, L., Kolodner, K., Williamson, P., Wright, S., & Kern, D. (2004). Faculty development in teaching skills: An intensive longitudinal model. *Academic Medicine, 79*(5), 469–480.

Davis, D., O'Brien, M., Freemantle, N., Wolf, F., Mazmanian, P., & Taylor-Vaisey, A. (1999). Impact of formal continuing medical education: Do conferences, workshops, rounds, and other traditional continuing education activities change physician behavior or health care outcomes? *Journal of the American Medical Association, 282*(9), 867–874.

Glick, T. (2002). How best to evaluate clinician-educators and teachers for promotion? *Academic Medicine, 77*(5), 392–397.

Gruppen, L., Frohna, A., Anderson, R., & Lowe, K. (2003). Faculty development for educational leadership and scholarship. *Academic Medicine, 78*(2), 137–141.

Holloway, R., Nesbit, K., Bordley, D., & Noyes, K. (2004). Teaching and evaluating first and second year medical students' practice of evidence-based medicine. *Medical Education, 38*, 868–878.

Kessenich, C., Guyatt, G., & DiCenso, A. (1997). Teaching nursing students evidence-based nursing. *Nurse Educator, 22*(6), 25–29.

Kirkpatrick, D. L. (1994). *Evaluating training programs: The four levels.* San Francisco: Berrett-Koehler.

Krugman, M. (2003). Evidence-based practice: The role of staff development. *Journal of Staff Development, 19*(6), 279–285.

Melnyk, B. M., Fineout-Overholt, E., Feinstein, N., Li, H. S., Small, L., Wilcox, L., & Kraus, R. (2004). Nurses' perceived knowledge, beliefs, skills, and needs regarding evidence-based practice: Implications for accelerating the paradigm shift. *Worldviews on Evidence-based Nursing, 1*(3), 185–193.

Munro, N. (2004). Evidence-based assessment: No more pride or prejudice. *AACN Clinical Issues, 15*(4), 501–505.

Parkes, J., Hyde, C., Deeks, J., & Milne, R. (2004). Teaching critical appraisal skills in health care settings. *The Cochrane Database of Systematic Reviews, 2*.

Pololi, L., Knight, S., Dennis, K., & Frankel, R. (2002). Helping medical school faculty realize their dreams: An innovative, collaborative mentoring program. *Academic Medicine, 77*(5), 377–384.

Sparks-Langer, G., & Colton, A. (1991). Synthesis of research on teachers' reflective thinking. *Educational Leadership, 48*, 37–44.

Part 3

Teaching/Learning Evidence-Based Practice in the Academic Setting

Introduction to Part 3

Harriet R. Feldman

The chapters that follow provide a number of innovative strategies that educators can use to facilitate learning in undergraduate and graduate students. If there is one thing we have learned as educators, it is that there is no such thing as a finished curriculum. The process of development is unending—to paraphrase Martha Rogers, curriculum is always evolving.

Chapter 11 is an example of how curriculum reform takes place. Also involving a graduate program, this chapter addresses the change process by bringing the faculty into the conversation. Through careful organization and orchestration, Krainovich-Miller and Haber were able to change the graduate curriculum at New York University. Once they recognized the need to implement EBP throughout the curriculum, they went about determining a model that would best suit their situation. This meant building faculty knowledge and alliances through meetings and faculty development workshops. The goal was to create a "paradigm shift from the faculty's point of view" and the focus was on the faculty's "EBP information literacy, critical appraisal, and statistical knowledge base." EBP experts were brought to these workshops and faculty members were asked to read selected articles in preparation for the visits. Agreement was reached about how to introduce EBP to graduate students and then ensure literacy in EBP throughout the curriculum. Once the groundwork was completed, the action plan was instituted with students, linking EBP assignments to PICO projects, debates, and case presentations in an effort to achieve intended outcomes.

Singleton, Truglio-Londrigan, and Allan focus in chapter 12 on getting faculty on board to reframe what and how they teach so that EBP is a guiding force in the graduate curriculum at Pace University. How do we change the mind-set of faculty? What strategies are effective? The Family Nurse Practitioner (FNP) program was among the first master's programs of its kind nationally and has been very successful over the years. In an effort to make sure that the program stayed on the cutting edge, the first two authors called upon a consultant, the third author, for assistance. Working together they were able to infuse EBP into all FNP coursework. The initiative began with reformation of the advanced research course (discussed in more depth in chapter 14), moving into the other core courses, which already had a strong foundation in EBP concepts, and then to the specialty or FNP clinical curriculum. There is also a discussion of course delivery in this chapter, with creative use of online lectures via discussion boards to develop students' ability to reflect on their own and colleagues' responses to posted questions. Last, a unique aspect of the chapter is a section entitled "Reflections of a Consultant," which speaks to the process of change.

In chapter 13 Grace focuses on the second-career population of students, a group whose numbers in nursing programs are on the rise nationally. These programs often are accelerated because although they are not already nurses, students generally have prior baccalaureate degrees in other fields. Some come to nursing with graduate degrees as well. The unique needs and challenges of this population call for new and creative teaching strategies; however, Grace makes the point that today's "traditional" student is often in a hurry, juggling responsibilities of family and job. EBP, in her view, makes research "particularly attractive" to this busy population, because "EBP strategies were developed to help the busy clinician efficiently find and apply research findings to the care of individual patients."

In chapter 14 Levin discusses EBP in undergraduate curriculum, but unlike Grace addresses the special circumstance of associate degree education where a course for nursing research is not traditionally taught. She asks the question: "Yet, are not ADN graduates also expected to base their nursing practice on the best evidence available?" and responds that EBP can be taught and learned in all nursing coursework, "whether or not students have had a research course first or ever." The chapter continues by discussing strategies for integrating EBP concepts into undergraduate didactic and clinical course content, and addresses such topics as what to do about the use of textbooks, often secondary sources that become quickly outdated as science is continuously developing; how to teach skills for clinical inquiry, how to handle nursing process papers within an EBP framework, in what context journal clubs might be useful, and the usefulness of clinical rounds to convey EBP content.

The next chapter focuses on nurses' diagnoses and their relationship to EBP. Cruz, Pimenta, and Lunney have done extensive research in this area and explain how the application of EBP principles to the diagnostic reasoning process improves the accuracy of nurses' diagnoses. They support the notion that though EBP is associated most often with research-focused courses, nonresearch sources are also valuable to making evidence-based decisions. They present the teaching strategy of case studies, which they see as an effective way to teach and learn, resulting in "the development of critical thinking and effective problem-solving skills." Through the case study, they are able to pose questions, identify cues, appraise evidence, and develop diagnostic hypotheses.

Another strategy to consider, based on a very different vantage point, is the use of nursing history as evidence for today's practice. In chapter 16, historian Sandy Lewenson describes her experiences with undergraduate and graduate students to help them understand the "historical antecedents to a procedure or clinical specialty, or theoretical basis for practice" with the hope that they will "make better decisions as nurses in the present." So as students examine primary sources, including early nursing journals, and interview a nursing leader or visit a school archive, they come to appreciate changes over time and can compare present with past issues in health care and nursing practice.

In the final chapter in this section, Valiga continues the conversation about teaching and learning, asking the question "What about the practice of teaching itself?" She takes the position that teaching is an advanced practice area of nursing and, thus, must be evidence-based. In order to be effective in the role of educator, she argues, the practice of teaching must be based on research and other forms of evidence. Practices that have characterized nursing education in the past may not be adequate to support new approaches to preparing practitioners for the present and future. In our past practice as clinicians and educators, we have heard countless times that "we have always done it that way" or "that is how I was taught." We have challenged these and similar points of view by showing practitioners and would-be practitioners that past practices and trial and error often do not yield the best outcomes. The same can be said of the practice of teaching—what we have done in the past does not always work with today's students. In fact, the technology associated with the current learning environment and the strengths and needs of our current student population challenge all of us daily to rethink the way we teach. In an effort to identify and validate new models of teaching, we owe it to our students and ourselves to use the best evidence available for teaching practices. This point is strongly made in this chapter: "nursing faculty must engage in thoughtful critique of that (education-focused) research and integrate or synthesize it to identify trends, patterns, and understandings."

Chapter 11

Transforming a Graduate Nursing Curriculum to Incorporate Evidence-Based Practice: The New York University Experience

Barbara Krainovich-Miller and Judith Haber

> The illiterate of the 21st century will not be those who cannot
> read and write, but those who cannot learn, unlearn, and relearn.
> —Alvin Toffler

The momentum in health care to improve the quality of patient care through EBP continues to escalate. "EBP" is now the international mantra of medicine, nursing, and other health professions. Interdisciplinary partnerships between and among researchers, practitioners, and educators are needed (Rosswurm & Larrabee, 1999; Stevens & Long, 1998). Nurse educators are challenged to prepare basic and advanced students to have core EBP competencies to use as the foundation of clinical practice. Faculty who are preparing nurse practitioners (NPs), clinical nurse specialists, midwives, educators, administrators, and informatics specialists are particularly challenged because advanced practice nurses will play a leadership role in supporting organizational change in implementing EBP. As such, EBP needs to be embedded in all graduate program curricula. A key ingredient for making a successful paradigm shift is securing the commitment of faculty, largely prepared in a traditional research paradigm, to acquire new competencies related to information literacy, critical appraisal, biostatistics, and teaching and learning strategies (Youngblut & Brooten, 2001).

RECOGNIZING THE NEED: NYU EXEMPLAR

In 2000, New York University's (NYU) Division of Nursing (DON) master's programs implemented a competency-based education outcomes framework (CBEO) (Lenburg, 1999) initiative. The overall aim of this initiative was to better prepare graduates for anticipated advanced practice workplace competencies and skills. The initial phase focused on converting program and course objectives to outcome statements and refining clinical evaluation tools to reflect essential competencies and skills for each program. As part of the DON's continuous quality improvement (CQI) process we examined the competencies of our NP clinical evaluation tools in light of feedback from preceptors and students.

Preceptors confirmed that they expected NP students to be clinically competent in developing and refining research-based practice protocols and guidelines (Haber, Feldman, Penney, Carter, Bidwell-Cerone, & Hott, 1994) and that clinical decision making needed to be based on the best available evidence (Sackett, Rosenberg, Gray, Haynes, & Richardson, 1996; Sackett, Straus, Richardson, Rosenberg & Haynes, 2000). A preliminary review of recent literature indicated that research-based protocols were now being referred to as evidence-based protocols or evidence-based nursing (EBN) protocols for advanced nursing practice (e.g., Grossman & Bautista, 2002).

Our evaluation further revealed that we had a strong nursing framework for our nurse practitioner, midwifery, and functional role master's programs (education, administration, and informatics) that addressed national accreditation criteria and included an expectation that advanced nursing practice was based on research. For example, programs addressed the American Association Colleges of Nursing (AACN, 1996) *Essentials of Master's Education,* National Organization of Nurse Practitioner Faculty's Task Force Guidelines (2002), the American Nurses Association (ANA, 2003b) *Social Policy Statement* and related specialty scope and standards (ANA, 1999, 2000a, 2000b, 2001a, 2001b, 2002, 2003c, 2004a, 2004b, 2004c), functional role national standards (e.g., ANA, 2000a), and ANA (2003a) guidelines for master's students' participation in nursing research.

Using a CBEO lens, however, our evaluation indicated that we lacked the specific EBP competencies and skills in the master's curriculum, in particular for the eight NP and midwifery programs. There was a definite need to update and refine these competencies to better reflect EBP principles and evidence-based decision making (Sackett et al., 2000). The faculty readily agreed that we needed to decide on and implement an EBP model so that our graduates would be prepared to assume leadership roles as "EBP work place change champions" (Titler, in press). Key to successfully implementing such a model would be faculty development in terms of EBP content as well as teaching strategies (Youngblut & Brooten, 2001).

Determining an EBP Model

In essence, our CBEO initiative uncovered the need to learn more about EBP from the perspectives of both evidence-based medicine (EBM) (Guyatt & Rennie, 2002; Sackett et al., 2000) and evidence-based nursing (EBN) (Ciliska, Cullum, & Marks, 2001; Ciliska, Pinelli, DiCenso, & Cullum, 2001). The initial Master's Work Group (MAWKG) meetings indicated that faculty were ready to implement an EBP thread throughout the master's curriculum. Although they were aware of EBP terminology from the literature and their respective advanced practice specialties, faculty did not have an in-depth command of the competencies, in particular how to teach the necessary information literacy and critical appraisal skills required for developing EBP products, such as EBP protocols, standards, care maps, critical pathways, or evidence summaries. Table 11.1 summarizes the initial action plan developed by graduate program faculty for implementing an EBP thread in the master's curriculum; Box 11.1 identifies initial master's student competencies for our EBP Model.

Developing EBP faculty and student competencies and curricular components was a major focus of Year 01 MAWKG bimonthly meetings and faculty development workshops. Specific outcomes were: (1) increased faculty EBP knowledge and skills; (2) identification through concept mapping of courses in the curriculum (description, outcomes, assignments) that currently addressed the use of theory and research for practice; and (3) targeting EBP content for specific courses in the core, advanced practice core, and specialty component courses. These presentations and workshops were conducted by local EBP experts as well as experts from McMaster's University School of Nursing in Canada.

TABLE 11.1   Three-Year Action Plan for Implementing EBP/EBN Threads in NYU's Master's Program Curricula

Overall Plan	Year 1	Year 2	Year 3
• Conduct electronic database search on EBP, EBM, and EBN literature. • Present critical appraisal of retrieved EBP, EBM, and EBN literature to faculty and preceptors. • Implement at least three EBN on-site workshops by McMaster's experts for faculty and preceptors over the next 3 academic years. • Identify EBP principles outcome competencies for NP and functional programs. • Identify curriculum courses that currently focus on theory and research for practice where EBP model can be integrated.	• Conduct a review of the literature on EBP, EBM, and EBN (fall semester). • Share with faculty results of the literature review (fall semester). • Form a Master's Workgroup (MAWG) task force to identify where EBP concepts could be introduced and what overall competencies were needed for EBP model (fall semester). • Provide a 2-day on-site hands-on workshop on EBP from nurse expert colleagues from McMaster's University, Canada (spring semester). • Concept map curriculum for evidence of related EBP concepts (spring semester).	• EBP presentation by faculty who attended summer McMaster's workshop to faculty and preceptors; emphasis on using EBP critical appraisal skills for critiquing individual studies and for systematic reviews, in particular meta-analyses (fall semester). • Faculty member who attended McMaster's summer workshop, agree to pilot the use of "asking clinical questions "and critiquing clinically relevant studies using EBP statistics in first specialty clinical practicum seminar course (fall semester).	• Level, implement, and evaluate information literacy competencies for core, advanced core, and specialty program courses (fall and spring semesters). • Evaluate relevancy of all course assignments in relation to EBP framework (e.g., research course requires critical appraisal of individual RCTs and systematic reviews using EBP framework). • Evaluate if 10 specialty programs' capstone projects reflect EBP framework. • Require Biostatistics course instead of Stats II course (fall semester).

TABLE 11.1 *(continued)*

Overall Plan	Year 1	Year 2	Year 3
• Determine EBP model based on review of literature and consensus of faculty. • Present derived EBP model to adjunct faculty and preceptors at annual workshop. • Infuse EBP model in all identified courses (description, outcomes/objectives, and assignment) of the curriculum by the end of year 2. • Evaluate annually, through CQI process, EBP model and enact any derived action plan.	• Implement agreed-upon EBP teaching strategies/initiatives identified by MAWG Task Force, e.g., Information Literacy (spring semester and ongoing). • Meet with health-science librarian for conducting information literacy competency workshop for faculty and students. • Request a clinical faculty member volunteer to attend summer workshop at McMaster's University, Canada, who would take a leadership role as an EBP resource person for faculty in the following academic year (spring semester).	• Meet with Statistics Department faculty to discuss the need for a different Statistics II course, one that will enhance students' competency in critiquing studies from an EBP framework (fall semester). • Implement task force–identified Information Literacy competency program (i.e., include in orientation sessions, core courses as required, library presentation, and assignments) and any other additional strategies needed for the development of EBP competencies (fall and spring semesters).	• Conduct 3rd EBP McMaster's on-site workshop for faculty and preceptors: emphasis on critically appraising systematic reviews (meta-analyses). • Disseminate implementation of EBP innovation through publications and presentations.

(continued)

TABLE 11.1   *(continued)*

Overall Plan	Year 1	Year 2	Year 3
		• McMaster's faculty conduct a second hands-on EBP workshop focusing on the use of the methodological critiquing criteria for individual studies and levels of evidence (spring semester). • Pilot and evaluate biostatistics course for increasing students' competency for critically appraising studies using EBP statistics.	

Inherent in the EBP paradigm shift from the faculty's point of view was the need to recognize that an academic assignment, whether for a core or specialty component clinical course, could no longer specify the number of research articles needed (e.g., reviewing 5 to 10 research articles on a clinical topic and synthesizing it for implications for practice). This type of assignment did not fit the EBP framework of acquiring the "best available evidence," whether it was provided by one systematic review or 15 individual research articles. We recognized, however, that changing from an academic exercise to a critical appraisal of all available research would require leveling expectations throughout the curriculum as well as changing how an advanced research course was taught. Clearly, faculty

Box 11.1
Initial EBP Student Competencies of EBP Model

Students will be able to demonstrate the following:

1. Information literacy competencies related to electronic searches format (Guyatt & Rennie, 2002; Sackett et al., 2001):

   - Formulate clinical questions related to patient clinical problems: patients or populations, interventions, comparison groups(s) or gold standard, outcome(s) of interest (PICO)

   - Use clinical questions to conduct electronic literature search

   - Use multiple scholarly electronic databases simultaneously for search

   - Retrieve research (data-based) articles of original research reports, including quantitative systematic reviews (meta-analyses) and national clinical guidelines

2. Conduct PICO projects

   - Summarize and critique individual studies using standardized critical appraisal totals related to quantitative and qualitative research

   - Critically appraise quantitative systematic reviews (meta-analyses) and qualitative systematic reviews using appropriate critiquing criteria (Cochrane Collaboration, 2001, 2003; Forbes & Clark, 2003; Stevens, 2001)

   - Synthesize a body of critiqued research to determine the best available evidence for a clinical question

   - Conduct critiques of specific types of studies in target courses (e.g., Advanced Pharmacology: prognosis research articles; Advanced Pathophysiology: causation articles; Specialty Clinical Management: therapy, prognosis, and harm articles)

3. Refine or develop evidence-based practice protocols

4. Conduct EBP debates

5. Conduct case study presentations using an EBP framework

also needed to sharpen their EBP information literacy, critical appraisal, and statistical knowledge base. Faculty needed to embrace EBP so that it could be embedded in the curriculum.

DEVELOPING AN EBP MODEL: KEY CONCEPTS PRESENTED TO FACULTY AND PRECEPTORS

Over several faculty development workshops, the history of the EBM movement was presented. The main points emphasized were as follows:

- EBM actually was begun in the United Kingdom in 1972 by Dr. Archie Cochrane, an epidemiologist, who severely criticized physicians for their lack of critical appraisal and synthesis of research, referred to as systematic reviews (Cochrane, 1972).

- Systematic reviews were essential to policy makers, health profession organizations, physicians, and the public, and the paucity of such reviews had a negative impact on health care outcomes (Cochrane, 1972).

- Cochrane recommended that a rigorous process for systematically reviewing several studies, in particular randomized controlled trials (RCTs) with periodic updates, was needed by physicians for quality diagnosing and treatment and in order for their patients to make an informed decision about whether to accept the diagnosis and treatment plan.

- Twenty years later Cochrane's recommendations were formally implemented at Oxford University and a year later the Cochrane Collaboration was established (Cochrane Collaboration, 2005). Today the Cochrane Collaboration is considered "the International 'virtual organization' " for systematic, up-to-date reviews of all relevant health care RCTs.

- Although more systematic reviews are produced in the UK, the United States is gaining momentum primarily due to the managed care movement, shift of clinical decision making from providers to payers, and a change in the medical and legal mind-set from defensive to offensive clinical practice (Pietranton, 2004).

- By the early 1990s, physician and nurse colleagues from the UK and Canada were leading the EBP movement. The actual term "evidence-based medicine" was coined around 1990 by Dr. Gordon Guyatt of McMaster University (Lang, 2004).

- Scholarly articles and meta-analyses were using or applying terms such as the "strength and quality of the evidence" and "levels of evidence" to refer to a basic framework for categorizing and rating research and then using rigorous criteria to produce systematic reviews.

- Most of the strength and quality of evidence frameworks consider quantitative meta-analyses (quantitative systematic reviews) of two or more RCTs Level I as the gold standard of best available evidence (e.g., American Heart Association-Emergency Cardiovascular Care Cummins & Hazinski, 2000; Oxford Centre for Evidence-based Medicine Levels of Evidence, 2001; Sackett et al., 2000; Stetler, 2001).

- In the United States, work of the Agency for Health Care Policy Research (AHCPR), which generated original evidence-based practice guidelines of the late 1980s and early 1990s, was part of this movement; several guidelines had nurse researchers chairing or functioning as members of guideline review panels.

- McMaster's University developed a leadership position in advancing the evidence-based nursing (EBN) movement through consultation and publications, including the journal *Evidence-Based Nursing* (DiCenso, 2003; DiCenso & Cullum, 1998).

OVERCOMING BARRIERS TO EBP

An extensive literature review revealed national and international barriers faced by the nursing profession when shifting from a research utilization (RU) to an EBP model. We deemed it important to present and discuss these barriers with faculty so that they could consider strategies for overcoming the specific barriers related to nursing faculty and students (Box 11.2).

Following the presentation of barriers, faculty agreed that a series of presentations embedded in faculty development workshops conducted by EBP experts would expedite implementing EBP content in graduate program curriculum. Prior to the workshops, presentation of EBP general concepts at MAWKGP meetings by local EBP experts helped to assess specific EBP concepts the experts needed to focus on at the workshops. An overall outcome for these meetings was to determine what aspects of the framework faculty were unfamiliar with and what concepts were confusing or misunderstood. Other outcomes would be to increase faculty's familiarity with (a) similarities and differences among the definitions

Box 11.2
Barriers for the Nursing Profession Shifting From an RU
to an EBP Nursing Model

- Newness of the EBM movement (Sackett et al., 2000)

- Faculty have not been trained in an EBM/EBN framework (e.g., Kessenich, Guyatt, & DiCenso, 1997; Stetler et al., 1998)

- Misconceptions about evidence-based practice by nurses (Di-Censo & Cullum, 1998; Jennings & Loan, 2001)

- Multiple models of levels of evidence and grades of recommendations to determine the quality of evidence of EMB (Centre for EBM, 2004; Melnyk, & Fineout-Overholt, 2005; Upshur, 2003) and lack of agreement by nursing on the hierarchy of research evidence to use (e.g., Swan & Boruch, 2004)

- Disagreement among nurses about whether EBN is a distinct construct or reflects too much of the medical model (e.g., Closs & Cheater, 1999; French, 2002; Ingersoll, 2000; Nagy, Lumby, McKinley, & Macfarlane, 2001; Stetler, 2001; Thompson, 2002; Zeitz & McCutcheon, 2003)

- Misconception that EBN is "cookbook" nursing (e.g., Di-Censo & Cullum, 1998)

- Terms being used interchangeably, for example, some nursing authors use the term EBM synonymously with EBP and switch to EBN as if synonymous with the other two terms (e.g., Gray et al., 2002; Steven & Harr, 2001)

- Faculty do not possess expert competency in information literacy (e.g., Kessenich, Guyatt, & DiCenso, 1997; Jacobs, Rosenfeld, & Haber, 2003; Shorten, Wallace, & Crooks, 2001)

- Lack of training in critical appraisal of research evidence (Kessenich, Guyatt, & DiCenso, 1997)

- Faculty lack of easy access to computerized databases (e.g., Bakken & McArthur, 2001; Kessenich, Guyatt, & DiCenso, 1997)

Box 11.2 *(continued)*

- "Lack of clinically relevant nursing research" (Kessenich, Guyatt, & DiCenso, 1997, p. 28) on a particular clinical topic that has been synthesized and published in a clinician-friendly format

- Gap between available nursing research in the form of systematic reviews and use by nurses for direct patient care (e.g., Feldman, Olberding, Shortridge, Toole, & Zappin, 1993; Stevens, 2001)

- Lack of health care agencies' organizational infrastructures to promote EBN practice (Foxcroft & Cole, 2004).

- Lack of academic agencies' organizational infrastructure to promote EBN as a framework for faculty development and course development

- Nurse educators not connecting quality patient outcomes to EBN (Deaton, 2001)

- Unclear distinctions between research utilization and EBN

- Not exposing undergraduate nursing students to EBN early in the curriculum in a research course so that EBN is then used and seen as critical to every subsequent course and then for future practice

of EBM, EBN, and EBP (Table 11.2); (b) critical EBP concepts, such as quantitative versus qualitative systematic reviews (Box 11.3); (c) differences between systematic and traditional literature reviews; (d) models for rating levels of evidence that judge the strength, quality, and consistency of research evidence) (Box 11.4); and (e) additional methodological critique criteria developed by the Evidence-Based Medicine Working Group (Box 11.5).

A synthesis of selected paradigm literature on the EBP movement (e.g., Sackett et al., 2000) was presented, including the major similarities and differences between EBP and RU (Stetler, 2001), and among definitions of EBM, EBN, and EBP. According to Jennings and Loan (2001), RU and EBP are used incorrectly at times as synonyms. It was determined through analysis of these definitions and related material that RU is not the same concept and in general EBP and EBN are subsets of the EBM

TABLE 11.2 Definitions Related to EBP Movement

Evidence-Based Medicine (EBM): "the process of integrating individual clinical expertise with the best available external clinical evidence from systematic research (Sackett et al., 1996, p. 71); "The conscientious, explicit and judicious use of current best evidence in making decisions about the care of individual patients. The practice of evidence-based medicine means integrating individual clinical expertise with the best available external clinical evidence from systematic research" (Sackett et al., 2000, p. 246).	Evidence-Based Practice (EBP): "integrating the best available research evidence with information about patient preferences, clinician skill level, and available resources to make decisions about patient care" (Ciliska et al., 2001, p. 520). "Process of finding, appraising and applying scientific evidence to the treatment and management of health care . . . discovery of underlying trends and principles developed from the accumulation and refinement of a large body of studies" (Ledbetter & Stevens, 2000, p. 98); "refers to a decision making approach based on integrating clinical expertise with the best available evidence from systematic research" (Kim, 2000, p. 4).	Evidence-Based Nursing (EBN): "a term [that] emerged fairly recently . . . evolved from the initial concept of evidence-based medicine (Sackett et al., 2000, p. 246); EBN has a broader meaning than research utilization. Its practice involves the following steps: (1) formulation of an answerable question to address a specific patient problem or situation; (2) systematic searching for the research evidence that could be used to answer the question; (3) appraisal of the validity, relevance, and applicability of the research evidence; (4) decision making regarding the change in practice; (5) implementation of the evidence-based practice decision; and (6) evaluation of the decision outcome" (Ciliska, Cullum et al., 2001).

movement. For the purposes of the presented model, the Ciliska, Pinelli et al. (2001) definition of EBP was used (Table 11.2).

In preparation for the workshop, three readings were given to faculty, one on teaching nursing students EBN (Kessenich, Guyatt, & DiCenso, 1987) and focusing on undergraduate students but with implications for graduate students. The second emphasized the need for faculty to introduce undergraduate and graduate students to systematic reviews (Stevens & Long, 1998). The third focused on what constituted systematic

Box 11.3
Major Characteristics of Systematic Reviews

Quantitative Systematic Reviews (meta-analyses):

- Cochrane Collaboration coined the term *systematic reviews* for meta-analyses, which employs statistical methods to combine the findings of at least two or more studies (also referred to as *quantitative systematic reviews)* (Krainovich-Miller, in press).

- Referred to as "evidence synthesis" by the Agency for Healthcare Research and Quality (AHRQ) and use the Cochrane rigorous process of systematic review "as outlined in the Cochrane Reviewers' Handbook" (Stevens, 2001, p. 530).

- "Adhere to a strict scientific design in order to make them more comprehensive, to minimize the chance of bias, and so ensure their reliability" (Systematic Reviews, 2001, pp. 3–7).

- "Use explicit and rigourous methods to identify, critically appraise, and synthesize relevant [primary/original] studies" (Mulrow, Cook, & Davidoff, 1997, p.389).

- Use statistical methods that maximize the estimation of treatment effect generated by multiple studies that meet inclusion criteria (Stevens, 2001).

- Referred to as "evidence summarizations" that produce the best available objective evidence on a topic (Albanese & Norcini, 2002).

- Offer clinicians the best available evidence to make sound clinical judgments for their patients (Krainovich-Miller, in press).

- Key to developing evidence-based practice protocols (Krainovich-Miller, in press).

- "Are a primary distinguishing feature that defines today's new paradigm of evidence-based practice as distinct from prior efforts in research utilization" (Stevens, 2001, p. 531).

(continued)

Box 11.3 (continued)

Qualitative Systematic Reviews:

- Do not use statistical methods to combine the findings but adhere to a systematic process for retrieving sources, selection, and critiquing for synthesizing findings called meta-syntheses.

Quantitative and Qualitative Systematic Reviews share the following characteristics:

- They are explicit: indicate the question the review will address, the method of retrieving primary sources, selection and critiquing criteria, and techniques to be used to synthesize the findings.

- They are reproducible: the use of explicit criteria enables another researcher to use the criteria and draw the same conclusion.

- They are efficient: an essential information management tool, condensing large amounts of primary/original studies into a manageable objective format.

Integrative Reviews:

Similar to and with similar characteristics of a qualitative systematic review, but a "broader, sometimes less rigorous, method used to systematically combine results from a body of studies' (Stevens, 2002, p. 530).

---

reviews and their relevance for EBP (Stevens, 2001). Faculty found these articles very useful to understand the major concepts of EBP.

Additional areas of concern for faculty were levels of evidence and differences among types of systematic reviews. Faculty communicated that the idea of using hierarchical models for rating the strength, quality, or consistency of research evidence was confusing. The literature revealed multiple models that originated from medical sources, which used from four to eight levels for rating the strength of evidence as well as additional sublevels for rating quality and consistency of evidence. There are also nursing models, some of which do not indicate the source of these levels.

Box 11.4
Levels of Evidence*

Level I: Evidence from a [quantitative] systematic review or meta-analysis of all relevant randomized controlled trials (RCTs), or evidence-based clinical practice guidelines based on systematic reviews of RCTs.

Level II: Evidence obtained from a least one well-designed RCT

Level III: Evidence obtained from well-designed controlled trials without randomization

Level IV: Evidence from well-designed case-control and cohort studies

Level V: Evidence from systematic reviews of descriptive and qualitative studies

Level VI: Evidence from a single descriptive or qualitative study

Level VII: Evidence from the opinion of authorities or reports of expert committees

*Source: Melnyk & Fineout-Overholt, 2005, p. 10: Levels modified from Guyatt & Rennie, 2002; Harris et al., 2001.

Box 11.5
Evidence-Based Medicine Working Group (1992) Methodological Criteria Required for Different Types of Studies

Etiology (causation of illness)

Therapy (effectiveness of interventions)

Harm

Diagnostic tests

Assessment tools

Prevalence

Prognosis

Quality of care

Overviews

Faculty agreed that levels of evidence was an important EBP concept and for several years, Stetler's evidence hierarchy (Stetler, 1998; Stetler et al., 2001) was used. Currently, the Melnyk and Fineout-Overholt (2005) levels of evidence hierarchy, presented in Box 11.4, is used because of the clarity of categories for ranking the types of research designs. Although students are presented with other models (e.g., U.S. Preventive Task Force; Agency for Health, Research, and Quality [AHRQ]), faculty and students found Melnyk and Fineout-Overholt's model very easy to understand and to apply as a critical appraisal tool.

Faculty also indicated that although they were familiar with meta-analyses, they were unfamiliar with differences among systematic reviews and how they differed from traditional literature reviews. A brief overview of the literature on this topic was presented to faculty. The Cochrane Collaboration Group coined the term *systematic review*. Faculty were referred to Rutledge, DePalma, and Cunningham's (2004) article, *A Process Model for Evidence-Based Literature Syntheses,* which clearly mirrors the criteria of systematic reviews. Their model indicates that systematic reviews are conducted by a team and that team members spent what was equivalent to full-time work during the year in order to conduct a systematic review. Systematic reviews are not conducted by a single individual and certainly are not an expectation of a master's or doctoral student's individual work. Systematic reviews that use the quantitative statistical design (meta-analysis) are considered a quantitative research method (see chapter 7).

The major differences between systematic reviews and traditional literature reviews were presented and the various types of systematic reviews were analyzed by faculty (Box 11.3). It was noted that although systematic reviews are considered to provide level-one evidence, even this type of evidence must be put through an EBP quality filter. This means that evidence from a systematic review, derived through the researchers' critical analysis and synthesis, must be integrated with other available best evidence from individual studies as well as the individual clinician's expertise and patient preferences (DiCenso, 2003; Sackett et al., 2000; Stevens & Long, 1998). Faculty indicated that quantitative systematic review and qualitative meta-syntheses (see chapter 6) and their critical appraisal criteria needed to be included in the graduate-level research course to core research competencies that could then be used and developed further in the advanced practice core and specialty component courses.

Another interesting discussion centered around specific domain criteria used for critically appraising individual research articles, using a therapy, diagnosis, prognosis, harm, or causality domain and determining their applicability to practice (Box 11.5). Some faculty thought that these criteria replaced the traditional critiquing criteria for quantitative and qualitative studies (LoBiondo-Wood & Haber, in press). Faculty were reassured that domain-specific critical appraisal criteria were actually more complementary and sophisticated than traditional quantitative and qualitative critique criteria. It was concluded that at the first planned faculty development workshop, domain-specific critical appraisal criteria would be covered in-depth by EBP experts. Faculty also agreed with the presented conclusion that the master's core (e.g., research and stats 2), advanced practice core (e.g., pharmacology, health assessment, strategies), and specialty component (e.g., NP Practicum theory II and III courses; NP Practicum II and III courses) did not reveal course outcomes and content that specifically addressed EBP concepts and terminology, evaluation methods, and related clinical competencies. Faculty expressed interest in pursuing this topic more formally through workshops so they could develop their own knowledge base and competencies and implement EBP in the overall curriculum and teaching and learning strategies, which included a major information literacy project.

INFORMATION LITERACY: KEY TO SUCCESSFUL IMPLEMENTATION OF EBP IN CURRICULUM

Prior to faculty development workshops on appraising research from an EBP framework, it was critical to make sure faculty were up-to-date on their electronic search skills. An NYU health science librarian, who is a nurse, conducted a brief overview of the latest on information literacy and reviewed the basic steps of "effective" electronic search strategies. It was clear that from an EBP framework, information literacy focused on the need to secure databased (research) articles, in particular quantitative systematic reviews, using a number of search strategies. Information literacy presumes a capacity to choose appropriate technological tools to obtain information. Even the most basic search of the scholarly literature should involve selecting at least two reputable electronic databases, using appropriate search terms for each database, "navigating myriad pathways to electronic journals or library catalogs of print holdings, as well as managing software for printing, saving, e-mailing bibliographic records" (Jacobs, Rosenfeld, & Haber, 2003, p. 321). In addition, it was stressed that using electronic databases, such as the Cochrane Review, is critical to retrieve systematic reviews, especially meta-analyses, as well as by appraising national organization practice guidelines.

The faculty agreed that it was essential to include information literacy in the master's students' orientation as well as assignments that would require electronic database searches in the core, advanced core, and specialty component courses (see examples in Table 11.3). All core courses required that students complete an online information literacy tutorial and attend an information literacy session on developing a specific information literacy competency (e.g., searches using epidemiological databases, such as the Centers for Disease Control [CDC], for the population-focused care core course and searches using databases to locate systematic reviews, such as Cochrane Collaboration or AHRQ for the research course. Students were encouraged to make individual appointments with the health science librarian to refine their search strategies. It also was recommended that biostatistics and research be taken as initial courses so that EBP critical appraisal skills are introduced and acquired early for use in subsequent core courses. (Table 11.3 also indicates EBP competencies and related teaching and learning activities to be developed at specific points in the curriculum related to course outcomes.)

Faculty assumed that students who had recently completed an undergraduate program had been introduced to electronic database searching from an information literacy perspective. Also presumed was that perhaps students were more computer savvy than some faculty were. In addition, faculty recognized that students are used to receiving information instantly through the World Wide Web, using a search engine such as Google or other search engines. Therefore, it would be necessary to stress from orientation on that they must learn to differentiate between scholarly and consumer searches.

This project assumed that students would increase their search skills one step at a time; yet it was also recognized that active hands-on experience, coupled with students' technological computer savvy, might very well accelerate mastery of information literacy competencies. Older graduate students who completed undergraduate programs 10 or more years ago, however, most likely would require more assistance. Therefore, we anticipated that the information literacy learning curve most likely would vary and require specific search strategies for each core course. Both a positive and negative consequence of electronic searches is the tremendous amount of material that is retrieved, which tends to overwhelm students at first until they learn how to sort and filter material with a quick read of the abstracts (Krainovich-Miller, in press). Included in the initial appraisal of material (citations) retrieved from this type of search are recognition of the types or levels of evidence (Box 11.4) from an EBP framework, the inherent value of each type, and the need to use filtering criteria. See Jacobs et al. (2003) for a complete presentation of the information literacy aspect of this EBP initiative.

TABLE 11.3 Examples of Information Literacy and Related EBP Competency* for Master's Curriculum Course Assignments

Core Course: Nursing Research	Advanced Core Course: Advanced Pharmacology	Specialty Component Course
• Formulate a clinical question (PICO). • Conduct an electronic search using at least two electronic scholarly databases with related search terms for a clinical topic denoting "only research" articles from the past 5 years; include Cochrane Database of Systematic Reviews as one of the databases. • Conduct another search for nationally recognized clinical guidelines related to clinical question. • Preevaluate search by skimming abstracts to determine articles are databased (research). • Conduct a critical appraisal using traditional critiquing criteria and a related EBP appraisal skill e.g., "numbers to treat."	• Formulate a clinical question related to pharmacology treatment. • Conduct an electronic search using at least three electronic scholarly databases with related search terms for a clinical topic denoting "only research" articles from the past 5 years; include Cochrane Database of Systematic Reviews as one of the databases. • Conduct another search for nationally recognized clinical guidelines related to clinical question. • Preevaluate search by skimming abstracts to determine articles are databased (research). • Compare any meta-analyses studies with findings from individual studies and pharmaceutical literature.*	• Formulate a clinical question related to clinical practice guideline retrieved from clinical practicum health care agency. • Conduct an electronic search using at least three electronic scholarly databases with related search terms for a clinical topic denoting "only research" articles from the past number of years from the last study indicated in a practice guideline; include Cochrane Database of Systematic Reviews as one of the databases. • Conduct another search for nationally recognized clinical guidelines related to clinical question. • Preevaluate search by skimming abstracts to determine articles are databased (research). • Conduct a critical appraisal with appropriate EBP appraisal criteria.* • Refine the clinical practice guideline based on the best available evidence from EBP framework.*

*Indicates an EBP competency versus a purely Information Literacy Competency. In our model we emphasize that Information Literacy Competencies are needed in order to effectively search the literature and obtain the literature to be appraised from an EBP competency framework.

OUTCOMES AND RECOMMENDATIONS

Overall, our EBP Action Plan was implemented without major barriers. Feedback from faculty, preceptors, and students indicate that a number of outcomes were achieved (Box 11.6). Based on our experience with introducing EBP into a graduate program, we recommend that organizational resources be provided for a 5-year action plan to allow for sufficient faculty to develop EBP competencies, because EBP requires a faculty culture change as well as knowledge and skill acquisition. In addition, we recommend that sufficient time be spent on leveling information literacy competencies throughout the initial courses and that these become a part of EBP competencies that are specifically linked to EBP course assignments, for example, PICO projects, evidence debates, and case presentations. We suggest that programs investigate changing their required master's statistics course, which emphasizes traditional statistics and learning the SPSS statistical package, to a biostatisics course, which emphasizes understanding treatment effectiveness formulas and their meaning as research evidence. As previously indicated, students need to complete their biostatistics and research courses early in the program in order to develop initial EBP competencies and skills necessary for critically appraising and synthesizing all types of evidence for all required courses.

Faculty acknowledged the need to give students feedback on their electronic searches as a necessary component of determining students' level of information literacy as well as their ability to critically analyze research reports. Faculty recognized that it was impossible to determine if a student has adequately summarized and critiqued a study unless the faculty member reads the study. Therefore, we recommend that students submit their electronic searches as well as copies of their research articles with each assignment. Another strategy to assist students in their synthesis of evidence is to have them prepare a table or grid of essential critical appraisal components for each study. For example, a critique would address the strengths and weaknesses of a study's research design, type and size of sample, type of data analysis, findings, and conclusion, and indicate whether the author of a study indicated limitations, and if any other limitations exist. This type of critique puts students in a position to rate the strength, quality, and perhaps consistency of the evidence provided and to determine applicability of findings for their clinical practice.

To be successful in implementing EBP into a graduate curriculum it is critical to have administrative support for this culture change, including faculty development resources. It is also crucial to establish a good relationship with, and acquire the necessary resources from, an expert

Box 11.6
Outcomes of EBP Action Plan

1. Faculty, students and preceptors (all) were more knowledgeable about the EBP movement and the need for making clinical decisions based on the best available evidence.

2. Students indicated an increase in information literacy competencies for conducting efficient comprehensive electronic searches to retrieve databased (research) literature including systematic reviews.

3. Faculty, students, and preceptors indicated they are much more confident in critically appraising individual studies, especially RCTs, as well as critically appraising systematic reviews using an EBP perspective.

4. Students indicated more confidence in refining or developing EBP protocols and for making evidence-based clinical decisions.

5. Students reported increased competence in determining applicability of research findings to practice.

6. Evaluation methods were developed to assess mastery of EBP targeted competencies.

7. Students indicated they wished that faculty teaching the research course would do the following: devote more class time to helping them critically appraise studies from a traditional and EBP framework, provide models of "good" summary and critical appraisal and a synthesis of several studies, and provide written feedback on a summary/critique and synthesis earlier in the semester so that they would have a better understanding of the expectation for a scholarly master's level paper.

8. The graduate research course was reorganized and taught from an EBP framework.

9. An EBP content unit was implemented in the final core course Population Focused Care.

10. Students who took biostatistics and research as their initial core courses indicated they were more confident critically appraising research articles in subsequent core courses compared to other students who did not take these courses; they indicated it was due to being able to use the newly acquired EBP competencies in their next core course.

(continued)

Box 11.6 (continued)

11. Faculty acknowledged that in large classes the workload of grading scholarly EBP assignments can be quite overwhelming.

12. Faculty requested further workshops on teaching strategies for implementing an EBP framework, especially with large core and advanced core classes.

13. Faculty are now including in the criteria for written assignments that students must provide evidence of the search that was conducted as well as submit a copy of the article that was critiqued.

14. Faculty requested assistance in developing strategies to determine appropriate EBP assignments for varying levels of courses throughout the curriculum. For example, an assignment in the final core course Population Focused Care should require students to perform an electronic search using at least two databases to retrieve databased (research) articles, including the Cochrane database; that is, retrieve, critically appraise, and synthesize articles to determine the best available evidence on a population focused topic.

15. Faculty determined that students should be given the option of deciding on a clinical topic for their capstone project very early in the curriculum so that they can build in-depth evidence-based knowledge on the topic.

librarian and faculty in the statistics department. In addition, we highly recommend that faculty review the top seven mistakes (Sackett et al., 2000, p. 205) to determine what errors they initially made or saw others make when trying to teach EBM (material in parentheses refers to Sackett et al.; additional suggestions appear in brackets):

- Teaching learners how to do research (rather than how to use it) [the reason why we changed the focus of our research course to critiquing for practice application].

- Teaching learners how to perform statistical analyses (rather than how to interpret them). [At our institution, Stats II emphasized performing statistical analyses using SPSS; we now require a biostatistics course that emphasizes interpretation of statistical tests for the appraisal of research.]

- Teaching a preset series of content topics (rather than have content determined by patient's problems). [Starting in the core courses, especially the research course, we attempt to have students develop "clinical questions" per the PICO EBP approach, which drives the search for best available evidence for answering the clinical questions.]

- Evaluating learners on the basis of their retention of facts (rather than on their skills in obtaining, appraising, and applying "facts" to patients).

- Insisting on sticking to the teaching schedule when the clinical service is swamped.

- Striving for closure by the end of every session (rather than leaving plenty to think about between sessions).

- Devaluing team members for asking "stupid" questions or providing "ridiculous" answers.

Implementing an EBP model requires a CQI process in order to evaluate effectiveness continuously and congruence with program outcomes. Student and preceptor feedback is key to this process. We began implementing our model, recognizing barriers to implementing an EBP curriculum framework; we concluded with examples of what we found to be some of the facilitators. The following were considered positive factors for implementing an EBP-model nursing master's program initiative:

- A strong nursing framework for the curriculum.

- A strong and flexible faculty who knew what they didn't know and who were willing to learn and try new teaching strategies.

- A CQI process that included master's students and preceptors in the development and evaluation of initiatives.

- Implementing a competency-based education outcomes initiative.

- Using the resources of a strong health-science librarian who could "talk the talk" for establishing information literacy competencies.

- Taking seriously Sackett et al.'s (2000) top seven mistakes when implementing EBP.

Graduate nursing education in the twenty-first century faces many challenges; EBP provides an educational challenge that capitalizes on the essence of advanced practice nursing, that is, critical appraisal of the best available evidence examined in light of clinical expertise and patient preferences to inform evidence-based decision making, and ultimately, improve patient outcomes.

REFERENCES

Albanese, M. A., & Norcini, J. (2002). Systematic reviews: What are they and why should we care? *Advances in Health Sciences Education, 7,* 147–151.

American Association Colleges of Nursing. (1996). *Essentials of master's education.* Washington, DC: Author.

American Heart Association-Emergency Cardiovascular Care Criteria. (1998). Retrieved January 31, 2005, from www.musckids.com/~ann.bald/ebm/1998_aha_ecc_levels_of_evidence.pdf

American Nurses Association. (1999). *Scope and standards of home health nursing practice.* Washington, DC: Author.

American Nurses Association. (2000a). *Scope and standards of practice for nursing professional development.* Washington, DC: Author.

American Nurses Association. (2000b). *Scope and standards of psychiatric-mental health nursing practice.* Washington, DC: Author.

American Nurses Association. (2001a). *Scope and standards for gerontological practice.* Washington, DC: Author.

American Nurses Association. (2001b). *Scope and standards of nursing informatics practice.* Washington, DC: Author.

American Nurses Association. (2002). *Scope and standards of hospice and palliative nursing practice.* Washington, DC: Author.

American Nurses Association. (2003a). *Education for participation in nursing research.* Washington, DC: Author.

American Nurses Association. (2003b). *Nursing's social policy statement.* Washington, DC: Author.

American Nurses Association. (2003c). *Scope and standards of pediatric nursing practice.* Washington, DC: Author.

American Nurses Association. (2004a). *Nursing: Scope and standards of practice.* Washington, DC: Author.

American Nurses Association. (2004b). *Scope and standards for nurse administrators* (2nd ed.). Washington, DC: Author.

American Nurses Association (2004c). *Scope and standards of addictions nursing practice.* Washington, DC: Author.

Bakken, S., & McArthur, J. (2001). Evidence-based nursing practice: A call to action for nursing informatics. *Journal of the American Medical Informatics Association, 8*(3), 289–290.

Centre for Evidence-Based Medicine, Institute of Health Sciences. (2001). *Oxford Centre for Evidence-based Medicine levels of evidence*. Retrieved January 31, 2004, from http://www.cebm.net/levels_of_evidence.asp#levels

Ciliska, D., Cullum, N., & Marks, S. (2001). EBN users' guide: Evaluation of systematic reviews of treatment or prevention interventions. *Evidence-Based Nursing, 4*, 100–104.

Ciliska, D. K., Pinelli, J., DiCenso, A., & Cullum, N. (2001). Resources to enhance evidence-based nursing practice. *AACN Clinical Issues: Advanced Practice in Acute and Critical Care, 12*(4), 520–528.

Closs, S. J., & Cheater, F. M. (1999). Evidence for nursing practice: A clarification of the issues. *Journal of Advanced Nursing, 30*(1), 10–17.

Cochrane, A. L. (1972). *Effectiveness and efficacy: Random reflections on health services*. London: Nuffield Provincial Hospitals Trust.

Cochrane Collaboration. (2001). *The Cochrane collaboration: Preparing, maintaining and promoting the accessibility of systematic reviews of the effects of health care interventions*. Oxford, UK: Author.

Cochrane Collaboration. (2003). *Cochrane reviewers' handbook*. Oxford, UK: Author.

Cochrane Collaboration. (2005). *Cochrane collaboration brochure*. Retrieved August 25, 2005, from http://www.cochrane.org/software/docs/newbroch.pdf

Cummins, R. O., & Hazinski, M. F. (2000). *The most important changes in the international ECC and CPR guidelines 2000*. American Heart Association. http://circ.ahajournals.org/cgi/content/full/102/suppl_1/I-371.

Deaton, C. (2001). Outcomes measurement and evidence-based nursing practice. *Journal of Cardiovascular Nursing, 15*(2), 83–86.

DiCenso, A. (2003). Leadership perspectives: Evidence-based nursing practice: How to get there from here. *Canadian Journal of Nursing Leadership, 16*(4), 20–26.

DiCenso, A., & Cullum, N. (1998). Implementation forum: Implementing evidence-based nursing: Some misconceptions. *Evidence-Based Nursing, 1*(2), 38–40.

Evidence-Based Medicine Working Group. (1992). Evidence-based medicine: A new approach to teaching the practice of medicine. *Journal of the American Medical Association, 268*(17), 2420–2425.

Feldman, C., Olberding, L., Shortridge, L., Toole, K., & Zappin, P. (1993). Decision making in case management of home healthcare clients. *Journal of Nursing Administration, 23*(1), 33–38.

Forbes, D., & Clark, K. (2003). The Cochrane library can answer your nursing care effectiveness questions. *Canadian Journal of Nursing Research, 35*(3), 18–25.

Foxcroft, D. R., & Cole, N. (2004). Organizational infrastructures to promote evidence based nursing practice. *The Cochrane Database of Systematic Reviews, 4*.

French, P. (2002). What is the evidence on evidence-based nursing? An epistemological concern. *Journal of Advanced Nursing, 37*(3), 250–257.

Gray, M., Bliss, D. Z., Bookout, K., Colwell, J., Dutcher, J. A., Engberg, S., et al., (2002). Evidence-based report card from the center for clinical investigation:

Evidence-based nursing practice: A primer for the WOC nurse. *Journal of Wound, Ostomy, and Continence Nursing, 29*(6), 283–286.

Grossman, S., & Bautista, C. (2002). Collaboration yields cost-effective, evidence-based nursing protocols. *Orthopedic Nursing, 21*(3), 30–36.

Guyatt, G. H., & Rennie, D. (Eds.). (2002). *Users' guides to the medical literature: A manual for evidence-based clinical practice.* Chicago: AMA Press.

Haber, J., Feldman, H. R., Penney, N., Carter, E., Bidwell-Cerone, S., & Hott, J. R. (1994). Shaping nursing practice through research-based protocols. *Journal of the New York State Nurses Association, 25*(3), 4–12.

Ingersoll, G. L. (2000). Evidence-based nursing: What it is and what it isn't. *Nursing Outlook, 48*(4), 151–152.

International Nurses Society on Addictions. (2004). *Nursing: Scope and standards of addictions nursing practice* (Rev. ed.). Washington, DC: American Nurses Association.

Jacobs, S. K., Rosenfeld, P., & Haber, J. (2003). Information literacy as the foundation for evidence-based practice in graduate nursing education: A curriculum-integrated approach. *Journal of Professional Nursing, 19*(5), 320–328.

Jennings, B. M., & Loan, L. A. (2001). Misconceptions among nurses about evidence-based practice. *Journal of Nursing Scholarship, 33*(2), 121–127.

Kessenich, C. R., Guyatt, G. H., & DiCenso, A. (1997). Teaching nursing students evidence-based nursing. *Nurse Educator, 22*(6), 25–29.

Kim, M. (2000). Evidence-based nursing: Connecting knowledge to practice. *Chart, 97*(9), 4–6.

Krainovich-Miller, B. (in press). Review of the literature. In G. LoBiondo-Wood & J. Haber (Eds.), *Nursing research: Methods and critical appraisal for evidence-based practice* (6th ed.). Philadelphia: Elsevier.

Lang, E. (2004). Feature review: The why and the how of evidence-based medicine. *McGill Journal of Medicine, 8,* 90–94.

Ledbetter, C. A., & Stevens, K. R. (2000). Basics of evidence-based practice part 2: Unscrambling the terms and processes. *Seminars in Perioperative Nursing, 9*(3), 98–104.

Lenburg, C. B. (1999, September 30). The framework, concepts and methods of the Competency Outcomes and Performance Assessment (COPA) Model. *Online Journal of Issues in Nursing.* Retrieved January 12, 2005, from http://www.ana.org/ojin/topic10/tpc10_2.htm

LoBiondo-Wood, G., & Haber, J. (in press) *Nursing research: Methods and critical appraisal for evidence-based practice* (6th ed., chap. 3–18). Philadelphia: Elsevier.

Melnyk, B. M., & Fineout-Overholt, E. (2005). *Evidence-based practice in nursing and healthcare.* Philadelphia: Lippincott.

Mulrow, C. D., Cook, D. J., & Davidoff, F. (1997). Systematic reviews: Critical links in the great chain of evidence. *Annals of Internal Medicine, 126*(5), 389–391.

Nagy, S., Lumby, J., McKinley, S., & Macfarlane, C. (2001). Nurses' beliefs about the conditions that hinder or support evidence-based nursing. *International Journal of Nursing Practice, 7*(5), 314–321.

National Task Force on Quality Nurse Practitioner Education. (2002). *Criteria for the evaluation of nurse practitioner programs* (2nd ed.). Washington, DC: Author.

Rosswurm, M. A., & Larrabee, J. H. (1999). A model for change to evidence-based practice. *Image, 31*(4), 317–322.

Rutledge, D. N., DePalma, J. A., & Cunningham, M. (2004). A process model for evidence-based literature syntheses. *Oncology Nursing Forum, 31*(3), 543–550.

Sackett, D. L., Rosenberg, W. M. C., Gray, J. A. M., Haynes, R. B., & Richardson, W. S. (1996). Evidence-based medicine: What it is and what it isn't. *British Medical Journal, 312*(7023), 71–72.

Sackett, D. L., Straus, S. E., Richardson, W. S., Rosenberg, W., & Haynes, R. B. (2000). *Evidenced-based medicine: How to teach and practice EBM* (2nd ed.). Edinburgh, Scotland: Churchill Livingston.

Shorten, A., Wallace, M. C., & Crookes, P. A. (2001) Developing information literacy: A key to evidence-based nursing. *International Nursing Review, 48*(2), 86–92.

Stetler, C. B. (2001). Evidence-based nursing: What it is and what it isn't. *Nursing Outlook, 49*(6), 286.

Stetler, C. B., Morsi, D., Rucki, S., Broughton, S., Corrigan, B., Fitzgerald, J., et al. (1998). Utilization-focused integrative reviews in a nursing service. *Applied Nursing Research, 11*(4), 195–206.

Stevens, K. R. (2001). Systematic reviews: The heart of evidence-based practice. *AACN Clinical Issues: Advanced Practice in Acute and Critical Care, 12*(4), 529–538.

Stevens, K. R., & Long, J. D. (1998). Incorporating systematic reviews into nursing education. *Online Journal of Knowledge Synthesis for Nursing, 5*(7).

Swan, B. A., & Boruch, R. F. (2004). Quality of evidence: Usefulness in measuring the quality of health care. *Med Care, 42*(2), 12–20.

Systematic reviews: Historical background: What are they and why are they useful? (p. 1). Retrieved December 12, 2004, from http://www.shef.ac.uk/scharr/ir/units/systrev/historical.htm

Thompson, D. R. (2002). Faking a difference: Evidence-based nursing and the illusion of diversity. *Nurse Education Today, 22*(4), 271–272.

Titler, M. G. (in press). Developing an evidence-based practice. In G. LoBiondo-Wood & J. Haber (Eds.), *Nursing research: Methods and critical appraisal for evidence-based practice* (6th ed.). Philadelphia: Elsevier.

Upshur, R. E. (2003). Are all evidence-based practices alike? Problems in the ranking of evidence. *Canadian Medical Association Journal, 169*(7), 672–673.

Youngblut, J. M., & Brooten, D. (2001). Evidence-based nursing practice: Why is it important? *AACN Clinical Issues, 12*, 468–476.

Zeitz, K., & McCutcheon, H. (2003). Evidence-based practice: To be or not to be, this is the question! *International Journal of Nursing Practice, 9*(5), 272–279.

Chapter 12

Incorporating Evidence-Based Practice Into Clinical Education for Nurse Practitioners: The Pace University Experience

Joanne K. Singleton, Marie Truglio-Londrigan, and Janet Allan

> If nothing ever changed, there'd be no butterflies.
> —Anonymous

Pace University has six colleges and schools that offer a wide range of programs for a diverse population of nearly 15,000 students. The Lienhard School of Nursing (LSN), established in 1966, focuses on education, research, and practice in primary health care. Students may enroll in the 4-year BS; BS completion program for RNs; Combined Degree Program for nonnurse college graduates; accelerated BS/MS program for RNs; bridge program to the master's for nurses with baccalaureate degrees outside of nursing; MS degrees in specialty areas such as Family Nurse Practitioner (FNP), Nursing Informatics, and Psychiatric Nurse Practitioner; and an MA in Nursing Leadership with foundational areas in educator and administrator roles.

The school has a history of clinical affiliations and partnerships. The Lienhard School of Nursing Center for Nursing Research, Clinical Practice, and International Affairs (CNRCPIA) was established in 1982. Primary Health Care Associates (PHCA), a unit of CNRCPIA, was established in 1997 in response to requests for services and partnerships from the outside community to serve uninsured and underserved populations.

As a leader in educational innovation and excellence, LSN traditionally has been on the cutting edge of nursing education. The FNP program is more than 30 years old and long has been nationally known and replicated. Though research-based practice is not a new concept in our graduate curriculum, sweeping quality initiatives in health care required us to do more. The graduate faculty decided to focus first on our FNP curriculum. As part of this change, we needed not only to systematically identify where and how EBP was already being taught across our graduate curriculum, but also the graduate faculty had to discuss and debate our own values, assumptions, and beliefs about EBP, and whether it should be a framework for the FNP curriculum. The integration of EBP in the curriculum was a challenge that graduate faculty assumed with the notion of transforming how nurses engage in clinical practice by creating an evidence-based educational framework and learning environment.

THE FOUNDATION: CONTENT AND FACULTY

Content: What Do We Do Now?

In systematically assessing across the graduate curriculum, we identified a strong foundation of EBP teaching and learning in two graduate core courses, Decision Making in Health Care Systems, and Advanced Nursing Research, and developed a model of EBP across FNP clinical courses. This foundation has been in place since the 2001–2002 academic year.

The Core Curriculum

Decision-Making in Health Care Systems is one of the first courses taken by students across the graduate curriculum. This course focuses on the decision-making process within the health care system in the United States from a primary health care perspective. Students are introduced to LSN's primary health care nursing philosophy and various decision-making models. Emphasis is on gaining an understanding of frameworks and the use of self-reflection to enhance the practitioner's decision-making skills. EBP is introduced as one of the frameworks to solve clinical problems in everyday practice. Upon completion of the course, it is expected that students will understand EBP in relation to clinical-based problems from a primary health care perspective.

EBP content is presented in the Blackboard electronic platform to allow for nontraditional educational opportunities. This platform facilitates adult learning that is student led. Students have one full week to complete all of the required readings and participate in the discussion board.

The online EBP session is divided into three sections. The first section presents for students required readings in the selected area of interest. In this instance required readings on EBP are electronically posted. The second section is an online lecture that is required reading. The online lecture shapes readings so that students begin to understand EBP and the overall rationale for its existence. An introduction to the principles of EBP is presented, including (1) development of an answerable question, (2) gathering the best evidence to answer the question, (3) appraising the evidence for validity and usefulness, (4) application of the intervention strategy to clinical practice, and (5) evaluation of the application of the evidence in the clinical setting (Sackett, Straus, Richardson, Rosenberg, & Haynes, 2000). In the third section, students turn to the electronic discussion board using the Blackboard platform. The student who accesses the discussion board responds to the question posted on the Blackboard discussion board (see Figure 12.1).

As students post their answers using the discussion board, they must review each other's postings and are required to respond to each other. This request is made in the following way:

> Once you have posted your own response take some time to reflect upon your colleagues' responses. Share your reflections with others in the class. Respond to one another and feel free to ask questions that others may answer for you.

The outcome of this online discussion has been very interesting and rewarding. Many students identify that at a fundamental level they do not practice within an EBP framework. For example, in many postings students identify that they do not gather day-to-day subjective and objective information obtained from their clients. Because of this, either a lack of information or sometimes misinformation may prevent them from practicing in a quality-driven, efficient, and effective manner. Students also have identified that certain policies within their clinical practice area have been developed based on tradition and not based in evidence. This

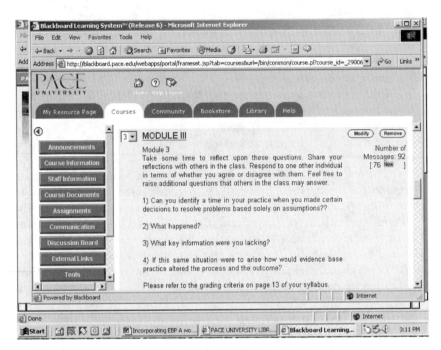

FIGURE 12.1   Blackboard snapshot of EBP discussion board.

may be seen with clinical intervention strategies or intervention strategies developed to assist the institutions to function more efficiently. For example, one registered nurse relayed a situation that transpired at her facility. The hospital administration decided they no longer wanted visiting hours in their intensive care unit (ICU). Rather, they wanted family and friends to have 24-hour visiting access. ICU staff was immediately concerned. No input was requested from them and there was no tracking down of best evidence that 24-hour visiting in the ICU was a strategy that proved effective either for families or the institution. Information pertaining to best practices on implementing such a policy change was also lacking. Completing the online module supports the overriding notion of always practicing with a question in mind.

The purpose of the discussion board is to have students realize that some professional practice is not based in evidence but rather in traditions carried over from one generation to the next. Along with this discussion there is the realization that decisions must be made with relevant evidence that is derived from valid research, clinical expertise, and patient values (Sackett et al., 2000). This understanding forms the foundation for the next core course, Advanced Nursing Research. In this course, students work with faculty on identifying clinical practice questions and to develop an ability to appraise evidence for clinical action.

The purpose of the EBP-focused research course is to use research as a tool to enhance practice. Specifically, students focus on clinical problems and designs along with the application of best evidence to clinical problems and focus on treatment effectiveness and clinical significance (see Table 12.1 for Web addresses to access clinical practice guidelines). Students are requested to focus on a searchable, answerable clinical question and then to synthesize the available evidence related to their clinical question. Appraising the available evidence for validity is an important part of the process, as well as evaluating findings for applicability to practice. For example, to demonstrate the user-friendly nature of EBP and to "make it real," students are requested to identify a practice protocol from their clinical practice and to evaluate the practice protocol for its validity, the evidence from which it was developed, and clinical significance. Students essentially ask a question about the protocol and then follow the EBP process to find answers to the question that may lead to a change in the protocol.

FNP Clinical Curriculum

Our FNP clinical curriculum consists of four 6-credit courses, taken sequentially. Students begin with Advanced Health Evaluation, which has a lab component, and progress through Family Nurse Practitioner: Advanced Theory and Practice I, II, and III, each of which has precepted clinical hours. Across these courses, EBP was modeled by teaching students to search for and use clinical practice guidelines, and through case studies that required students to use an EBP approach in the treatment and management of case patients.

TABLE 12.1 Examples of Web Addresses for Accessing Clinical Practice Guidelines

National Guideline Clearing House	http://www.guideline.gov
Guide to Clinical Preventive Services	http://www.ahrq.gov/clinic/
American College of Cardiology	http://www.acc.org/clinical/ statements.htm
American Heart Association	http://american heart.org/presenter. jhtml?
American Cancer Society	http://cancer.org

Graduate Faculty: What Is Our Vision?

Over the course of the past several years since beginning to incorporate EBP into the graduate curriculum, the graduate faculty has had the opportunity to discuss, debate, and expand their knowledge of and experience with EBP. This is a necessary ongoing process, facilitated through discussions at monthly faculty association meetings, graduate curriculum meetings, and teaching colloquia, and through visiting scholars and consultants. Several faculty have current publications and presentations on EBP and are engaged in related research. As we discussed our initial EBP curriculum efforts, debated EBP concepts and definitions, and became more engaged with EBP, our shared vision of EBP as a framework for the FNP curriculum became clear.

Architects of a Curriculum: Where Do We Wish to Go?

Reaching consensus on revision of the FNP curriculum offered both opportunity and challenge. The graduate faculty decided that a curriculum revision was necessary. This revision was led by the lead FNP faculty, presently consisting of the chairperson of the Department of Graduate Studies Curriculum Committee and chairperson of the Department of Graduate Studies. Ongoing input from graduate faculty and information from past student course evaluations as well as data from focus groups conducted with graduate students was used. In addition, a curriculum consultant was engaged.[1]

In preparation for curriculum revision, we did content mapping of clinical assessment and management courses to make certain we were covering all FNP content areas, as well as those for the FNP (ANCC) certification exam. Indeed we cover all content, and in fact, go well beyond in order to prepare highly qualified FNPs. Our curriculum is comprehensive; however, the way it was laid out needed some adjusting. In Advanced Health Assessment, we do not address comprehensive histories and physicals, as students take a three-part exam to be placed into this course. Advanced Health Assessment focuses instead on histories and

---

[1]There are several luminaries in EBP and Dr. Janet Allan is one of them. Presently vice-chairperson of the U.S. Preventive Task Force, Dr. Allan is an adult nurse practitioner and has been a leader in EBP at the advanced practice level. She has extensive publications and presentations on EBP, and in her current and former deanships has been instrumental in promoting and supporting EBP curricula. Dr. Allan provided consultation to Dr. Singleton, lead FNP faculty, on the integration of evidence-based concepts into all aspects of the FNP specialty curriculum.

physicals, special populations, and advanced assessment. The next course, FNP Theory and Practice I, focused on acute problems across the life span and across systems. This was followed by FNP Theory and Practice II, which focused on chronic and comorbid conditions across the life span and across systems. The last course, FNP Theory and Practice III, continued with chronic and comorbid conditions, and also addressed the nurse practitioner's role and responsibilities. Although we discussed EBP, it was not a framework for the curriculum.

OUR REVISED FNP CURRICULUM

EBP is now our framework. Course descriptions and objectives have been changed to reflect EBP as part of our culture (see course descriptions in Table 12.2 and course objectives in Table 12.3). The new model for teaching will be action-based. Faculty will use modeling and mentoring to guide and facilitate students in active participation. The Advanced

TABLE 12.2 Example of Course Description Before and After EBP Curriculum Revision

Previous Course Description Advance Health Assessment	Revised Course Description Advance Health Assessment
This course is designed to assist the student to become proficient in culturally sensitive health assessment and to develop skills in health evaluation consistent with advanced nursing practice for health promotion and health restoration. Students will practice advanced health-evaluation techniques, including individual, family, and cultural assessment, laboratory tests, diagnostic studies and interpretation, and documentation of the findings.	This course is designed to assist the student to gain proficiency in comprehensive health evaluation across the life span within the context of family and community. Using an EBP framework, the student will develop skills in history taking, family assessment, cultural assessment, risk assessment, basic laboratory procedures and diagnostic studies, health promotion/disease prevention planning, and appropriate documentation. This skill set will enable the student to begin to develop diagnostic reasoning skills consistent with advanced practice nursing and will assist the student to progress to a problem-focused history and physical.

TABLE 12.3 Example of Course Objectives Before and After EBP Curriculum Revision

Previous Course Objectives Family Nurse Practitioner: Advanced Theory And Practice I	Revised Course Objectives Family Nurse Practitioner: Advanced Theory And Practice I
1. Synthesize major concepts from a wide range of disciplines to develop a theoretical base for advanced primary health care nursing practice with individuals within the context of families and communities who need health promotion/maintenance, illness prevention, and care of acute and chronic conditions.	1. Demonstrate clinical reasoning ability in formulating patient assessments.
2. Critically analyze research related to primary health care nursing for the development of advanced practice. strategies for use with individuals within the context of families and communities who need health promotion/maintenance, illness prevention, and care of acute and chronic conditions.	2. Implement a plan of care according to patient and family needs based on current standards of practice.
3. Implement advanced primary health care nursing strategies for individuals within the context of families and communities who need health. promotion/maintenance, illness prevention, and care of acute and chronic conditions.	3. Evaluate the effectiveness of the plan of care for the patient and family.
4. Evaluate advanced primary health care nursing strategies for individuals within the context of families and communities who need health promotion/maintenance, illness prevention, and care of acute and chronic conditions.	4. Analyze research to facilitate best practice. Establish collaborative and consultative relationships within the interdisciplinary health-care system.
5. Establish collaborative and consultative relationships with interdisciplinary health-care systems for provision of care to individuals in need of health. promotion/maintenance, illness prevention, and care of acute and chronic conditions.	5. Demonstrate accountability for ethical and culturally sensitive care through peer review and quality assurance.
6. Demonstrate accountability for ethical and culturally sensitive care through peer review and quality assurance.	

Health Assessment course has been revised and will now include complete head-to-toe assessment. In Advanced Health Assessment, faculty will model using EBP and show students how this applies to risk assessments and health promotion/disease prevention planning. The FNP Theory and Practice courses will use a systems approach to create a more logical curriculum, and will address acute and chronic/comorbid conditions across the life span by system. In FNP Theory and Practice I, faculty will show students how to access and use treatment guidelines and will require them to begin to use EBP with their case patients. In their next course, FNP Theory and Practice II, faculty will do the same as FNP Theory and Practice I, but expect students to show increased mastery. A developmental model will be used to evaluate students in Theory and Practice I and II. Further, students will be evaluated on midterm case studies and a final multiple-choice exam. Midterm case studies will be evaluated using the same set of criteria, but a rubric will be developed for grading to show how students have gained proficiency in responding to their case patients. We also are evaluating using computer-simulated case patients by course that will allow us to increase the expected performance level of students. In the final FNP Theory and Practice course, students will be required to put EBP into action, bringing them full circle. Faculty will continue in the same fashion but we will then have students look at the needs of a practice population. Based on identified needs, they will select an evidence-based guideline for prevention or treatment and implement it at their practice site (Table 12.4).

Some strategies for the new curriculum will include (1) beginning each course with a review of EBP, discussing how it works and asking students to reflect on their developing understanding of EBP; (2)

TABLE 12.4   EBP Project

Putting Evidence Into Practice Project

- Students will implement an EBP guideline at their clinical site.
- In collaboration with the clinical preceptor, the student will work with clinicians at their practice setting to identify a need for their practice population for health promotion or treatment.
- The student will follow the steps identified by the U.S. Preventive Task force for the implementation of an EBP guideline.
- The student will submit a project report and will respond to the following criteria: process for the identification of the practice population need; the identified need; the EBP guideline that was implemented; the implementation process; and preliminary implementation outcomes.

interactive teaching with an Internet connection to access databases, Web sites, articles, and guidelines during class; (3) moderated small-group work on aspects of EBP in the classroom; (4) moderated in-class discussions of EBP in students' clinical precepted experience and how to access and use evidence at their practice sites; (5) in-class instruction and ongoing support as necessary from our highly skilled reference librarians on database searches; (6) as previously discussed, EBP treatment and management of case patients; and (7) an EBP implementation project in their final course.

Although the current research course is not prerequisite to FNP Theory and Practice I, it has been recommended and will be acted on soon. We will also evaluate the introduction of EBP in the fourth graduate core course, Concepts of Primary Health Care for Advanced Practice Nursing. In addition, we will continue to assess and adjust as necessary the EBP foundation provided in core courses.

As part of the school-wide continuous quality improvement (CQI) plan, each revised course will be evaluated and will be compared by campus and across campus. The Associate Dean for academic affairs and chair of the Department of Graduate Studies will work with the director of our funded Joan M. Stout, RN EBP Initiative to assess all faculty who will be teaching the FNP clinical courses to determine their knowledge and experience with EBP and to develop a plan for one-on-one mentoring to prepare them for teaching the new curriculum.

REFLECTIONS OF A CONSULTANT—DR. JANET ALLAN

For me, serving as a consultant is always an honor and ever enlightening. Academic programs engage consultants for many reasons that may include providing external review of a program for validation, revision, or deletion; offering content expertise related to a specific area; or assessing and developing a plan for dealing with problematic communication and leadership issues in a program or teaching group. My specific role as a consultant for the LSN FNP program was to provide validation and additional content expertise. This role has been a pleasure to fulfill and easy to enact. Two major factors greatly facilitated my role: (1) the commitment and vision of the dean and graduate faculty to integrating EBP into the entire graduate curriculum; and (2) the depth of expertise in concepts of EBP of the lead FNP faculty (first author of this chapter), who is also the chairperson of the Department of Graduate Studies Curriculum Committee. In my view, these two factors were essential for the success of the curriculum transformation.

How We Proceeded

The lead graduate faculty and I developed a very effective process. We used a combination of e-mail and phone appointments over a 3-month period to assess all FNP specialty courses (descriptions/objectives, content outlines, assignments, and evaluations, including clinical projects and evaluations and teaching strategies). This dialoguing process enabled me to review and re-review evolving course material and provide suggestions for additional objectives, content, learning experiences, and references. This dialoguing process facilitated my understanding of the philosophy, direction, and culture of the school that underpinned this curricular reform and enabled me to tailor my advice appropriately.

The success of any change must be measured by the outcomes produced. EBP has been integrated into the FNP courses and implementation of these courses was to begin in fall 2004. These courses are the forerunners of other graduate courses that were being revised during the 2004–2005 academic year. The next challenge for the faculty will be the evaluation of the outcomes of this curriculum innovation. Because integrating EBP into nursing curricula is relatively new, there are few well-defined measures of success. Another contribution that the LSN graduate program will make is to provide leadership in the development of generalizable outcomes by which we can measure the success of integrating EBP into nursing courses and curricula.

PUTTING IT INTO PRACTICE

The Institute of Medicine's 2001 report entitled *Crossing the Quality Chasm: A New Health Care System for the 21st Century* strongly recommended that health professionals provide evidence-based care. This is a major challenge to nurse providers and to those who educate those providers. As nurse educators we must accept the challenge to integrate the essential knowledge, skills, and values about EBP into our curricula. To do this, we must reeducate ourselves and take the necessary steps to help our colleagues embrace EBP. We know that EBP is the future of nursing and a major way to improve the quality of care that nurses provide.

Living and breathing an EBP curriculum is a challenge that LSN graduate faculty have agreed to take on because of a shared vision and belief that through this framework we will be able to support the development of reflective practitioners. EBP is reshaping practice and our students need to be socialized into EBP.

REFERENCES

Institute of Medicine. (2001). *Crossing the quality chasm: A new health system for the 21st century*. National Academy Press: Washington, D.C.

Sackett, S. L., Strauss, S. E., Richardson, W. S., Rosenberg, W., & Haynes, R. B. (2000). *Evidence-based medicine: How to practice and teach EBM* (2nd ed.). Edinburgh, Scotland: Churchill Livingstone.

Chapter 13

Teaching Evidence-Based Practice to Second-Career Nursing Students

Jeanne T. Grace

A prudent question is one-half of wisdom.

—Frances Bacon

Students in accelerated baccalaureate programs for nonnurses present unique educational challenges. Each cohort includes individuals with diverse life experiences and previous undergraduate majors. What these students have in common is their desire to become nurses and their willingness to engage a rigorous program to accomplish that goal in the shortest time possible. These are students in a hurry. Because of the condensed time frame of their nursing program, they are particularly sensitive to any course work that does not appear to have immediate relevance to their goal of professional competence. The traditional undergraduate nursing research course, with its semester-long approach to understanding all the elements of a research project, often fails to meet these students' immediate relevance test. Nor are accelerated program students the only undergraduates in a hurry—an increasing number of adults balance nursing education with jobs and family responsibilities and do not have the luxury of time to waste.

TRADITIONAL UNDERGRADUATE RESEARCH COURSES: WHAT'S WRONG?

As a teacher of nursing research courses for traditional undergraduates, RN/BS completion students, and now accelerated program students, I am also aware of growing inconsistencies between the traditional under-graduate nursing research course content and the practice environment for which we are preparing our students. These inconsistencies exist for all our undergraduate students, not just accelerated program students. The focus of the traditional course, organized according to the sections of the research report, is identifying the elements of research design and understanding the research producer's design choices. The format for research report critique outlined in undergraduate research texts is pri-marily descriptive, with little guidance for evaluating whether strengths outweigh weaknesses. Application takes the form of research utilization, a deliberate, structured, time-consuming institutional/group process.

Synthesis is an advanced skill: it is unrealistic to expect an undergrad-uate nursing student to be able to evaluate and resolve ambiguities in a study's design or in findings between studies, or to place an individual study in the context of the existing body of literature in a field. These are appropriate expectations for graduate education (Millor, Levin, Carter, Doswell, Jacobson, & Shortridge, 1991). Successful students I have taught in traditional undergraduate nursing research courses tell me they're no longer afraid to read a research article, but they don't trust their indepen-dent ability to judge the merits of the study or its potential application for practice.

The growth of the EBP movement has resulted in an increasing number of resources to assist baccalaureate nurses with precisely this dilemma. Reputable organizations like the Cochrane Collaboration select and synthesize worthy individual studies and publish conclusions about the body of findings as systematic reviews. Other governmental and professional organizations evaluate the available literature and produce evidence-based clinical practice guidelines. Secondary appraisal journals select and critically review both individual studies and meta-analyses, reporting evidence that matters for patient care (Box 13.1). The traditional undergraduate nursing course, however, rarely teaches as central skills the strategies for finding and using these valuable research summary products. When I've introduced these "shortcuts" late in the semester to

Box 13.1
Examples of Preappraised Evidence for Practice

Systematic Reviews

Cochrane Collaboration (http://www.cochrane.org). Abstracts for Cochrane systematic reviews can be searched online and are indexed in MEDLINE. Reviews are updated as new research becomes available. Full text for the reviews is available online by subscription.

Examples of recently released review topics:

- community-based interventions for the prevention of burns and scalds in children

- effect of longer-term modest salt reduction on blood pressure

- exercise-based rehabilitation for heart failure

- exercise therapy for chronic fatigue syndrome

The Cochrane Collaboration also maintains the Database of Abstracts of Reviews of Effectiveness (DARE), a central listing of meta-analyses and systematic reviews published elsewhere that meet the Cochrane standards for rigor.

Clinical Evidence (http://www.clinicalevidence.com). Published by the BMJ Publishing Group, *Clinical Evidence* reviews bodies of evidence supporting various therapies and concludes whether the evidence supports or refutes use of that therapy. *Clinical Evidence* is organized by disease entities.

Secondary Appraisal Journals

ACP Journal Club (formerly called *Best Evidence*; http://www. acpjc.org). Indexed in MEDLINE.

Evidence-Based Nursing, Evidence-Based Midwifery, Evidence-Based Mental Health, Evidence-Based Medicine all published by BMJ Publishing Group. Table of contents, abstracts, and selected articles are available online without subscription. Web site for *Evidence-Based Nursing* is http://ebn.bmjjournals.com/

(continued)

Box 13.1 (continued)

Clinical Practice Guidelines

Professional organization: The Association of Women's Health, Obstetric and Neonatal Nurses (AWHONN) publishes a series of EBP resources. Titles include Neonatal Skin Care (2001) and Promotion of Emotional Well-Being During Midlife (2001). The Web site for AWHONN is http://www.awhonn.org

These guidelines are also included and indexed in the National Guidelines Clearinghouse, discussed below.

Government: The Agency for Healthcare Research and Quality (AHRQ) makes available EPC evidence reports on the AHRQ Web site http://www.ahrq.gov

Titles include Blood Pressure Monitoring and Mind-Body Interventions, Gastrointestinal Conditions.

The National Guidelines Clearinghouse (http://www.guidelines. gov) collects guidelines from professional organizations and governmental bodies in one searchable Web site.

students in traditional undergraduate nursing research courses, I find myself wondering why the students and I have spent the majority of the course developing identification skills for elements of research design, instead of best-evidence search and application skills.

EBP FOR UNDERGRADUATES?

For undergraduate students in a hurry, the evidence-based approach to research is particularly attractive. EBP strategies were developed to help the busy clinician efficiently find and apply research findings to the care of individual patients (Guyatt & Rennie, 2002). EBP embodies an explicit understanding that it is impossible to stay current with all the practice-relevant research and an expectation that clinicians will look for specific research in the literature to address clinical problems as those problems arise. Further, EBP is firmly rooted in the context of clinical care. Each learning exercise begins with a patient care scenario and concludes with the consideration of how the evidence can be applied in that scenario. The process of appraising evidence for practice is well delineated, with detailed guidelines and work sheets available to assist the novice (see Guyatt & Rennie [2002] for examples).

In some ways, however, undergraduate nursing students do not match the practicing physicians and medical residents who were the original audience for EBP approaches. Until very recently, the focus of evidence-based student materials has been medical: the diagnosis, prognosis, and therapy of disease. Although these examples may be relevant for advanced practice nurses and graduate nurse-practitioner students, they provide less guidance for the core activities of staff nurses. EBP, moreover, incorporates the clinician's assessment skills as well as the patient's values and preferences with research evidence as clinical decisions are made. For undergraduate nursing students, these assessment skills are also under development, complicating the application process.

EBP distinguishes between foreground questions (for which evidence can be immediately applied to the care of the patient) and background questions (for example, basic understanding of the pathophysiology of a disease). In their clinical rotations, undergraduate nursing students are still mastering background questions and their implications for patient assessment and care: this is particularly true for students in accelerated programs. It is more difficult to frame a meaningful foreground question when background knowledge is not yet secure. Yet if students do not have the opportunity to rehearse EBP during their basic education, how can we expect them to incorporate evidence into practice as graduates?

Given the potential benefits and challenges of EBP for undergraduate students in a hurry, how should we reform the teaching of undergraduate nursing research? First, we need to identify the skills students will need to apply evidence to practice, and reconstruct our course objectives and content accordingly. Second, we need to assure that we apply EBP strategies in ways that emphasize their relevance for nursing core concepts and problems. Finally, we need to define what portion of the vast research literature we expect undergraduate students to be able to apply as evidence.

WHAT IS THE MINIMUM SKILL SET FOR EBP?

EBP starts with the ability to recognize a clinical dilemma and frame the elements in the form of an answerable question. For the best-developed body of evidence—that related to questions of therapy—the question format is defined by the acronym PICO: patient/population of interest, intervention, comparison to the intervention, and outcome. Format variations exist for other types of questions. Framing the question is not just a classification exercise. Students must categorize the type of question they're asking, identify the most salient characteristics of the patient population, define the priority outcome, and often generate a hypothesis about a potential nursing intervention to complete a well-formed question.

The terms used to frame the question then transfer as key search terms for the next step, locating the best evidence. This skill involves accessing electronic resources, combining search terms, and using limits, filters, and available high-yield databases to conduct a literature search that is both sensitive and specific for best evidence. Additional aspects of this skill include the ability to recognize a relevant citation by inspecting the abstract and key words online, and the ability to retrieve the full text of relevant citations in some form.

Once the potential evidence has been retrieved, the student must be able to appraise it. Guided by the EBP work sheets (Centre for Health Evidence, 2004), appraisal has three major components. First, the validity of the results is evaluated, using criteria specific to the type of question being asked and the strongest research designs available to answer questions of that type. Second, the study results are explicitly stated and measures of clinical meaningfulness are applied. Finally, the student must compare the characteristics of the study participants to the patient in the original clinical dilemma, in order to determine if the results would be applicable. When preappraised evidence is available, the student has substantial help accomplishing the first and second tasks.

Interpreting the evidence comes next. The student must be able to translate the appraised findings into proposed actions or ways of thinking that can be applied in practice and is expected to address the clinical dilemma. This skill represents the vital connection between research and the nursing process—it is essential to both. Continuing the nursing process, the proposed nursing action then can be applied and the outcomes evaluated. This completes both the nursing process and the evidence use cycle, tying research course skills firmly to clinical experiences.

The EBP minimum skill set intersects, but is not identical with, the content of a traditional undergraduate nursing research course. Information about specific study designs is only relevant to the extent it helps the student understand why some designs provide stronger evidence than others for specific types of questions. Fluency in research terminology is not an inherent EBP goal. Weighted mean differences and odds ratios are the most commonly occurring "traditional" statistics, and there is an emphasis on confidence intervals, as opposed to hypothesis testing.

ASSURING RELEVANCE FOR UNDERGRADUATE NURSING STUDENTS

The EBP approach to research use must address nursing concerns and core clinical problems comprehensively for application by undergraduate nursing students. Because the evidence-based health care movement originated with our medical colleagues, the four identified domains of foreground question—diagnosis, therapy, prognosis, and harm—reflect a disease-oriented discipline. Nurses have broader concerns, and require two additional domains of foreground question: human response and meaning. These domains facilitate the incorporation of qualitative, as well as quantitative, descriptive research designs.

Human-response questions address how persons process and manage health issues in their everyday lives, including encounters with systems and providers. Examples of human responses would be coping and therapy adherence. Depending on the state of knowledge about a specific human response, best evidence might be a quantitative descriptive study with reliable and valid measures or a qualitative inquiry, particularly from a grounded theory framework. Meaning questions address both the personal beliefs of persons dealing with health concerns and also the ethical, social, and cultural contexts that shape their values and decisions. The strongest evidence for these questions will be qualitative studies, particularly those conducted from ethnographic and phenomenological perspectives.

In order to fully incorporate nursing question domains into EBP, undergraduate students need the same sort of appraisal tools for human response and meaning questions that have been developed for therapy, diagnosis, prognosis, and harm. At the University of Rochester School of Nursing, we have drafted these critical-appraisal work sheets. Validity is appraised according to the relevance of research participants to the research question and the appropriateness and rigor of data collection and analysis strategies. Our work sheet for human response guides students to consider how the research aids in understanding the patient's response to health issues, with practice implications for assessment and management (including counseling). The critical-appraisal work sheet for meaning guides students to consider how the research aids in understanding patient values, a crucial requisite for applying evidence to practice.

MAKING THE TASK MANAGEABLE FOR UNDERGRADUATES

If we can't expect undergraduate students independently to critique and synthesize bodies of research literature, how do we help them develop initiative as evidence-based practitioners? One fundamental strategy is to focus their activities on best evidence—systematic reviews and individual studies that have been preappraised by reliable sources. In essence, we teach students to start at the top of each question domain's strength of evidence pyramid (Figure 13.1) and to discontinue efforts to apply evidence if best evidence cannot be found. This allows students to develop and enact a restricted skill set for EBP.

The minimum skill set necessary to frame the clinical question (as described above) remains the same, but the skill set for locating evidence is somewhat modified. Students follow a search strategy that is carefully designed to retrieve systematic reviews and secondary appraisals of evidence first. If these are unavailable, the final steps of the strategy are designed to identify original studies that pass through the OVID evidence-based filters in MEDLINE and CINAHL (Box 13.2).

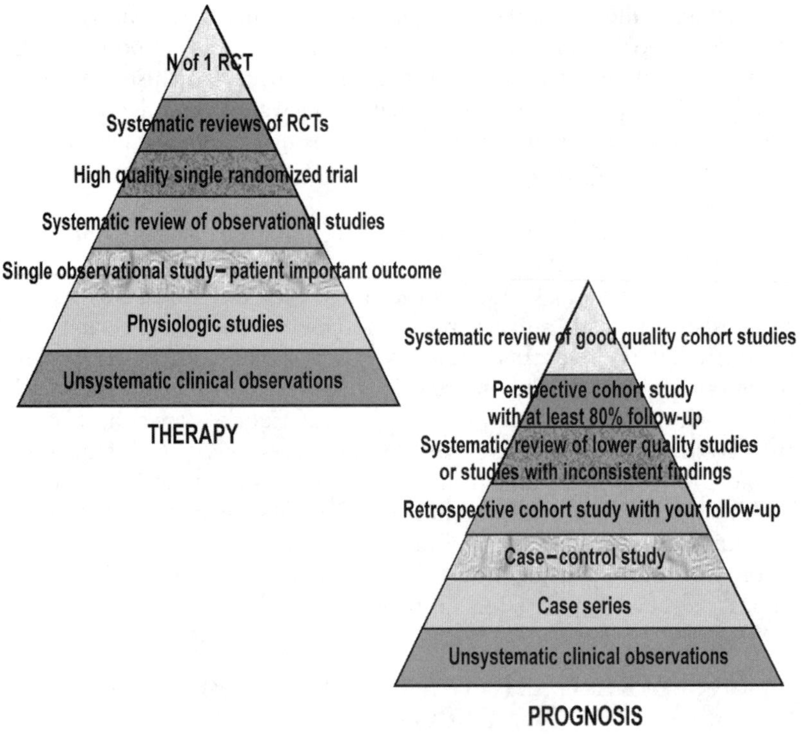

FIGURE 13.1 Examples of strength of evidence pyramids.
Based on M. H. Ebell, J. Siwek, B. D. Weiss, S. H. Woolf, J. Susman, B. Ewignman, & M. Bowman (2004); and G. Guyatt & D. Rennie (2002).

Box 13.2
Evidence-Based Literature Search Filters

Evidence-based filters in OVID (there is a set for CINAHL and a separate set for MEDLINE) search for and combine all studies that contain terms consistent with best-evidence designs to answer diagnosis, prognosis, harm, or therapy questions. The filters are accessed by selecting the Run Saved Search button below the search term dialog box on the main search page of OVID. This opens a menu of stored searches: CINAHL therapy, diagnosis, prognosis, harm, and qualitative filters; and MEDLINE therapy, diagnosis, prognosis, and harm filters. These filters have also been adapted for use in the PubMed search engine.

After the selected search runs in OVID, the final line of the search history contains all the citations in CINAHL or MEDLINE that use terms consistent with desirable study design for the specified type of clinical question. Combining this line (use AND) with the line in the OVID search that represents all the citations assembled by use of keywords and subject headings results in a list of only those citations relevant to the clinical problem for studies that "talk the talk" of best evidence.

More information on the construction of EB filters is available at http://www.urmc.rochester.edu/HSLT/Miner/digital_library/tip_shee ts/OVID_eb_filters.pdf

Students are held accountable for reading and appraising the original research, as well as the secondary appraisal. The availability of a secondary appraisal from a reputable source, however, serves to identify the study as potentially worthy. The secondary appraisal also assists the student by providing an informed opinion about the validity and clinical meaningfulness of results. This allows the student to focus on the salient details for comparing the evidence's subjects and setting with the student's clinical problem of interest.

STRATEGIES FOR SUCCESS

Converting an undergraduate nursing research course to an evidence use course is a paradigm shift. Conceptually, the most crucial understanding for students is distinguishing the types or domains of foreground question because the domain determines what is considered best evidence and what guidelines apply for critical appraisal. It makes sense, therefore, to use the question domains as organizing topics for the course and to provide ample practice in recognizing and formulating questions in each domain at the beginning of the course.

The therapy question domain has the best-developed body of evidence in both medicine and nursing, and so is a reasonable place to start. Students tend to generate therapy questions from their clinical experiences more easily than they generate other domains of questions, and they are also more likely to be able to find relevant best evidence. The body of therapy evidence also contains most of the systematic reviews and meta-analyses (collectively referred to as overviews). Starting at the top of the evidence pyramid for therapy suggests that we teach students to understand, appraise, and apply these overviews before we teach them the skills to analyze individual studies. The guidelines for appraising individual therapy studies provide an opportunity to introduce students to the concepts of causality, bias, and the implications of both for study design. The guidelines further require an understanding of the ways outcomes can be quantified, for example, frequency percentage change for categorical outcomes and effect sizes for continuous outcomes (descriptive statistics). The necessity to estimate the precision of both types of outcomes with confidence intervals provides an opportunity to review statistical inference.

Human-response questions are central to nursing practice, so it would be strategic to address this domain next. Best evidence for the human-response domain consists of descriptive studies, both quantitative and qualitative. Measurement concepts—reliability and validity of quantitative instruments and truth value of qualitative findings—provide context for the appraisal of human response evidence. The discussion of meaning questions provides an opportunity to revisit the appraisal of qualitative studies. The diagnosis, prognosis, and harm domains of foreground questions reflect the epidemiologic origins of EBP. Understandings of appropriate sample choice provide context for appraising evidence that addresses all these questions. Appraisal of diagnosis evidence further requires a familiarity with sensitivity, specificity, and test predictive value (Box 13.3).

We promote the habits of evidence best by providing repeated opportunities to practice them. For students in a hurry, this suggests minimizing textbook reading about evidence and instead maximizing the reading of evidence itself. As a class, we read, appraise, and discuss application of evidence for each foreground question domain. Each student then formulates a question of personal interest from that domain, searches for evidence, appraises the evidence, and proposes a clinical application and

Box 13.3
Diagnosis Accuracy Terms

Sensitivity—the percentage of cases with a positive diagnosis of some condition that are correctly detected by a diagnostic test (true positive test results divided by the total number of cases of the condition). A negative test result on a highly sensitive test excludes the diagnosis with a high degree of confidence.

Specificity—the percentage of cases that do not have some condition that are correctly detected as not having the condition by a diagnostic test (true negative test results divided by the total number of cases without the condition). A positive test result on a highly specific test confirms the diagnosis with a high degree of confidence.

Positive predictive value—the percentage of positive results on some diagnostic test that actually represent cases of some condition (true positive test results divided by the total number of positive test results). Unlike sensitivity and specificity, positive and negative predictive values reflect the prevalence of the diagnosis in the population. For a test of given sensitivity and specificity, the positive predictive value will be higher for a commonly occurring diagnosis than for a rare diagnosis.

Negative predictive value—the percentage of negative results on some diagnostic test that actually represent persons without the diagnosis (true negative test results divided by the total number of negative test results).

evaluation strategy for the evidence. Because students' ability to recognize best evidence develops during the semester, they receive feedback on their question, evidence search, and selection of evidence before they begin the appraisal process for each question domain (Box 13.4).

Relevance is central to the choice of evidence that is to be assigned as class reading: The topics need to be of interest for basic nursing practice, and it wouldn't hurt if they reflected the content of the clinical courses most students are taking concurrently. I have asked my colleagues who teach those courses to let me know if there is specific evidence they would like me to read with their students. For instance, we have read a systematic review of smoking-cessation nursing interventions at the request of the psychiatric/mental health course faculty. Because the evidence use cycle

Box 13.4
Steps in an Evidence Use Cycle Assignment

Step 1—Framing the Question

Write a brief description of a patient care dilemma you encountered in your clinical experience. Identify a foreground question that when answered would help you address the dilemma. Identify the domain (therapy, human response, meaning, diagnosis, prognosis, harm) of your foreground question. Frame your question using the PICO strategy appropriate to a question of that domain.

Step2—Searching for Evidence

Using the PICO terms of your question as keywords and guides to subject headings, conduct a search for best evidence for your question, using the strategies and databases discussed in class. Document your search strategy. Identify one or more single studies or systematic reviews that appear to be relevant to your clinical dilemma and report the citations for those sources in APA format.

Step 3—Appraising the Evidence

Read and reread the evidence source until you understand it. Using the critical appraisal work sheet for the domain of your question (or the outline guides available at the Centre for Health Evidence Web site, http://www.cche.net/usersguides/main.asp), answer the three main questions:

- are these results valid?

- what are the results?

- how can I apply the results to patient care?

and the specific subquestions for the domain of your question.

Step 4—Interpreting the Evidence

Return to your original clinical dilemma. Considering your setting and your patient's values and preferences, propose a specific plan for applying this evidence to practice in the clinical dilemma.

Step 5—Evaluating Your Application of Evidence

How will you know if your application of evidence is successful in resolving your clinical dilemma? What information will you need to collect to decide? Propose a specific plan for evaluating your application of evidence to practice.

is so intertwined with nursing process, I have also provided my colleagues with the dates during the semester when they can expect our mutual students to demonstrate specific skills in evidence use. I hope my colleagues will incorporate those expectations into their assignments (Box 13.5). Our accelerated program offers a part-time option, and part-timers take the nursing research course before they begin any of their clinical courses. When students have no current clinical context, they experience some difficulty in framing foreground questions for purposes of

Box 13.5
Sharing Expectations of Evidence-Based Skills With Other Faculty— Example of a Timeline

---

Timeline for Fall 2004

By these dates, expect the students to have these skills:

- 10/4—Formulate a clinical question in PICO format, identify question domain (e.g. harm).

- 10/11—Conduct an efficient and effective literature search for therapy best evidence.

- 10/25—Appraise a therapy systematic review or meta-analysis to answer a therapy question, propose application to practice and evaluation.

- 11/8—Appraise a therapy individual study, propose application to practice and evaluation.

- 11/15—Conduct an efficient and effective literature search for human-response best evidence.

- 11/22—Appraise a human response individual study, propose application to practice and evaluation.

- 11/29—Conduct an efficient and effective literature search for meaning best evidence.

- 12/6—Appraise a meaning individual study, propose application to practice and evaluation.

- 12/16—Conduct an efficient and effective literature search for diagnosis best evidence. Appraise a diagnosis individual study, propose application to practice and evaluation.

assignments. I suggest to these students that they frame a question based on an encounter they or a family member has had with health care, or that they pursue a health promotion issue of interest. A recent student appraised the evidence comparing low-fat and low-carbohydrate diets for weight loss.

Adopting an EBP approach for accelerated students should provide them with information and skills for research use that have immediate relevance in their clinical experience. It is important, however, to be clear about what this approach will not provide. The successful student in this course will not be prepared to design a research study or to evaluate weak evidence. Students will be able to assess studies for utility in practice, but not necessarily for conceptual or design elegance. We are currently realigning the content of our master's-level research courses to reflect the different research competencies that evidence-prepared undergraduate students will bring to graduate study.

Finally, the EBP approach explicitly reminds us about the limits of evidence and research. For background questions, it is more efficient to consult a textbook or a literature review article than to search the literature for appraised evidence, even though the textbook is a time capsule for knowledge. Background questions do not have direct practice implications, and textbooks and literature reviews are the synthesis products for this type of basic knowledge (Guyatt & Rennie, 2002). Within the scope of basic nursing practice, there are many areas where best evidence does not yet exist. When there is insufficient evidence to support a clinical decision, that decision must still be made on the basis of expert opinion, tradition, or individual experience. Baccalaureate-prepared nurses who are habitual evidence users at least will be aware of their bases for practice in these areas and able to identify clinical questions requiring further study.

REFERENCES

Centre for Health Evidence. (2004). *Users' guides to evidence-based practice.* Retrieved September 17, 2004,* from http://www.cche.net/usersguides/main.asp

Ebell, M. H., Siwek, J., Weiss, B. D., Woolf, S. H., Susman, J., Ewignman, B., & Bowman, M. (2004). Strength of recommendation taxonomy (SORT):

---

*Note: This Web site provides the content for the worksheets for critical appraisal of diagnosis, harm, overview, practice guidelines, prognosis, and therapy studies, among others, in outline form. Interactive worksheets incorporating this content are available by subscription at http://www.usersguides.org

A patient-centered approach to grading evidence in the medical literature. *American Family Physician, 69*(3), 548. Retrieved September 6, 2004, from http://www.aafp.org/afp/20040201/548.html

Guyatt, G., & Rennie, D. (2002). *Users' guides to the medical literature. Essentials of evidence-based clinical practice.* Chicago: AMA Press.

Millor, G. K., Levin, R. F., Carter, E., Doswell, W., Jacobson, L., & Shortridge, L. M. (1991). Cognitive skills and development competencies for conducting research critiques. *Journal of the New York State Nurses Association, 22,* 12–16.

Chapter 14

Teaching Evidence-Based Practice Throughout an Undergraduate Curriculum: Here, There, and Everywhere

Rona F. Levin

A prudent question is one-half of wisdom.

—Francis Bacon

What comes first, the chicken or the egg? In the case of nursing curricula, the question might be rephrased as, What comes first, research courses or clinical courses? As with the chicken-or-egg conundrum, there is really no one right answer to the latter question. We need to help students learn the information contained in both types of courses, but the order may be irrelevant. There are advantages and disadvantages to either sequence. In the case of offering research prior to clinical courses, students can gain a knowledge of the scientific method and concepts of EBP, which (we say) they are then able to apply in clinical courses. On the other hand, without knowledge of clinical content, students will find that asking burning clinical questions about practice is quite difficult. This is not to mean that the rich clinical examples of research principles in action, which make a research course palatable for most students, and the purported need to base practice on best evidence will not have meaning. Now the chicken-or-egg question is only a conundrum in baccalaureate and higher degree nursing curricula. Interesting is the case of associate degree nursing (ADN) education in which there is no research course in the curriculum to grapple with. Yet, are not ADN graduates also expected to base their nursing practice on the best evidence available?

My answer to the above questions is that teaching and learning strategies for helping students to practice nursing from an evidence-based perspective may take place in any course, whether or not students have had a research course first or ever. Under any circumstances, clinical courses need to weave EBP concepts into course content and clinical practica—here, there, and everywhere.

STRATEGIES FOR INTEGRATING EBP CONCEPTS INTO CLINICAL CURRICULA

Should We Throw Out the Textbooks?

According to Sackett and colleagues (2000), we should "burn the textbooks" (p. 31). Why? Because they are outdated the moment they are published. Given the increasing rapidity with which new information is disseminated these days, reliance on textbooks for knowledge about clinical practice means that the clinician is not making decisions based on the latest and best evidence. Sackett and colleagues suggest three criteria for deciding on whether or not to use a textbook:

1. The edition has been published within the last year. (Anything older is outdated.)
2. References are plentiful, especially in relation to recommendations for diagnosis and management.
3. Principles of evidence are used by the authors to support their statements.

Think about how heavily we all have come to rely on textbooks in the courses we teach. In lieu of throwing them all out, however, perhaps we need to help students to use them critically. One learning activity I have used to accomplish this objective is to have students select any nursing

intervention, technique, or protocol from a nursing textbook and determine the evidence the author used to support the recommended practice
behavior (see Box 14.1). This activity may be used as an exercise or
assignment in an introductory research or EBP course, or in any clinical
course in the curriculum. My recommendation would be to use this
exercise in the first clinical course in the curriculum.

How Do We Teach Skills for Clinical Inquiry?

Helping students to develop a questioning mind-set is the teacher's most
important job. The legacy of the wizard in chapter 1 suggests that we
model curiosity and support the value and necessity of constantly questioning our practice as strategies that can be used in any course, in any
setting, at any time there is a teachable moment. When teaching an
introductory class on EBP to students at any educational level or to
practicing nurses, one effective teaching strategy is to provide evidence
that suggests a commonly accepted and/or used practice has not been
supported by evidence. As an example, many faculty teach the use of
alternative (also known as complementary or holistic therapies) for pain
management. These alternative therapies include therapeutic touch, various relaxation techniques, aromatherapy, acupuncture and acupressure,
and biofeedback among others. Two recent systematic reviews, one a
narrative review and the other a meta-analysis have suggested that support
for the effectiveness of some of these therapies is lacking. For example,
in a meta-analysis (see chapter 7) to answer a question about the effectiveness of alternative therapies for labor pain, Smith, Collins, Cyna, and
Crowther (2003) found that acupuncture and hypnosis may help relieve
labour pain, but that there is insufficient evidence about the benefits of
music, white noise, aromatherapy or biofeedback, and no evidence about
the effectiveness of massage or other complementary therapies. In another
article about the evidence related to therapeutic touch, O'Mathuna (2000)
found that many authors inaccurately represented the findings of studies
about the effectiveness of therapeutic touch and concluded that there is
not substantial evidence to support the effectiveness of therapeutic touch
for achieving pain relief in comparison to other therapies.

The point of this dialogue with students is to help them understand
the need to question their practice, any practice, even what often is
thought of as the most routine or assumed to be of benefit to patients.
And as teachers we need to share with students the evidence that supports
the substantive content we include in our courses. As a matter of fact,
we may even want to supplement our textbooks with the latest evidence
available on a clinical topic, such as the systematic reviews cited above.

Box 14.1
Learning Activity for the Critical Evaluation of Textbooks

Objectives

- Determine whether recommended practices are based on evidence.

- Suggest potential problems that may arise from using non-evidence–based textbooks.

Directions for Implementation: Have students select a nursing technique or protocol from one of their clinical textbooks and answer the following questions:

1. In what year was the textbook published?
2. Does the author cite any references in the narrative or protocol for the technique or protocol described?
3. Is the citation contained in a reference list or bibliography in the textbook?
4. If the answer to questions 2 or 3 is yes, list the references and identify:
   (a) whether the reference is a primary or secondary source;
   (b) the type of publication represented (e.g., nursing journal, textbook, clinical practice guideline); and
   (c) the kind of evidence this source represents.

Students either may submit their findings in writing or present them orally in class, or both. Follow-up discussion is recommended. During the discussion, the following questions help students to achieve the learning objectives for this activity:

1. What references, if any, did you find for the selected technique or protocol?
2. If there was no reference to support the recommended technique, what is the author's recommendation based on? How do you know it is valid practice recommendation?
3. What is the value of evidence for nursing practice?

Adapted from H. R. Feldman & R. F. Levin, 2002, *Instructor's resource manual to accompany nursing research: Methods, critical appraisal, and utilization* (5th ed., pp. 5–7). Philadelphia: Mosby.

Another strategy to facilitate students' developing a critical, questioning mind-set is to require them to come up with one burning clinical question for every clinical experience. Students may then discuss their questions in a postconference and determine first if the question is a background or foreground question, and then decide how to proceed in finding the answer. Perhaps students could take turns during a semester to find evidence that bears on their question and then share it with other students during a seminar or postconference the following week. Another approach would be for all students to agree on trying to answer one of the questions presented in postconference for the following week. In this case, each student would locate a study or other type of evidence related to that question. Students do not have to have had a research course to find a study related to their question. Learning to read studies at a very basic level at this point may, in fact, help students to value research more once they get to take a course in it. And in an ADN curriculum, where there is no research or specific EBP course in the curriculum, this type of strategy is essential to incorporate an appreciation and basic understanding of the value of research for practice and the necessity of using the best available evidence to guide practice.

What About Nursing Process Papers?

I would guess that most clinical faculty still require nursing process papers from students. We can use these to develop EBP awareness in our students in every single clinical course. Instead of asking students to provide a purely theoretical rationale for their nursing decisions and actions, or a quote from their textbook to support the practice, ask them to provide a source of evidence from the literature for their nursing diagnoses and interventions. (See chapter 15 for a discussion of using evidence to support nursing diagnoses.) In developing a nursing process paper, the integrative review on intramuscular injections might be used as an example to support the students' choice of injection site for a patient the student cared for during a clinical experience.

Are Journal Clubs Setting-Specific?

It is interesting that there are two chapters in this book (18 and 20) that refer to journal clubs as a strategy for introducing EBP in the clinical setting. Why not use them as an academic strategy to promote students' understanding of research principles and the EBP process? Depending on the number of students in a course, students could work independently or in small groups to assume responsibility for finding a study to answer a specific clinical question and facilitating the discussion about the validity and relevance of the study to their question. In lower-level courses, this question might even be generated by the teacher to make sure the clinical topics in the syllabus are covered. I envision this strategy being used in postconferences or as a monthly 1-hour session in clinical courses about a topic on the syllabus in lieu of a didactic lecture. (No, we don't have to cover every single item on the NCLEX-RN. And, yes, there is life after NCLEX-RN.)

What About EBP Rounds?

In a recent article on *Strategies for Advancing EBP in Clinical Settings*, Fineout-Overholt, Levin, and Melnyk (2005) discuss rounds as a strategy for introducing EBP in the clinical arena. This is another promising strategy for integrating EBP into clinical courses. Rounds would go something like this:

1. Instructor makes EBP rounds with students during each clinical practicum (or specifically designated practica).
2. Students are asked to come up with at least one clinical question for each patient seen.
3. Select one or two of these questions to serve as a postconference topic.
4. Have students get together in pairs to search for evidence to answer the clinical question, which they are to present at a postconference the following week.
5. Facilitate the discussion of how this evidence would be combined with the clinical expertise of the practitioner and the specific patient's values and preferences.
6. Ask students how they might evaluate the introduction of change in practice based on the preceding discussion.

These rounds may be used at any level in any clinical course.

If Not EBP Rounds, What About CATs?

Another clinical strategy suggested by Fineout-Overholt and colleagues (2005) when there may not be enough time for EBP rounds is a technique called CATs (critically appraised topics). An assignment for students in a clinical course would go something like this:

1. Choose a nursing intervention or practice you have discussed in class.
2. Ask students to present (or hand in) a one-page paper, summarizing the evidence on this particular intervention.
3. Depending on the level of the course and whether or not students have had an EBP, statistics, or research course focusing on treatment effectiveness formulas (e.g, NNT, RR), ask students to write a one-page summary (or two if you want double spacing) of the evidence that bears on the nursing intervention and the recommendations for practice that are based on this review.
4. Results of the students' work may be presented to the entire class in a postconference or class.

SO WHERE ARE WE GOING?

The whole point of this chapter is to get you to think creatively. Stretch your imagination! Take a risk! Go for it! Chances are whatever new teaching and learning strategies you introduce at least will get the students' attention because those strategies are different from the norm. Try it; play with it! That is what makes teaching exciting for us educators, and what makes learning exciting for our students, here, there, and everywhere.

REFERENCES

Feldman, H. R., & Levin, R. F. (2002). *Instructor's resource manual to accompany nursing research: Methods, critical appraisal, and utilization* (5th ed.). Philadelphia: Mosby.

Fineout-Overholt, E., Levin, R. F., & Melnyk, B. M. (fall/winter 2004/2005). Strategies for advancing evidence-based practice in the clinical setting. *Journal of the New York State Nursing Association, 35*(2), 28–32.

O'Mathuna, D. P. (2000). Evidence-based reviews and reviews of therapeutic touch. *Journal of Nursing Scholarship, 32*(3), 279–285.

Sackett, D. L., Straus, S. E., Richardson, W. S., Rosenberg, W., & Haynes, R. B. (2000). *Evidence-based medicine: How to practice and teach EBM.* London: Churchill Livingstone.

Smith, C. A., Collins, C. T., Cyna, A. M., & Crowther, C. A. (2003). Complementary and alternative therapies for pain management in labour. *The Cochrane Database of Systematic Reviews* 2003, Issue 2. Art. No.: CD003521. DOI:10.1002/14651858.CD003521.

Chapter 15

Teaching How to Make Accurate Nurses' Diagnoses Using an Evidence-Based Practice Model

Diná de Almeida Lopes Monteiro da Cruz,
Cibele Andrucioli de Mattos Pimenta, and Margaret Lunney

> The teacher is one who made two ideas grow where only one
> grew before.
> —Elbert Hubbard

The interpretation of human responses is a complex nursing task that serves as the basis for selecting nursing interventions. This complexity is one of the sources of varying levels of accuracy of nurses' diagnoses (Lunney, 1990). A review of accuracy studies since the 1960s showed that in all studies, accuracy of nurses' diagnoses varied widely from low to high (Lunney, 2001). For example, in a clinical study in which nurses knew they were being judged for accuracy, almost 34% of nurses averaged below 3 on a 5-point scale of accuracy (Lunney, Karlik, Kiss, & Murphy, 1997). This is a dilemma for nursing because even the best evidence-supported interventions will be risky for patients and a waste of time and resources if diagnoses are inaccurate.

When the principles of EBP are applied to the diagnostic reasoning process, the accuracy of nurses' diagnoses is likely to be improved. Case study analysis is a useful strategy to face such challenges. In this chapter, we explain the relationship of accuracy of nurses' diagnoses and EBP and demonstrate use of case studies as a strategy for teaching EBP as it relates to diagnostic reasoning.

ACCURACY OF NURSES' DIAGNOSES AND EBP

Diagnosis in nursing is focused on human responses to health problems and life processes (NANDA International, 2003). The validity of associations made between the manifestations presented by patients—that is, subjective and objective data and diagnostic decisions—is an essential factor for accuracy of nursing diagnoses. Accuracy of nursing diagnosis is defined as "a rater's judgment of the degree to which a diagnostic statement matches the cues in a patient situation" (Lunney, 1990, p. 14). Use of EBP principles can improve diagnostic accuracy by providing research and other evidence to judge the validity of associations between observations and diagnostic statements.

Achieving accuracy of nurses' diagnoses is challenging for many reasons. One reason is that nurses often need to make diagnostic decisions based on limited amounts of patient data. Patients do not present with all defining characteristics and the overlap of defining characteristics among human responses to health problems and life processes—for example, fear, anxiety, and ineffective coping—further complicates the diagnostic reasoning process.

In developing EBP protocols, the concept of evidence has to be explored and refined continuously. Although the term *evidence* is frequently associated with research findings, research and nonresearch sources can and should be used by nurses when making evidence-based decisions (Goode, 2000; Melnyk & Fineout-Overholt, 2005; Sackett, Straus, Richardson, Rosenberg, & Haynes, 2000). Nonresearch sources may be theoretical or anecdotal. Patient preferences should always be included as a source of evidence and even may conflict with research-based evidence (Sackett et al.). In EBP, the goal is to use the best available evidence, with patient preferences being a priority. Frequently, the best evidence available is not the strongest evidence possible but evidence-based decisions are still possible (Muir-Gray, 2004).

EBP requires availability of computerized systems to conduct literature searches and identify relevant information in adequate time periods.

Nurses need to perform literature searches, select relevant publications, and appraise the evidence for application to current clinical situations. Literature searches are mainly performed using electronic databases such as CINAHL (general base for nurses and allied health professionals), MEDLINE (general base), and EMBASE (McKibon & Marks, 1998). These databases provide access to citations published in health-related literature sources and frequently to the abstracts of studies and revisions of study findings. Use of these three databases is elsewhere described from the perspective of nursing (Burnham & Shearer, 1993). Electronic databases are very large, so appropriate information retrieval requires familiarity with Boolean searching systems in order to keep the number of identified sources to manageable quantities (McKibon & Marks, 1998).

Based on the premise that evidence-based principles can help nurses to improve the accuracy of diagnosing human responses, Levin, Lunney, and Krainovich-Miller (2004) developed the PCD format to guide the application of these principles to diagnostic reasoning. The PCD format has three components: Patient population, Comparison, and Differential diagnosis. Given clinical situations in which the issue is to make the most accurate diagnoses, the first component of the PCD format refers to the *population* that the patient represents. The second component—*comparison*—is concerned with matching the patient cues with the identified defining characteristics of diagnoses such as those developed by NANDA International (2003). The third component—*differential diagnosis*—is concerned with choosing the best explanation among the diagnostic hypotheses derived during the previous steps. Each component of the PCD format is subdivided in three subcomponents: (1) asking answerable questions, (2) searching for evidence, and (3) appraising evidence. The content of the answerable question is unique for each component. Figure 15.1 synthesizes the PCD format and integrates the main content of each component.

USE OF CASE STUDIES AS A TEACHING STRATEGY

Case studies can be powerful tools in teaching and learning, because they "provide a process of participatory learning that facilitates active and reflective learning and results in the development of critical thinking and effective problem-solving skills. This develops self-directed lifelong learners" (Tomey, 2003, p. 34). Case studies have been used in preparing lawyers and physicians since the turn of the nineteenth century, and currently other disciplines also use case studies for teaching (Carter, 1999). Although the question of what constitutes a case is not completely

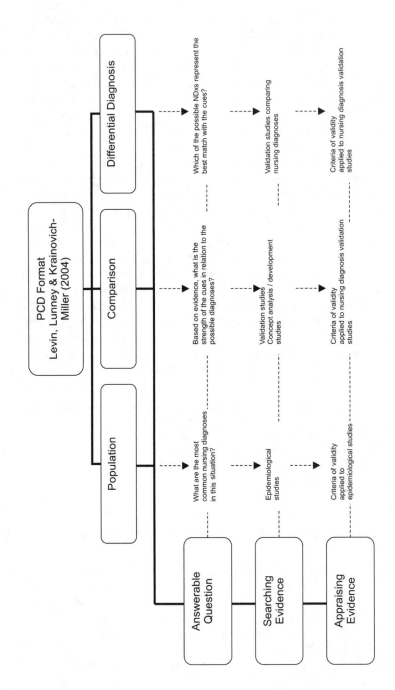

FIGURE 15.1 PCD Format

answered (Carter, 1999), the definition provided by Herreid (1997) is simple and represents major ideas shared by many disciplines. "Cases are stories with a message. They are not simply narratives for entertainment. They are stories to educate" (p. 92). Cases can be used as exemplars or problem situations (Carter, 1999) to help learners integrate knowledge and develop problem-solving skills.

In actual learning situations, learners are provided with both the case study and directions for how to use the case study. The directions guide learners in completing the tasks of evidence-based practice and facilitate immersion in the clinical situation. Directions may include objectives related to the case study as a learning strategy, the results expected with the case completion, and a time frame. Completing these tasks requires access to online literature databases, and time to perform the tasks inherent in the PCD format. If the results of individually performed tasks are discussed in groups, students benefit from each others' discoveries. Use of groups with no more than five or seven participants reinforces the learning process and assures conditions for everyone to express their ideas. A nurturing environment facilitates expression of ideas and the assignment of a group leader helps the group stay focused (Carlson-Catalano, 2001).

CASE STUDY

The following case is an exemplar of applying evidence-based principles to diagnostic reasoning when learners are familiar with evidence-based principles and diagnostic reasoning. The results of the tasks learners should perform will be presented to exemplify use of the PCD format. The results presented here are not absolute or definitive. Additional evidence may have become available after this chapter was prepared.

Directions

The objective of this case study analysis is to apply the PCD format to make the most accurate diagnosis. Students should read the clinical description carefully and they should each imagine being the nurse in the scenario. They are expected to state the nursing diagnosis that best explains the patient's situation by applying the PCD format. For each component—patient population, comparison, and differential diagnosis—students perform the three activities of asking answerable questions, searching the evidence, and appraising the evidence. Results of these three activities for each step should be integrated as the evidence for the diagnostic statement.

A Patient in Respiratory Critical Care (Perry, 2001)*

Mrs. H, 70 years old, was admitted to a respiratory medical unit because she presented with increasing shortness of breath over several days and had a history of chronic obstructive pulmonary disease (COPD). Soon after her arrival, her shortness of breath became progressively worse and she was transferred to a critical care unit for possible intubation. She said she had been intubated during a previous hospitalization and expressed reluctance to be intubated again. She spoke about her living will, the seriousness of her illness, and the implications of being intubated. Mrs. H's physician explained that this acute exacerbation of COPD was treatable, so Mrs. H consented to intubation. She was nasally intubated and placed on a ventilator.

During the first week in the unit, Mrs. H repeatedly asked staff members who were working with the ventilator what they were doing. When suctioning was indicated, she grimaced and gripped the side rails. She made frequent inquires about how she was doing. The primary nurse explained what was happening to her, including attempts to wean her from the ventilator. During that week, Mrs. H participated in her personal care as much as possible. Weaning trials were not successful during the first week.

Mrs. H had good support from her daughter, who visited each day during her lunch break. Mother and daughter communicated well and were obviously close. Mrs. H's daughter often read to her mother from the Bible.

During the second week, Mrs. H developed sinusitis from the nasal intubation. This setback discouraged her. She often wrote or mouthed the words, "I'm not getting better." As each day went by, Mrs. H's statements became fewer and more negative, such as, "I can't get off this ventilator" or "I want to be done with this."

During the third week of intubation, Mrs. H's participation in her care and use of the call bell lessened. She no longer inquired what the nurses or therapists were doing at the ventilator. Mrs. H slept during the day and often during her daughter's visits.

---

*Reprinted with Permission of NANDA International

Analysis

Component 1: Population

The answerable question for *population* is, What are the most common nursing diagnoses in the population this patient represents? If this is the area of students' experience, they will have a mind-set for the answer. The second activity is to search the research evidence to answer this question. Table 15.1 presents the number of references found in CINAHL and MEDLINE, according to the subject headings or keywords used in the search.

The subject headings that produced the most manageable number of references are listed in S5, S6, and S7 of Table 15.1. By reading the abstracts, students select the references that are descriptive studies on nursing diagnoses of critical care patients. Four articles were selected from CINAHL: Logan and Jenny (1991), Roberts, Madigan, Anthony, and Pabst (1996), Asencio (1997), Wang and Lee (2002); and four were selected from MEDLINE: Wieseke, Twibell, Bennett, Marine, and Schoger (1994), Gordon and Hiltunen (1995), Alorda et al. (1996), Pasini, Alvim, Kanda, Mendes, and Cruz (1996). These articles have to be read by students with the aim of answering the question: Which are the most common nursing diagnoses among critical care patients? Students should expect these articles to present research results about the prevalence of nursing diagnoses in critical care patients. These results constitute evidence.

TABLE 15.1   Number of Articles Retrieved According to Subject Search for *Population* Question

Subject search	Number of articles	
	CINAHL	MEDLINE
S1: Nursing diagnosis	2537	1661
S2: Critical care	2574	7252
S3: Intensive care	–	6371
S4: Critically ill patient/critical illness	2054	4825
S5: S1 and S2	4	64
S6: S1 and S3	–	15
S7: S1 and S4 / Limit: research	10/3	4/NA*

Note: *Not applicable

There are many questions to be posed in relation to this evidence, and the goal in this phase, as in other phases, is to choose the best available evidence. Students should apply evidence-based principles even if the best available evidence is not as strong as desired. In order to appraise the validity of evidence for the population, the teacher or group leader should ask questions about study designs. In this component, students should appraise prevalence studies. The following are some possible questions: Is the population similar to the population of the case study patient? Are there any study reports in which the results were applied to similar patients? How were the samples drawn? Did the sampling methods assure for a varied range of clinical situations in critical care nursing? Other appropriate questions for prevalence studies are related to data collection procedures and results. These are as follows: How were the data collected? Were the nursing diagnoses collected from the chart or by investigators? Did data collection cover varying domains of human responses? How was accuracy of nursing diagnoses assured?

A final question in component 1 is, Are the results valid and reliable? The answer to this question is based on the previous answers about sampling and data collection. Validity and reliability are continuous properties, so students need to think in terms of more or less valid; more or less reliable. To complete component 1, students need to select the most valid and reliable results found among the studies appraised.

Analysis

Component 2: Comparison

For *comparison*, the question is, Based on evidence, what is the strength of the cues in relation to possible alternative diagnoses? As in component 1, students need to search the evidence in literature databases such as CINAHL and MEDLINE for studies on the diagnostic hypotheses being considered. For *comparison*, it is important to include as evidence specific content from a classification system that indicates which cues are accepted for the diagnoses being considered. The classification of NANDA International (2003) meets this characteristic.

In component 2, students should return to the situation and ask which data are cues to possible nursing diagnoses, and which are highly relevant to explain the patient situation. In Perry's (2001) case study, cues to possible nursing diagnoses could be: decreased participation in care, decreased use of the call bell, decreased interest in providers' actions, increased sleep, and decreased communication with daughter (who used to read from the Bible to her). Students may point out some other cues, but strong agreement is expected on these mentioned cues. Possible diagnostic explanations for these cues could be fear, powerlessness, hopelessness, and spiritual distress. If students have any other explanations, those should be included in the analysis.

By performing CINAHL and MEDLINE searches with the diagnostic labels and the term *validation* as subject headings or keywords, the authors found 15 articles on fear; none on hopelessness, 12 on hope, 3 on powerlessness, and 7 on spiritual distress (Table 15.2). Note that only CINAHL generated articles with this combination of subject headings. Five articles were selected for full reading, according to the abstract content. These were Beyea and Peters (1987), Hensley (1994), Bufe and Abdul-Hamid (1995), Twibell, Wieseke, Marine, and Schoger (1996) and Whitley (1997). The articles were read to appraise the validity of the evidence they presented, with a goal of choosing the best available evidence.

In order to appraise the validity of evidence for the *comparison* question, the following aspects are helpful. For validation studies, the questions on study design are as follows: Were the defining characteristics judged by a panel of experts or were they identified through clinical validation studies? Were control groups used, that is, were the defining characteristics compared between patients with and without the diagnoses? Is the sample of the study similar to the patient population? Would the sampling method include patients similar to the patient of the case

TABLE 15.2 Number of Articles Retrieved According to Subject Search for *Comparison* Question

Subject search	Number of articles	
	CINAHL	MEDLINE
S1: Fear (and validation studies)	1202 (15)	4736 (0)
S2: Hopelessness (and validation studies)	175 (0)	(0)
S3: Hope (and validation studies)	870 (12)	(0)
S4: Powerlessness (and validation studies)	251 (3)	(0)
S5: Spiritual distress NANDA (and validation studies)	25 (7)	(0)
S6: S1 and S3	–	15
S7: S1 and S4 / Limit: research	10/3	4/NA*

Note: *Not applicable

study? The questions on data collection are, Did the instruments applied contain a wide variation of defining characteristics of the diagnoses being considered? Did the authors develop operational definitions for the defining characteristics? Were the instruments tested for validity and reliability? The questions on results are, Were the results valid and reliable? How do the results apply to the patient of the case study?

Studies on concept analyses can also provide evidences for *comparison*. The following are questions that can be asked: What is the purpose of the study (identification, development, clarification)? Are the methods consistent with the purposes of the studies? Are the results valid, reliable, and applicable to the patient in the case study?

The components of the diagnostic hypotheses should also be compared to information from NANDA International (Table 15.3). It is important to read carefully the definition, the defining characteristics, and the related factors of diagnostic hypotheses.

Analysis

Component 3: Differential Diagnosis

In component 3, students make decisions about the best explanation(s) for case study situations. Students need to choose the diagnosis(es) that best matches with the cues. Students should reconsider the evidences from the validation studies and NANDA International (2003) or other classification systems. The literature databases to be used are the same as the previous components. Students should answer questions on differential diagnosis comparing each possible diagnosis against the other ones. In order to appraise the evidence for *differential diagnosis*, the questions to be asked are similar to the questions in component 2, comparison. Students should proceed with the questions if they find studies that compare diagnostic hypotheses.

For Perry's (2001) case study, research findings that compared two or more of the hypotheses being considered were not found. The best available evidence for the comparison was the information from NANDA International that is presented here for each diagnostic hypothesis (Table 15.3). Some cues are shared by two or more nursing diagnoses but examination of the definitions of each diagnosis, consideration of possible interventions for each diagnosis, and anticipation of the desired outcomes for each diagnosis facilitated a decision that *hopelessness* was the best diagnosis supported by the evidence. This was also the diagnosis that Perry (2001) stated in her analysis (pp. 140–142). Students can be invited

TABLE 15.3 Selected Nursing Diagnoses*

Label	Fear (pp. 75–76)	Powerlessness (p. 141)	Hopelessness (p. 90)	Spiritual Distress (pp. 177–178)
Definition	Response to perceived threat that is consciously recognized as a danger	Perception that one's own action will not significantly affect an outcome; a perceived lack of control over a current situation or immediate happening	Subjective state in which an individual sees limited or no alternatives or personal choices available and is unable to mobilize energy on own behalf	Impaired ability to experience and integrate meaning and purpose in life through a person's connectedness with self, others, art, music, literature, nature, or a power greater than oneself

(continued)

TABLE 15.3 (continued)

Label	Fear (pp. 75–76)	Powerlessness (p. 141)	Hopelessness (p. 90)	Spiritual Distress (pp. 177–178)
Defining Characteristics	*Report of* apprehension, increased tension, decreased self-assurance; excitement, being scared, jitteriness, dread, alarm terror panic *Cognitive:* Identifies object of fear; stimulus believed to be a threat; diminished productivity, learning ability, problem-solving ability *Behaviors:* Increased alertness; avoidance or attack behaviors; impulsiveness; narrowed focus on "it" (i.e., the focus of the fear)	*Low:* expressions of uncertainty about fluctuating energy levels; passivity *Moderate:* nonparticipation in care or decision making when opportunities are provided; resentment, anger, guilt; reluctance to express true feelings; passivity; dependence on others that may result in irritability; fearing alienation from caregivers; expressions of dissatisfaction and frustration over inability to perform previous tasks/activities; expression of doubt regarding role performance; does not monitor progress; does not defend self-care practices when challenged; inability to seek information regarding care	Passivity, decreased verbalization; decreased affect; verbal cues (e.g., despondent content, "I can't," sighing); closing eyes; decreased appetite; decreased response to stimuli; increased/decreased sleep; lack of initiative; lack of involvement in care/passively allowing care; shrugging in response to speaker; turning away from speaker	*Connections to self:* express lack of hope, meaning and purpose in life, peace/serenity; acceptance, love, forgiveness of self, courage; anger; guilt; poor coping *Connections with others:* refuses interactions with spiritual leaders; refuses interactions with friends, family; verbalizes being separated from their support system; expresses alienation

TABLE 15.3 (continued)

Label	Fear (pp. 75–76)	Powerlessness (p. 141)	Hopelessness (p. 90)	Spiritual Distress (pp. 177–178)
	Physiological: increased pulse; anorexia; nausea; vomiting; diarrhea; muscle tightness; fatigue; increased respiratory rate and shortness of breath; pallor; increased perspiration; increased systolic blood pressure; pupil dilatation; dry mouth	*Severe:* verbal expressions of having no control over self-care or influence over situation, or influence over outcome; apathy; depression over physical deterioration that occurs despite patient compliance with regimens. *Connections with art, music, literature, nature:* inability to express previous state of creativity (singing/listening to music, writing); no interest in nature; no interest in reading spiritual literature		*Connections with power greater than self:* inability to pray; inability to participate in religious activities; expresses being abandoned by or having anger toward God; inability to experience the transcendent, requests to see a religious leader; sudden changes in spiritual practices; inability to be introspective/inward turning; expresses being without hope, suffering.

(continued)

TABLE 15.3 *(continued)*

Label	Fear (pp. 75–76)	Powerlessness (p. 141)	Hopelessness (p. 90)	Spiritual Distress (pp. 177–178)
Related Factors	Natural/innate origin (e.g., sudden noise pain, loss of physical support); Learned response (e.g., conditioning, modeling from or identification with others); separation from support system in potentially stressful situation (e.g., hospitalization, hospital procedures); Unfamiliarity with environmental experience(s); language barrier; sensory impairment; innate releasers (neurotransmitters); Phobic stimulus.	health care environment; illness-related regimen; interpersonal interaction; lifestyle of helplessness	abandonment; prolonged activity restriction creating isolation; lost belief in transcendent values/God; long-term stress; failing or deteriorating physiological condition	self-alienation; loneliness/social alienation; anxiety; sociocultural deprivation; death and dying of self or others; pain; life change; chronic illness of self or others

Source: NANDA International. *Nursing Diagnoses: Definitions and Classification 2003–2004.* (2003). Philadelphia: Author.

to check whether their conclusions, after applying the PCD format, are the same or similar to Perry's.

In actual patient situations, depending on the diagnosis and the patient's condition, nurses should ask patients to consider their diagnostic hypotheses and state their preferences or beliefs. This would constitute strong evidence to support diagnostic decisions.

CONCLUSIONS

The PCD format (Levin et al., 2004) was designed as a guide to apply principles of EBP in diagnostic reasoning. Case studies are useful as tools for teaching the integration of EBP to achieve highly accurate diagnoses. For each component of the PCD format, *population, comparison,* and *differential diagnosis*, learners are directed to ask answerable questions, search available evidence, and appraise the evidence for applicability to the specific clinical situation. The goal is to make the most accurate diagnoses using the best available evidence, including patient preferences.

Applying principles of EBP to nurses' interpretations of patients' responses is a challenge, considering the current state of clinical nursing research. Following the PCD format proposed for the case study, the best available evidence (for almost every aspect) was located in the NANDA International classification. This evidence, however, is not considered strong evidence. Additional clinical studies are needed to develop stronger evidence for diagnosis in nursing. Further work is also needed to develop and refine the criteria for appraising evidence for nursing diagnoses and improving the usefulness of literature databases for an EBP perspective on nursing diagnoses. Measurement tools need to be developed for specific nursing diagnoses and nurses need to be taught the skills for searching and appraising diagnostic-related evidence.

REFERENCES

Alorda, C., Garau, J. M., Frau, J. M., Esteban, M. M., Bover, A., Vidal, C., & Artigas, B. (1996). [Functional health patterns and nursing diagnosis in intensive care units]. Patrones funcionales de salud y diagnósticos de enfermería en las unidades de medicina intensiva. *Enfermeria Intensiv, 7*(1), 3–8.

Asencio, J. M. M. (1997). Evaluation of a critical patient according to the degree of nursing dependence. *Enfermeria Clinica, 7*(1), 9–15.

Beyea, S. C., & Peters, D. D. (1987). Hopelessness and its defining characteristics. In A. M. McLane (Ed.), *Classification of nursing diagnoses: Proceedings of the seventh conference* (pp. 186–188). Saint Louis: Mosby.

Bufe, G. M., & Abdul-Hamid, M. (1995). Identification of depression, anxiety, and powerlessness in medical patients. In M. J. Rantz (Ed.), *Classification of nursing diagnoses: Proceedings of the eleventh conference* (pp. 242–243). Glendale, CA: CINAHL.

Burnham, J., & Shearer, B. (1993). Comparison of CINAHL, EMBASE, and MEDLINE databases for the nurse researcher. *Medicine Reference Services Quarterly, 12*(3), 45–57.

Carter, K. (1999). What is a case? What is not a case? In M. A. Lundeberg, B. B. Levin, & H. L. Harrington (Eds.), *Who learns what from cases and how?* (pp. 165–178). Mahwah, NJ: Erlbaum.

Carlson-Catalano, J. (2001). A teaching method for diagnostic skill development. In M. Lunney, *Critical thinking and nursing diagnosis: Case studies and analysis* (pp. 44–65). Philadelphia: NANDA.

NANDA International. (2003). *Nursing diagnoses: Definitions and classification 2003–2004*. Philadelphia: Author.

Goode, C. J. (2000). What constitutes the 'evidence' in EBP. *Applied Nursing Research, 13*(4), 222–225.

Gordon, M., & Hiltunen, E. (1995). High frequency: Treatment priority nursing diagnoses in critical care. *Nursing Diagnosis, 6*(4), 143–154.

Hensley, L. D. (1994). Spiritual distress: A validation study. In R. M. Carroll-Johnson (Ed.), *Classification of nursing diagnoses: Proceedings of the tenth conference* (pp. 200–202). Philadelphia: Lippincott.

Herreid, C. F. (1997). What is a case? Bringing to science education the established teaching tool of law and medicine. *Journal of College Science Teaching, 27*(2), 92–94.

Levin, R., Lunney, M., & Krainovich-Miller, B. K. (2004). Improving diagnostic accuracy using an evidence-based nursing model. *International Journal of Nursing Terminologies and Classifications, 15*(4), 114–122.

Logan, J., & Jenny, J. (1991). Interventions for the nursing diagnosis dysfunctional ventilatory weaning response: A qualitative study. In R. M. Carroll-Johnson (Ed.), *Classification of nursing diagnoses: Proceedings of the ninth conference* (pp. 141–147). Philadelphia: Lippincott.

Lunney, M. (1990). Accuracy of nursing diagnoses: Concept development. *Nursing Diagnosis, 1*(1), 12–17.

Lunney, M. (2001). *Critical thinking and nursing diagnosis: Case studies and analyses*. Philadelphia: NANDA.

Lunney, M., Karlik, B., Kiss, M., & Murphy, P. (1997). Accuracy of nurses' diagnoses of psychosocial responses. *Nursing Diagnosis, 8*(4), 157–166.

McKibon, K. A., & Marks, S. (1998). Searching for the best evidence. Part 1: Where to look. *Evidence-Based Nursing, 1*(3), 68–70.

Melnyk, B. M., & Fineout-Overholt (Eds.). (2005). *EBP in nursing and healthcare: A guide to best practice*. Philadelphia: Lippincott Williams & Wilkins.

Muir-Gray, J. A. (2004). *Evidence-based healthcare* (2nd ed.). Edinburgh, Scotland: Churchill Livingstone.

Pasini, D., Alvim, I., Kanda, L., Mendes, R. S., & Cruz, D. A. L. M. (1996). [Nursing diagnosis in patients in intensive care units]. Diagnósticos de enfermagem de pacientes em unidades de terapia intensiva. *Revista da Escola de Enfermagem da USP, 30,* 501–518.

Perry, K. (2001). A patient in respiratory critical care. In M. Lunney, *Critical thinking and nursing diagnosis: Case studies and analyses* (pp. 74, 140–142). Philadelphia: NANDA.

Roberts, B. L., Madigan, E. A., Anthony, M. K., & Pabst, S. L. (1996). The congruence of nursing diagnoses and supporting clinical evidence. *Nursing Diagnosis, 7*(3), 108–115.

Sackett, D. L., Straus, S. E., Richardson, W. S., Rosenberg, W., & Haynes, R. B. (2000). *Evidence-based medicine* (2nd ed.). Edinburgh, Scotland: Churchill Livingstone.

Tomey, A. M. (2003). Learning with cases. *Journal of Continuing Education in Nursing, 34*(1), 34–38.

Twibell, R. S., Wieseke, A. W., Marine, M., & Schoger, J. (1996). Spiritual and coping needs of critically ill patients: Validation of nursing diagnoses. *Dimensions of Critical Care Nursing, 15*(5), 245–253.

Wang, L. T., & Lee, C. (2002). Respiratory intensive care unit resource use and outcomes in Taiwan. *Journal of Professional Nursing, 18*(6), 336.

Whitley, G. G. (1997). Three phases of research in validating nursing diagnoses. *Western Journal of Nursing Research, 19*(3), 379–399.

Wieseke, A., Twibell, K. R., Bennett, S., Marine, M., & Schoger, J. (1994). A content validation study of five nursing diagnoses by critical care nurses. *Heart & Lung, 23*(4), 345–351.

Chapter 16

Learning From the Past: Using Nursing History as Evidence

Sandra B. Lewenson

Education is not the filling of a pail, but the lighting of a fire.
—William Butler Yeats

History goes beyond one's own experience and provides evidence for practice. It lets one view the experience of others and the myriad of possibilities that created past outcomes, and lets one use this understanding as the basis for practice. Lynaugh (1996) said it plainly enough when she wrote that "history is our source of identity, our cultural DNA" (p. 1). To ground students in the profession, they need to know what has gone on before. If all nursing actions have a historical antecedent, then it is imperative that history be uncovered, studied, and taught to the next generation of nurses. In this way, the experience of others in nursing is part of the evolutionary progress that propels the profession to improve and advance.

Early in the twentieth century nursing educators believed that a standard curriculum would assure the quality of nursing education and practice. The National League of Nursing Education (NLNE) (which began in 1893 as the American Society of Superintendents of Training Schools for Nurses, renamed the NLNE in 1912, and finally renamed the National League for Nursing in 1952) published a curriculum guide in 1917, 1927, and 1937 for nursing schools to use throughout the United States. Nursing history held a valued place in the curriculum in all of these guides. Each guide suggested that nursing schools offer a separate course in nursing history that would teach students about the history of nursing, highlighting the struggle to professionalize nursing care and accept social responsibility to provide that care. The purpose of the history course recommended in the 1937 guide was to "help the student nurse find herself in her new vocation and appreciate the social responsibilities which she inherits when she identifies herself with nursing as a profession" (NLNE, 1937, p. 237). Early nursing leaders recognized the importance of passing on past wisdom and knowledge about nursing to new recruits into the profession, thereby assuring continuity of practice and professional ideals. History provided the evidence to support the work of new generations of nurses (Lewenson, 2004).

Over time, nursing curricula changed to accommodate the ever expanding knowledge base that nurses needed to use in the changing health care environment. Curriculum reforms, changes in accreditation criteria for nursing programs, and the increased responsibilities nurses assumed in a variety of clinical settings, such as in the newly formed coronary care units in the 1960s (Keeling, 2004), required nursing curricula to meet these demands for more content. Additionally, the efforts of nursing leaders to move nursing education away from the hospital apprenticeship model toward a university-based educational model required changes in what was taught and how it was taught.

As a result of the demand to teach more specialized and clinically relevant content, nursing history and thus historical evidence is rarely included in teaching nursing students. At best, history is integrated into the curriculum and left to individual faculty to determine what in the past is of value and how to impart that knowledge (Lewenson, 2004). Evidence of how nurses did things in the past, whether it be clinical, social, or political, often loses out to content that faculty identify as more important because of the pressure of succeeding on prelicensure exams, certification requirements, and other measurable outcomes that schools are expected to meet. Given these restraints, faculty need help to identify the kinds of historical evidence that support their teaching efforts.

This chapter describes some strategies faculty can use that will enable students to understand the relevance of historical antecedents to a procedure or clinical specialty or theoretical basis for practice. Although not meant to provide historical or methodological content, this chapter can provide insights about the possibilities of what and how to explore history as an evidential basis for course content. A further goal is to assist faculty in determining what "evidence" from the past is needed to help students make better decisions as nurses in the present. Also, I hope that the perspectives brought forward can help nurses to understand and respect their rich clinical backgrounds and avoid what Nelson and Gordon (2004) call the "rhetoric of rupture," which is the separation from nursing's clinical past that causes nurses to continually reinvent themselves and their work. The devaluing of our rich clinical past contributes to the bias, or "nursism," that nurses experienced and continue to endure (Lewenson, 2004). And last, I hope to stimulate nursing educators to use historical research and integrate historical evidence into all their courses.

Lewenson (2004) said, "To advance evidence based practice, we need history to supply the data to understand the work" (p. 375). In 1978 nurse historians recognized the need to assist faculty to use historical research in their classrooms and to meet this need established the American Association for the History of Nursing (AAHN). The goal of the AAHN (2004) has been to "to foster the importance of history as relevant to understanding the past, defining the present, and influencing the future of nursing." In 2001, AAHN adopted a position paper entitled "Nursing History in the Curriculum: Preparing Nurses for the 21st Century," that

> advocates the inclusion of nursing history in the curricula of all undergraduate and graduate nursing programs. History content should be integrated into courses at the undergraduate and master's level. At the doctoral level, a history of nursing course based on the advanced scholarship of nurse historians, and exemplifying sound historical research methods, should be required.

STRATEGIES TO TEACH HISTORY AS EVIDENCE

Using history to provide the evidence or rationale to support nursing practice involves various approaches that can be used with the different levels of nursing students. The first gives undergraduate students a first-hand experience with examining primary sources, where students can read early textbooks or nursing journals. Students can visit archives, hospital libraries, museums, or Internet sites, or interview nurses on content being studied. Students studying leadership, for example, could interview a nursing leader about his or her experiences and relate it to the work students are doing in the class. Students can visit their own school's archives to learn about its history.

A second-level strategy requires the use of historical research by graduate students and involves critique and analysis of content, such as social, political, or economic factors, that broaden students' perspectives on topics studied. The knowledge gained from historical analysis of, for example, the coronary care unit, supports a student's clinical experience on such a unit, perhaps giving insight into changes in technology, physician-nurse relationships, and other factors relevant to coronary care. Using historical research supports student learning by fostering critical thinking and deepening understanding. An example I have used is having students in a community health course assess the same community in which they are practicing, but assess it using data from an earlier point in time. By examining an earlier time, students can compare and contrast morbidity and mortality rates, changes in demographics, immigration rates, communicable diseases, and other relevant community health factors that have shaped the health of that particular community during the current period of time. Data are collected from primary sources such as census data, police statistics, and newspapers depicting the years designated. Secondary sources may be books written about the community. Students may comb the data for clues about who lived in the community at that time, what their concerns were or what the politics were like, or ask how nurses interacted with the community. They may examine similarities and differences between earlier periods and the present, and ask other relevant questions that allow them to compare and contrast current issues in health care with the past. Thus critical-thinking skills are used and students are able to expand the way they think by examining historical data.

The third-level strategies are used with doctoral students. They can expand upon the second-level example by raising particular research questions and using a historical research method to answer these questions. Buck's (2004) recently published work is, in part, work completed for her dissertation; it represents a higher level of study of history than the previous two levels. In this instance, doctoral students use both primary and secondary sources to answer specific research questions raised in their practice that can be answered using historiography. Courses that doctoral level students take would also include historical elements that promote critique and analysis of relevant clinical issues.

Both undergraduate and graduate students may benefit from teaching strategies that use historical evidence from all three levels (see Table 16.1), depending on the depth and breadth required, level of student, and student's readiness to learn. An undergraduate student may be comfortable looking at earlier texts or nursing journals and become excited from reading what was done before. Nurse practitioner students may

TABLE 16.1 Examples of Levels of Strategies for Teaching Nursing History as Evidence for Nursing Practice

Examples	Level 1 : Undergraduate Students	Level 2: Graduate Students
	Use firsthand experience using primary sources, such as early nursing journals or textbooks; visit libraries, archives, museums, Internet sites	Use historical research, which supplies the critique and analysis of the content, such as social, political, or economic factors.
Community Health	Read historical materials such as: Eliza J. Moore (1900) article, "Visiting Nurse" published in the *American Journal of Nursing*; Wald's (1915) *The House on Henry Street,* or her later book written in 1934, *Windows on Henry Street.*	Read historical research studies such as Buhler-Wilkerson (2001), *No Place Like Home: A History of Nursing and Home Care in the United States*; Buck (2004), *Home Hospice Versus Home Health: Cooperation, Competition, and Cooptation.* Collect community assessment data from an earlier period, for example from 1893 on the Lower East Side of New York.
Nursing Clinical Skills	Examine nursing journals over a 20-year period for skills such as skin care, bed bath, dispensing of medication. Examine nursing textbooks such as Clara Weeks Shaw	Read historical studies related to clinical practice, such as Jones (2005), *Knowledge Systems in Conflict: The Regulation of African American Midwifery*; Keeling (2004), *Blurring the Boundaries*; Brush & Capezuti (2001), *Historical Analysis of Siderail Use in American Hospitals Between Medicine and Nursing: Coronary Care Nursing, Circa the 1960s.*
Leadership	Write a biographical sketch on a nursing leader, such as Lavinia Dock or Mabel Staupers. Interview a nurse who holds public office and ask about his or her background in nursing (see Feldman & Lewenson, 2000).	Select historical studies related to leadership such as Whelan (2005), *A Necessity in the Nursing World: The Chicago Nurses Professional Registry, 1913–1950.*

explore the historical research completed on a clinical topic and use findings to support their practice; a doctoral student may actually conduct historical research to better understand a question raised in nursing, requiring historical evidence to respond. Because this chapter focuses on undergraduate and master' students, the remaining discussion is limited to the first two levels. As learning is not linear, both levels will be integrated throughout.

STRATEGIES USING HISTORICAL EVIDENCE TO TEACH NURSING CONTENT

Teaching Community Health Content

Faculty can teach nursing content using history to both illustrate the past and better understand the present science. Faculty who teach undergraduate students about the role of the public health nurse might assign readings such as Lillian Wald's (1915) famous work, *The House on Henry Street,* or her later work published in 1934, *Windows on Henry Street.* These texts enable students to read firsthand how this noted public health nurse assessed the community and described the work of public health nurses living at the Henry Street Settlement on the Lower East Side of New York during the latter part of the nineteenth and early twentieth centuries. Reading Wald's (1915) words, in which she describes the condition of the streets in which she walked as she met a mother lying on blood-stained rags in the back room of a tenement, is compelling for students to read and respond to.

If locating the book for the whole class is problematic, then reading passages aloud in class (or posting it on the school's Web site) will allow students to "hear" the words and provide an opportunity for in-class or online discussion. Students learn that nursing back then was not as easy or simple as they may have thought, nor were the living conditions of the immigrant populations that Wald cared for too different from those of today. Students learn to discern the similarities and differences in care between and among, for example, nutritional patterns, health care practices, or the kinds of roles that nurses in the community developed. Changes over time become evident when students are encouraged to look at historical references from that period to better understand the nature of their work. Best practice changes over time depending on the kinds of data collected and interpretation of those data.

Wald (1934) collected data on the work at Henry Street using nursing records, patient anecdotes, studies on various areas affecting community health, and the cost of nursing service. In *Windows on Henry Street,* she speaks about the value of 24-hour visiting nurse service provided to maternity cases.

> In addressing a group of impoverished women from whom I wished to learn their evaluation of the different services available to them, I asked which of all the forms of relief were most prized. With one voice they said, "The nurse who comes when the baby comes." (p. 86)

Wald explains how the nurse visits the mother prior to the delivery of the newborn, assesses the home setting, and returns to the home to supervise a dignified delivery. Her explanation of the work of the visiting nurse in the community and the efforts that were made to support the mother and the family during childbirth provides students "evidence" on how Wald expected families to be supported and perhaps raises students' awareness of how families now should be supported during childbearing. Although historical background may not explain or predict what nurses do today, it provides context in which to assess a particular setting and helps the nurse make decisions about care.

Depending on the breadth and depth of the assignment and for which student population it is most appropriate, assigning additional readings in historical research can also expand students' knowledge about public health nursing in ways that solely learning contemporary roles cannot provide. One such example would be Karen Buhler Wilkerson's (2001) research and the award-winning book *No Place Like Home: A History of Nursing and Home Care in the United States.* Adding this type of historical evidence opens up the possibilities of seeing nursing within a social, political, and economic context that is different from the current view of nursing.

Historical research also provides the necessary critique of the people involved, the settings, their ideas, and the events that are essential to this type of research. The critique offers students another way of knowing and a useful decision-making tool. Recent historical studies, such as Buck's (2004) study of how society views death and dying and how hospice care offers a different alternative to hospital and home care. Buck studies the community-based services offered in Connecticut between 1965 and 1982 to people who were in the process of dying. In addition, Buck examines legislative issues related to home care reform and how these influenced the passage of important Medicare hospice-benefit legislation (p. 26). Students can use this study as a context for discussing how end-of-life care decisions are made today. Best evidence from the past, as presented in Buck's study, provides a way to understand the issues involved in care of the dying, such as cost, sociopolitical factors, and philosophical beliefs.

Another example of using historical evidence to understand community health nursing is having students compare community assessment data from an earlier period to data from the current time. By conducting a community assessment, students learn how to collect data about various demographic, social, political, educational, and other relevant factors. They learn to use Internet sources as well as library and archival materials, depending on the dates they select. At Pace University's Lienhard School of Nursing, a group of three master's students completed a community assessment of the Lower East Side using 1893 data, the year that Lillian Wald and Mary Brewster started the Henry Street Settlement. The students investigated specific components of the community assessment as a part of a larger study that was being conducted. One student looked at cultural health care behaviors of the Italian immigrant to New York City in 1893 and compared these behaviors with current health care behaviors of immigrant populations who reside in the same area more than 100 years later. Two other students gathered data about the 1893 demographics on the Lower East Side, including statistics on morbidity and mortality rates, safety, sanitation, education, communicable diseases, and other variables specific to a community assessment. These data became the evidence that supported both Wald's decision to open a nurses' settlement house in the area, and provided a basis for students to assess the health care needs of this same community in the present.

Although I used this second-level strategy with master's degree students, undergraduate students would benefit from searching for the evidence for a community assessment, using data from an earlier period. Research skills are developed along with the ability to compare and contrast evidence related to assessing community health and subsequent decision-making processes in order to enhance the health of the community.

Nursing Skills Content

Another teaching strategy to use when teaching the relevance of historical evidence to practice is to refer to earlier texts in nursing. One example is when teaching undergraduates about the use of hospital beds, including safety issues related to the use of side rails, turning and positioning of patients, prevention of decubuti, and the changes in types of hospital beds. Some interesting earlier texts include those by Clara Weeks-Shaw, who wrote one of the earliest nursing texts in 1885, entitled *Text-Book of Nursing,* and later nursing texts by Anna Caroline Maxwell and Amy

Elizabeth Pope who wrote *Practical Nursing: A Text-book for Nurses* first published in 1907. Weeks-Shaw warns students that

> crumbs in a bed constitute one of the minor miseries of sickness, and can not be too carefully looked out for. There should be a regular crumb hunt after each meal. A bed well cared for is evidence of a good nurse. From neglect or ignorance of its proper management very serious consequences may arise in the form of bed-sores. (p. 49)

Maxwell and Pope (1923) noted that the "principal means of preventing [bedsores] will be measures which will preclude pressure, friction, and the presence of moisture, and that will improve the circulation of blood and lymph in the parts" (p. 112). Maxwell and Pope list examples of measures that prevent bedsores from forming, including "keep the bed free from crumbs, and sheets, nightgowns, pads, and binders and the like free from wrinkles" (p. 112), along with several other recommendations, such as keeping the skin dry, maintaining skin integrity, relieving pressure on the skin, massaging surrounding areas, and other measures that we continue to address with our students today. Students can compare the literature of 1923 and 2005 to see which recommendations continue and which differ. What was the best evidence in 1923 versus the best evidence in 2005? How were decisions made about skin care? Were they simply learned and passed on year after year, or were they based on clinical observations, studies, or other evidence supporting the skill? Reading firsthand from these texts and earlier nursing journals allows students to see changes in care over time, reinforcing learning about the need to keep up with new evidence about the effectiveness of an intervention. It helps students learn content on nursing skills from a historical perspective and perhaps encourages valuing of past practices in nursing, thus avoiding constant "reinvention" of these practices (Nelson & Gordon, 2004). Although care has changed over time, the evidence produced by past practices paved the way for more informed practice today and a different way of understanding the content being taught.

Aside from using primary sources, such as early textbooks, use of historical research, for example, related to safety issues and the use of side rails, such as the one completed by Brush and Capezuti (2001), provides another venue for using history as evidence. Brush and Capezuti examined the social, economic, legal, and political ramifications leading to changes in the use of side rails affecting the safety of patients. Undergraduate and graduate students can use this research to understand the historical dimension of side rail use and incorporate the findings in their practice. Faculty can use the study to help identify resources they can use with students, such as the earlier texts that describe the types of beds used, ways to care for the patients in these beds, and the use of side rails and when they become first evident in nursing texts (Brush & Capezuti, 2001). They can trace changes in beds in hospitals and compare them with the types of beds used in hospitals today. Some of the questions that students can explore include the following: What did beds look like? What were the cost factors surrounding the purchase of beds? Who ordered the beds and equipment? What were the safety issues surrounding the use of beds and side rails? Brush and Capezuti's (2001) work, along with the textbooks and nursing journals, create a number of ways that faculty can look at historical evidence to explain phenomena taught today. Decisions about patient care and safety may be supported, interpreted, questioned, contradicted, or expanded upon by the evidence collected in reviewing past literature.

SUGGESTIONS FOR FACULTY PREPARATION

To teach history as evidence, faculty can familiarize themselves with available historical sources in their communities. For example, identifying retired nurses may offer a wealth of information for student assignments. Information about how medications were dispensed, what kinds of needles were used, and how nurses relate to pharmacy and other departments in a hospital or home care setting allows for nurses to better understand the historical antecedents of their actions today. Ask other faculty and nurses to identify nurses who have retired. With permission, students can interview them about their work as nurses. Some questions that students can ask include educational experiences that prepared them for their work, and some of the changes they saw while in practice. For example, two students at the Lienhard School of Nursing interviewed nurses who had worked for more than 25 years in the emergency room of a community hospital. The students were able to understand the changes in these nurses' roles and when triage was first implemented in the hospital and how it was implemented. Another source is hospital libraries and archives, especially those that may have had a school of nursing affiliation at one time; these often provide an excellent source of older texts and nursing journals. School libraries may also contain texts listed in a historical or "outdated" section along with classic texts in nursing. Faculty can also use texts they may have saved from their own nursing school experience and highlight similarities and differences in the nursing care provided. Instead of throwing out old journals in your attics, bring them in for students to use. Many journals from the 1960s and 1970s reveal the historical content for students that was once the current content for faculty.

The Web site at AAHN.org provides an important resource, offering lists of archives and centers containing important historical nursing collections; bibliographic references to books on historical method, historiographies, and other important historical texts in nursing history. The site directs users to other important Web sites for nursing history. The organization's journal, *Nursing History Review*, offers outstanding historical research that can be used in teaching history as evidence. Faculty using the Internet can explore sites like New York City's Tenement Museum (http://www.tenement.org/), housed a few blocks from the Henry Street Settlement, and students can take a virtual tour of the museum. The virtual tour enables students to "walk" through the museum and think about the kind of health care experienced by families who lived in the tenements. A student comment from an online discussion in a nursing history course that I taught revealed what was learned from the evidence gained by visiting the Tenement Museum. The student wrote:

> I viewed the virtual tour of the tenement homes. Although I see stark and overcrowded rooms, people lived in a close knit community. My grandmother grew up on the Lower East Side in the early 1900s. She spoke of sharing her bed with her sisters and brothers. Children were not accustomed to sleeping alone. Her aunts, uncles and other family members lived in the same building. I can imagine my great-grandmother finding comfort having her family close by in the "New World." I was told my great-grandmother did not speak English. Even though life in the tenement appears drab and awful, it may be possible that this life was not as awful compared with the people living at that time. My 11-year old thinks it's "horrible" that my family did not own a car (we lived in the city) we had one bathroom, no shower and one television (black and white). When we observe life in the past we compare it to our present life and cannot get a clear understanding of what it was like to live in the tenements in the early 1900s.

From this student's observations, much can be learned about the immigrant experience in the past and perhaps the relevance to current health care, family, and community health issues. By studying historical evidence, the experience takes on a deeper dimension and encourages students to look at current situations and issues from a different perspective.

CONCLUSIONS

History offers an understanding about people, places, processes, and ideas, providing the social, political, and economic context for explaining why something occurred. Though measured outcomes, clinical trials, and statistical data provide ways of examining an event, history allows one to explore factors that led up to the event and then subsequently to look at the resulting stream of possibilities that occurred following that event. History answers different kinds of questions about clinical practice than more quantitative methods, yet without the historical antecedents to practice, we risk the necessity of continually reinventing ourselves and not learning from the past (Nelson & Gordon, 2004). The ability to ask questions is the basis of the critical thinking that nurses must exercise in order to make clinical decisions. When studied and critically evaluated, the experiences of those who lived before tell a story that is part of the knowledge base from which to make decisions. When carefully mined, the historical experience offers data that can guide patient care. Moreover, these experiences help nurses reflect on and evaluate trends and issues that enable them to better confront the issues in the present. History provides evidence for practice, and thus it is essential that faculty include history as a way to develop the skills and strategies needed to impart this knowledge. Using history to create meaningful learning experiences for students is one way for faculty to think outside the box.

By offering students ways to study content based on historical materials and critique supports the development of decision-making skills. Evidence-based practice uses many forms of data to support the care nurses provide and has lent credence to the clinical work that nurses have always provided. Nurses need to examine historical data that reflects changes in practice in order to value, use, and redirect patient care today. Nelson and Gordon's (2004) most recent concern about the "rhetoric of rupture" and the loss of the historical aspects of nursing practice sums up my concern about the need to consider historical data as important evidence in nursing practice today:

> Rather than depicting itself as a profession that evolves and adapts to historical and scientific contingencies, developing and expanding on the contributions, knowledge and skill of the mass of practicing nurses, both historically and contemporaneously, nursing tends instead to deny these contributions and recast its skill and knowledge as novel and discontinuous. (p. 255)

Faculty need to impart the relevance of historical evidence to clinical practice today. In this way, we can give nurses the opportunity to value their past, appreciate the present, and help shape a better future by making decisions using the best evidence available.

REFERENCES

American Association for the History of Nursing. (2001). *Nursing history in the curriculum: Preparing nurses for the 21st century.* [Position paper.]. Retrieved June 7, 2004, from http://aahn.org/position.html

American Association for the History of Nursing. (2004). About AAHN. Retrieved August 11, 2004, from http://aahn.org

Brush, B. L., & Capezuti, E. (2001). Historical analysis of siderail use in American hospitals. *Journal of Nursing Scholarship, 33*(4), 381–385.

Buck, J. (2004). Home hospice versus home health: Cooperation, competition, and cooptation. *Nursing History Review, 12,* 25–46.

Buhler-Wilkerson, K. (2001). *No place like home: A history of nursing and home care in the United States.* Baltimore: Johns Hopkins University Press.

Feldman, H. R., & Lewenson, S. B. (2000). *Nurses in the political arena: The public face of nurses.* New York: Springer Publishing.

Guide for Integrating History into the Nursing Curriculum. (1999). Philadelphia: The Invitational History Conference and American Association for the History of Nursing.

Keeling, A. W. (2004). Blurring the boundaries between medicine and nursing: Coronary care nursing, circa the 1960s. *Nursing History Review, 12,* 139–164.

Lewenson, S. B. (2004). Integrating nursing history in the curriculum, *Journal of Professional Nursing, 20*(6), 374–380.

Lynaugh, J. E. (1996). Editorial. *Nursing History Review, 4,* 1.

Maxwell, A. C., & Pope, A. E. (1923). *Practical nursing: A text-book for nurses* (4th ed.). New York: Putnam.

Moore, E. J. (1900). Visiting nursing. *American Journal of Nursing, 1*(1), 17–21.

National League of Nursing Education, Committee on Curriculum. (1937). *A curriculum guide for schools of nursing.* New York: NLNE.

Nelson, S., & Gordon, S. (2004). The rhetoric of rupture: Nursing as a practice with a history? *Nursing Outlook, 52,* 255–261.

Wald, L. D. (1915). *The house on Henry Street.* New York: Henry Holt.

Wald, L. D. (1934). *Windows on Henry Street.* Boston: Little, Brown.

Weeks-Shaw, C. (1899). *A text-book of nursing: For the use of training schools, families, and private students* (2nd ed., rev.). New York: Appleton.

Whelan, J. D. (2005). A necessity in the nursing world: The Chicago Nurses Professional Registry, 1913–1950. *Nursing History Review, 13,* 49–75.

Chapter 17

Why We Need Evidence-Based Teaching Practices

Theresa M. Valiga

> The system in place in education has displayed a remarkable
> ability to take on the appearance of any number of reforms
> without changing in any substantial way. We have not yet learned
> the fundamental lesson: No substantial change can occur in edu-
> cation without a substantial change in the thinking of educators.
> —Richard Paul

This book is based on the need for, and value of, evidence-based clinical nursing practice and focuses on how educators can help students and practitioners learn about and engage in EBP. Yet what about the practice of teaching itself? Is there not a need for an evidence base to that area of nursing practice?

Just as direct patient care (provided by nurses working in hospitals, homes, rehabilitation centers, long-term care facilities, or any number of other settings) and the management of patient care (provided by nurse practitioners, nurse midwives, and nurse anesthetists) are considered practice roles, so too is the teaching of nursing (provided by faculty in schools of nursing and educators in practice settings) an *advanced practice role*. The recipients of that practice (e.g., students) and the settings in which that practice takes place (e.g., academic institutions) are quite different from those typically associated with nurses, but the practice is still nursing. And a similar case can be made for those involved in the administration of nursing services (i.e., nurse managers and executives), the systematic and scientific study of nursing (i.e., nurse researchers), and the future direction of the profession (i.e., professional nursing association staff, nurse public policy workers, nursing consultants, and others).

Thus, when we talk about advanced practice roles in nursing, we must not limit that discussion to direct care providers. This chapter, therefore, introduces the concept of evidence-based *teaching* practices (EBTP), discusses the meaning and relevance of that concept for the nurse educator in today's academic environment, describes one example of EBTP in action, and provides an overview of programs and resources currently in place to advance EBTP and the science of nursing education.

THE NEED FOR EVIDENCE-BASED TEACHING PRACTICES

For more than 100 years, thousands of nursing education programs have graduated millions of individuals who have assumed roles as care providers, teachers, administrators, researchers, leaders in the public policy arena, consultants, entrepreneurs, and other types of practitioners. And, for the most part, these graduates have been successful in providing safe quality care, and quality education. Yet the health care delivery system that now exists is vastly different from what it has been, and the graduates of all types of nursing education programs today must be armed with a different set of knowledge, skills, and values if they are to survive, and indeed thrive, in this new health care arena. Nursing education, therefore, needs to change dramatically.

Nursing education, however, is not the only profession that needs to face this challenge. During the 2002 Summit on the Education of Health Professionals (Institute of Medicine [IOM], 2003), it was acknowledged that "education for [all] the health professions is in need of a major overhaul" (p. 1) in order to achieve "an outcome-based education system that better prepares clinicians to meet both the needs of patients and the requirements of a changing health system" (p. 1). One of the areas in which all health professionals need to be prepared, according to the IOM, is the ability to engage in EBP where one integrates research findings with one's clinical expertise and the things the patient values in order to achieve optimum care (pp. 45–46).

If our educational systems are to change dramatically in order to accomplish the goals outlined by the IOM, nursing faculty must call into question the many traditions and sacred cows that characterize nursing education (e.g., rigid and highly sequential curricula, learning theory and clinical practice simultaneously, and teacher-centered practices), and nursing education itself must join the effort to advance EBP. In fact, faculty must be skilled in two areas: helping their students learn how to engage effectively in evidence-based nursing practice and developing and using an evidence base for their own practice of teaching.

Recent research has informed educators of how individuals learn, and there is a growing body of evidence to support ways in which faculty can enhance students' cognitive/intellectual development, promote their critical thinking and decision making, help them become more culturally competent, guide them in working effectively on intra- and interdisciplinary teams, and support them in their efforts to assume leadership roles. Because there is very little funding to support major educational studies (National League for Nursing [NLN], 2002), the evidence in these and other areas is not as conclusive as it is in some areas of clinical practice. But faculty must find ways to continually develop the scholarship of teaching (Boyer, 1990) and the science of nursing education so that our educational practices continue to produce graduates who can function effectively in today's chaotic, ambiguous, uncertain, and constantly changing health care, social, and political arenas.

In 1990, Boyer proposed an inclusive view of what it means to be a scholar and introduced the idea of the scholarship of teaching. He acknowledged that teaching is more than a routine function that almost anyone can do. It is, instead, "a dynamic endeavor involving all the analogies, metaphors, and images that build bridges between the teacher's understanding and the student's learning" (p. 23). Indeed, teachers need to be scholars, that is, individuals who are aware of the research in their field of practice (teaching/learning), ask significant questions about that practice (teaching), engage in scholarly activities to further understand that practice and be most effective in it, embrace change, and are always open to new perspectives.

The NLN Task Group on Nurse Educator Competencies reported recently (2004) on the core competencies of nurse educators, one of which is to "engage in scholarship." This report notes that to engage effectively in scholarship the nurse educator

- Draws on evidence-based literature to improve teaching.

- Exhibits a spirit of inquiry about teaching and learning.

- Designs and implements scholarly activities in an established area of expertise.

- Disseminates nursing and teaching expertise through various means and to a variety of audiences.

- Demonstrates skill in proposal writing for grants and other funding initiatives.

- Demonstrates qualities of a scholar: integrity, courage, perseverance, vitality and creativity. (p. 7)

One can see, then, that the practice of teaching is much more than merely transmitting what one knows to others and evaluating their retention of pieces of information through multiple-choice tests. It is, instead, a highly scholarly endeavor that requires an evidence base if it is to be credible and ever-evolving.

DEVELOPING AN EVIDENCE BASE
FOR NURSING EDUCATION

How does an evidence base for nursing education develop? How does an inclusive science of nursing education come to be created? The evidence base on which teaching practices in nursing must be built evolves from myriad scholarly activities undertaken by faculty in all types of nursing programs, by doctoral students preparing for the faculty/scholar role, and by master's students preparing to teach nursing. One element of this process is to identify the intended outcomes of the educational process, as those are informed by current and anticipated expectations of the nursing role. Program outcomes, therefore, must reflect the knowledge, skills, and values nurses need to practice in today's challenging health care arena.

It is critical that faculty be well informed about the education-focused research that has been reported in higher education, nursing, and other fields that could serve to inform their own teaching practices. For example, we now know a good deal about the value of student-centered learning and active involvement of the learner; our educational practices, then, need to be designed to reflect those insights. We also are coming to know about the value of using simple and highly sophisticated simulations to enhance learning; faculty, therefore, must design learning experiences that effectively incorporate these and other technologies.

In addition to being aware of the education-focused research being reported in our own and other fields, nursing faculty must engage in thoughtful critique of that research and integrate or synthesize it to identify trends, patterns, and understandings. Simultaneously, we must identify the gaps in our knowledge regarding how students learn nursing and how faculty can best facilitate that process. For example, we really do not know the best ways to assess what students truly have learned or what the experience is like of being a student of nursing in this age and time. These (and many more) are questions we must pose for research.

An inclusive science of nursing education will evolve if faculty engages in scholarly concept analyses of educational phenomena, such as what it means to succeed in nursing school, what it means to fail, student-teacher relationships, student-student relationships, learning in groups, and so on. "Experimenting" with innovation and major redesign of nursing education also will help us build a science of nursing. In fact, a national call has been issued for innovation and significant reform in nursing education (NLN, 2003), and faculty would do well to heed such a call if we are to produce graduates who will be successful in today's health care system and if we are to develop the evidence base for how best to engage those soon-to-be graduates most effectively in their current and lifelong learning experiences.

And, of course, faculty/scholars must design quality studies to examine the nursing education enterprise. Systematic inquiry, using a range of methods that evolve from various paradigms (e.g., scientific, feminist, critical, interpretive, and postmodern) is necessary if we are to develop an inclusive science of nursing education, and the studies that are undertaken must be multisite so that we can expand our understandings beyond the circumstances of a single school. Findings from these studies then need to be applied and their impact evaluated, and we must involve students themselves in the process. In fact, in a recent piece entitled "Building Pedagogical Intelligence," Hutchings (2005) noted that by involving students in examinations of teaching and learning, we teach them what to look for and expect regarding quality, we enhance their overall learning, we make them "better contributors to the improvement of teaching by raising the quality of the feedback they can offer" (p. 2), and we help them become "agents of their own learning" (p. 2).

Thus, there are many aspects of building an inclusive science of nursing education that would support EBTP, and all educator/scholars have a responsibility to contribute to this effort. All faculty members must employ a critical mind and a questioning spirit as they design curricula and appropriate evaluation methods, design learning experiences with students, develop collaborative initiatives with colleagues in the clinical setting, and fulfill the other responsibilities of the faculty role. Admittedly, this is no easy task, but it is being done, and there are programs and resources available to assist faculty as they advance EBTP and an inclusive science of nursing education. The following example illustrates how knowledge gained through research informed the design of teaching/learning and evaluation strategies used with first- and second-year students in a baccalaureate program.

AN EXAMPLE OF EVIDENCE-BASED TEACHING PRACTICES

A colleague and I drew upon the research of William Perry (1970) and those who used his cognitive/intellectual development model, including Knefelkamp and Slepitza (1976), and Touchton, Wertheimer, Cornfeld, and Harrison (1977), to redesign the following courses in the baccalaureate program in which we were teaching: Introduction to Professional Nursing I and II (two 1-credit, freshman-level courses), Health Assessment (a 3-credit, sophomore-level course with a laboratory component), and Basics of Nursing Practice (a 3-credit, sophomore-level course with a clinical component). Several sections of each of these courses were taught simultaneously; developmental instruction strategies were used in one section each semester, while the other sections were taught using more traditional strategies.

Research (cited in McGovern & Valiga, 1997) showed that in order to facilitate a student's advancement to higher levels of cognitive/intellectual development, a balance of "challenge" and "support" needed to be provided. The things that challenge students to develop in their thinking include diversity (of views, perspectives, approaches to managing problems, etc.) and vicarious learning (i.e., learning through the experiences of others). The things that support students in their current mode of thinking include structure (e.g., extensive directions from faculty, limited options to make decisions or choices regarding one's learning), and a high degree of personalism exhibited by the teacher (i.e., sharing of personal stories, knowing students' names and areas of interest). If there is too much challenge in the learning environment, students will be overwhelmed and retreat to more comfortable levels of thinking. Likewise, if there is too much support in the learning environment, students will remain stagnant and not progress.

Finding a healthy balance of challenge and support, therefore, was a goal of the faculty teaching these courses. Some of the strategies used to achieve this balance appear in Box 17.1. All of these strategies (and others) were crafted within the cognitive/intellectual development model and guidelines for developmental instruction strategies that evolved from it. Faculty, therefore, were basing their teaching practices on research rather than on tradition or long-held beliefs about the nature of schooling, teaching, and learning.

Box 17.1
Teaching Strategies to Achieve a "Healthy" Balance
of Challenge and Support

- Clear, written explanations were provided for all assignments (i.e., why students were being asked to complete them and what faculty hoped would be achieved by those activities), and criteria for grading were made explicit.

- Each student selected from among several options offered by faculty the assignments he or she wished to complete.

- Included in the options for assignments were some that reflected the faculty's growing interest in using the arts and humanities, for example, writing a poem or writing a short story, to facilitate learning and demonstrate what has been learned (Valiga & Bruderle, 1997).

- Several different textbooks, for example health assessment, were ordered and students were invited to select the book that most appealed to them.

- Students were actively involved in working with faculty to teach the course, and they were evaluated by their peers, as well as by the faculty.

- One-Minute Papers (Cross, 1981) were used weekly to get continual feedback on how the students were experiencing the course and what they were learning.

- Student/Faculty Dialogue Teams were established where student representatives and the faculty met biweekly to discuss each other's perceptions of how the course was progressing, discuss whether the expectations of each were being met, and outline mutually agreed-upon solutions if problems arose.

Although the quantitative measures of these teaching practices did not show significant differences between these students and those in other sections of the courses (see McGovern & Valiga, 1997), the qualitative experiences of students were quite different. Had the outcomes of these teaching practices been multimethod, rather than merely quantitative in nature, it is expected that "significant" differences would have been documented, and more meaningful contributions to the development of an inclusive science of nursing education would have been made. The faculty/scholars, however, did demonstrate the value of EBTP, and their work provides insights into how nursing education could be reformed if it were evidence based.

PROGRAMS AND RESOURCES THAT ADVANCE EBTP AND AN INCLUSIVE SCIENCE OF NURSING EDUCATION

"Cultivating the disciplines of asking questions and seeking evidence is time intensive" (Satya-Murti, 2000, p. 2382) and it requires dedication and support if faculty are to be successful with such "cultivation." Sadly, the amount of funds available to support pedagogical research has been severely limited in the past 10 to 20 years, as a disproportionate amount of funding has gone to support clinical studies. In addition, the number of graduate programs that prepare individuals for a teaching or educator/scholar role and the funding to support the development of such programs virtually vanished during the 1990s. Finally, although most academic institutions expect faculty to be competent as teachers and educational program architects (innovators, designers), what they reward is funded research; in nursing, *funded* research typically equates with *clinical* research. As a result of these and other factors, few supports are in place to encourage faculty who wish to advance EBTP and develop an inclusive science of nursing education.

Largely as the result of today's critical faculty shortage (American Association of Colleges of Nursing [AACN], 2003; NLN, 2004) many schools of nursing are opening or expanding graduate programs that are designed to prepare educators. It is wonderful that such preparatory programs once again are being recognized as valuable. Given the likelihood that so few current faculty have been formally prepared as educators themselves, however, one must question the foundation from which to teach these students. It is hoped that these teachers-to-be are learning about the newest research in education, learning, assessment, and so on, and that they are being assisted to develop their abilities to engage in EBTP.

Today also brings increasing calls from the higher education community for better preparation of individuals for the faculty role. Largely through the efforts of the Preparing Future Faculty initiative (DeNeef, 2002), colleges and universities are more aware of the need to focus preparation, ongoing development, and reward systems on excellence in teaching and fulfillment of the full scope of the faculty role, rather than solely or primarily on research skills. Many institutions have created centers for teaching and learning, centers for improving teaching, or centers of teaching excellence where faculty can come together to talk about innovations in teaching, the latest research about learning, and how to enhance student/teacher relationships. Such centers serve as a source of support for faculty and a means to their lifelong development as educator/scholars.

There are numerous journals now being published that include reports of education-focused research, and these are excellent resources for faculty who are committed to EBTP. A partial listing of these journals may be found in Box 17.2. In addition to these resources, faculty interested in becoming more expert in EBTP and in developing an inclusive science of nursing education might consider attending development programs offered by such organizations as the National League for Nursing, the American Association of Colleges of Nursing, one's nurses association, and Sigma Theta Tau International, as well as those offered through private companies dedicated to this purpose.

Funding for education-related research today is primarily limited to private foundations, individual schools, and FIPSE (Funds for Improvement

Box 17.2
Journals With Education-Focused Research Reports

Action Learning: Research and Practice

American Educational Research Journal

British Educational Research Journal

Community College Journal of Research and Practice

Educational Action Research

Educational Researcher

Journal of Curriculum Studies

Journal of Further and Higher Education

Journal of Nursing Education

National Forum of Applied Educational Research Journal

Nursing Education Perspectives

Studies in Higher Education

Teaching in Higher Education

of Post-Secondary Education). An example of support by a nursing organization is the National League for Nursing, which provides a grants program to support small studies and pilot studies for national, multisite projects. Unfortunately, most of the funding available from these kinds of sources is relatively small, and this limits the nature and scope of studies that can be undertaken. Despite limited resources to fund education-related research, there are nurse educator/scholars who are making an effort to advance evidence-based teaching and develop an inclusive science of nursing education.

CONCLUSIONS

It is clear that if nursing education is going to be more scholarly in nature, we will need a larger cadre of educator/scholars who engage in the scholarship of teaching. We also will need comprehensive funding to support multisite, multimethod, high-quality studies of teaching and learning in nursing. Further, our colleges and universities will be required to acknowledge the value of evidence-based teaching, provide support (e.g., centers of teaching and learning, small grants, and research assistants) for its pursuit, and institute the structures and practices necessary for rewarding these kinds of scholarly contributions.

Students in nursing programs today should expect that the teaching practices used by their faculty are evidence-based and not simply reflective of traditional practices and sacred cows. They should expect that at least some of their faculty are engaged in pedagogical research and are contributing to the development of an inclusive science of nursing education. And they should expect to be involved actively in the learning process and in evaluating themselves and their faculty.

Note: The perspectives expressed by the author are her own. They are not official perspectives of the National League for Nursing.

REFERENCES

American Association of Colleges of Nursing. (2003). *Faculty shortages in baccalaureate and graduate nursing programs: Scope of the problem and strategies for expanding the supply.* Washington, DC: Author.

Boyer, E. L. (1990). *Scholarship reconsidered: Priorities of the professoriate.* Princeton, NJ: The Carnegie Foundation for the Advancement of Teaching.

Cross, K. P. (1981). *Adults as learners.* San Francisco: Jossey-Bass.

DeNeef, A. L. (2002). *The Preparing Future Faculty program: What difference does it make?* Washington, DC: Association of American Colleges and Universities.

Institute of Medicine, Committee on Health Professions Education Summit. (2003). *Health professions education: A bridge to quality* (Quality Chasm Series). Washington, DC: The National Academies Press.

Hutchings, P. (2005). Building pedagogical intelligence. *Carnegie Conversations.* Retrieved January 12, 2005, from http://perspectives.carnegiefoundation.org/

Knefelkamp, L. L., & Slepitza, R. (1976). A cognitive-developmental model of career development: An adaptation of the Perry scheme. *Counseling Psychologist, 6*(3), 53–58.

McGovern, M., & Valiga, T. M. (1997). Promoting the cognitive development of freshman nursing students. *Journal of Nursing Education, 36*(1), 29–35.

National League for Nursing. (2002). *Funding for nursing education research* [Position statement]. New York: Author. Retrieved February 3, 2005, from http://www.nln.org/aboutnln/PositionStatements/fundfornursed02.htm

National League for Nursing. (2003). *Innovation in nursing education: A call to reform* [Position statement]. New York: Author. Retrieved February 3, 2005, from http://www.nln.org/aboutnln/PositionStatements/innovation.htm

National League for Nursing. (2004, September). *The nursing faculty shortage: A national perspective.* Presentation at Congressional Briefing, Washington, DC. Retrieved February 3, 2005, from http://www.nln.org/New/congressional briefing090804.pdf

National League for Nursing Task Group on Nurse Educator Competencies. (2004). *Core competencies of nurse educators.* Retrieved February 3, 2005, from http://www.nln.org/profdev/competency.htm

Perry, W. G. (1970). *Forms of intellectual and ethical development in the college years: A scheme.* New York: Holt, Rinehart and Winston.

Satya-Murti, S. (2000). Review of "Evidence-based medicine: How to practice and teach EBM." *Journal of the American Medical Association, 284,* 2382–2383.

Touchton, J., Wertheimer, L., Cornfeld, J., & Harrison, K. (1977). Career planning and decision-making: A developmental approach to the classroom. *Counseling Psychologist, 6*(4), 42–47.

Valiga, T. M., & Bruderle, E. R. (1997). *Using the arts and humanities to teach nursing.* New York: Springer.

Part 4

Teaching/Learning Evidence-Based Practice in the Clinical Setting

Introduction to Part 4

Harriet R. Feldman

The clinical setting is at the heart of nursing because this is where we apply the knowledge and skills that influence patient care. The interesting and diverse strategies that follow are designed to prepare nurses to implement EBP effectively in the work setting. The goal of doing so, of course, is to improve patient outcomes. The message of the chapters in this section is that using individual and group strategies, educators and staff directly involved in patient care activities should roll up their sleeves, with the goal of implementing EBP practices in their work settings.

In chapter 18 Quinlan presents an array of strategies to teach EBP in the hospital setting. These include journal clubs, nursing practice councils, use of performance-improvement models, and nursing peer review. An important point made is that many practicing nurses never have had a research course and entered nursing at a time when EBP as a concept in nursing did not exist, so their learning needs are very different from those who entered later. This presents a special challenge in determining the kinds of strategies that will be implemented in the workplace setting. To meet this challenge Quinlan states, "The nurse educator or coordinator can provide staff with the forum and materials to do what nurses do naturally and competently, that is, critically appraise what they observe and read. The educator's role is to raise the bar so that nurses may reach for the best evidence and provide the means to get there." Another challenge is organizational culture. Because of the intensity and acuity of the acute care setting, where staffing often is not optimal, there is little time for focused learning. Therefore, any efforts to engage staff must be flexible and be both supported and rewarded by the organizational leaders.

In chapter 19, Everett and Titler provide an extensive discussion of how they have implemented EBP in their clinical setting, University of Iowa Hospitals and Clinics. They include a comprehensive base of published work to support what they have been doing. The Iowa model is described as "an example of an EBP practice model" that has been widely disseminated over the past few years. A team approach is advocated; for example, staff members must be involved in selecting a topic to focus on because they will be at the front line of implementing potential changes in practice. Once a topic is selected, its fit with the organization and its priorities must be determined. Actual team formation follows, including determining who the stakeholders will be, because one needs to know the topic in order to select the appropriate stakeholders. Evidence retrieval is the next step in implementing their model, followed by conversations about the feasibility of applying the evidence to practice. Prior to adopting the evidence in practice, the approach is piloted. A variety of strategies to implement the new evidence is discussed in this chapter, as well as the support needed within the institution just to get the pilot up and running. Last, the role of nursing staff in various positions is discussed, from chief nurse executive to nurse managers, to staff nurses, to nursing assistive personnel, to educators. All are important resources for moving EBP forward in the practice setting.

In chapters 20 and 21, Fineout-Overholt and Worral, respectively, present two focused and practical strategies—the journal club and traveling posters. In the first of these chapters, journal clubs are viewed as a teaching/learning strategy that can facilitate "understanding of the EBP process and increase use of best evidence for clinical decision making." The idea of a journal club is not new; however, the evidence shows that it remains an effective approach in general. Fineout-Overholt describes not only the purposes and benefits of a journal club, but also the infrastructure necessary and methods to develop and conduct it, and how outcomes can be evaluated to determine its effectiveness. Of course, the need for facilitators or mentors, considered "champions," is critical to this endeavor and includes committed leadership. She sees the main benefits of a journal club as follows: Every level of practitioner can participate; all providers can be assisted to gain skills in asking questions and finding and appraising evidence; students can be introduced through this venue to professional practice; ideas can stimulate research or quality improvement initiatives; and participants can gain continuing education units.

Worral writes about the importance of commitment by nursing staff to engage in EBP-related conversations at the point where care is delivered and then use the results of evidence reviews directly on the nursing units. The traveling poster facilitates this process by establishing a physical presence on the unit to engage nurses in active learning about EBP. One outcome of this approach to learning EBP is the following: "Among the 60 nurses who completed the test included with the poster, all achieved a score of 80% or higher, indicating that those nurses who did read the poster and complete the test were able to demonstrate adequate point-in-time understanding of the basics of EBP." An actual poster setup is included in this chapter to give you a sense of what it really looks like.

Engaging faculty and students in the learning process can only serve to advance knowledge in nursing education and practice.

Chapter 18

Teaching Evidence-Based Practice in a Hospital Setting: Bringing It to the Bedside

Patricia Quinlan

> Changes may not happen right away, but with effort even the difficult may become easy.
>
> —Bill Blackman

The ability to access research and translate it into practice is increasingly essential to nursing in an environment that demands care that is current, competent, and cost-effective. Today, students who enter academic nursing programs can expect to receive some type of practical training on how to access evidence as well as critically analyze research designs and methods of application. Nurses in leadership positions and those providing direct patient care would agree about the importance of developing practice protocols that are supported by research and other evidence. Strategies are needed to address the learning needs of practicing nurses who entered the field before the EBP movement and have not had prior exposure to access and application of best evidence. Implementing these strategies in a climate of workforce shortages, increasing technology, and consumerism certainly presents a challenge to today's nurse administrators and educators.

Recent studies demonstrate that nursing practice (Potter et al., 2004) is nonlinear, and therefore learning to use evidence should be an adaptive and flexible process that ensures every path to knowledge is traveled. In the hospital setting, pathways to learning are more likely to be found within a professional practice model that is founded on principles of shared governance. Shared governance is a "structural model" through which nurses can express and manage their practice with a high level of professional autonomy" (Porter-O'Grady, 2003). Hess (2004) views shared governance as not just a structural framework but also a process whereby staff nurses play an active role in unit operations. The basic components of a shared governance model described by Anthony (2004) are autonomy, independence in practice, accountability, empowerment, participation, and collaboration.

Learning to make evidence-based decisions belongs within the shared governance model designed to facilitate clinically sound and autonomous professional practice. The structural configurations within a shared-governance practice model can channel the dynamic flow associated with creating and perfecting practice standards, managerial strategies, and the quality improvement process. Educators have noted little indication that teaching EBP leads to sustained changes in behavior (Holloway, Nesbit, Bordley, & Noyes, 2004). Teaching EBP within practice model structures serves to facilitate sustained use of evidence because the skills needed to retrieve and appraise the evidence are permanently integrated into the model structure. Learned skills are embedded within the practice model structures and hence repeatedly applied in the field. The shared governance model structures suggested in this chapter are (1) professional development, (2) nursing practice council/committee, (3) performance improvement council/ committee, and (4) nursing peer review. The interdependence among the model structures centered on EBP standards is shown in Figure 18.1.

The professional development structure serves to facilitate methods of nursing education. The method chosen within this structure to demonstrate applied evidence-based learning is the journal club. Journal clubs are particularly useful because a primary function of the club is critical analysis of published research. The second structure chosen to integrate evidence-based learning is nursing practice council/committee, which is a forum to research, craft, and revise practice standards. The third structure to be presented is performance improvement council/committee, which focuses on analysis and improvement of care. The last structure pertains to nursing peer review. Peer review, a process wherein nurses

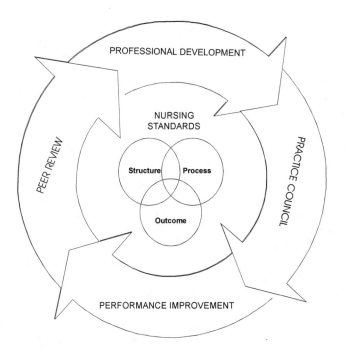

FIGURE 18.1   Professional practice model diagram.

review the practice of other nurses and compare actual practice to evidence-based professional standards, can be conducted within an organized committee or case study framework.

Essential resources for evidence-based learning through any of the suggested model components are as follows:

- Availability of a nurse researcher who is adept at research methodological design; although onsite access is ideal, offsite availability for consultation is a workable alternative;

- Full-service library with subscriptions to databases that contain high-level EBP sources, such as the Cochrane Library;

- Experts such as quality or clinical specialists or nurse educators to bridge the gaps between how to access, interpret, implement, and evaluate evidence-based decisions;

- Active participation by RN staff, recruiting RNs who have had previous education can provide a "train-the-trainer" foundation; and

- Coordination of administrative details, for example, designated responsibility to schedule meetings, arrange for meeting places or classes at the library, and provide copies of materials needed for learning sessions.

The strategies described in this chapter are specific to the hospital setting but may have relevance to community-based settings.

JOURNAL CLUB

Journal clubs will be described in more detail in chapter 20, but we will introduce them briefly here. A journal club is an appropriate forum to educate staff about clinical evidence (Goodfellow, 2004). The term *club* has connotations of collegiality, common purpose, and connection. The club structure is likely to motivate staff participation because it elevates a routine staff meeting agenda to a privileged, intellectual exercise. Though the conduct and organization of a journal club can and should be directed by staff, the club requires facilitation by nurses who are proficient in both accessing and evaluating evidence. Clinical and quality specialists as well as nurse educators can assume this role if they are experienced in appraising the research literature. Consultation and review of articles with a doctorally prepared nurse scholar in advance of the meeting is another way to adjust for knowledge deficits of club members, as these experts can facilitate understanding and provide mentorship to group leaders.

The degree to which journal club "ground-rules" need to be established depends on the interests, personalities, and dynamics of the group. Although the frequency of club meetings will depend on the level of enthusiasm and commitment of participating members, ideally frequency should be every 1 to 2 weeks. Frequency may have to be adjusted, depending on the availability of participants, and is often impacted by organizational workforce characteristics, for example, 12-hour shifts. At any given time, competing patient care needs can preclude a prescheduled journal club time slot, resulting in a cancelled meeting. Cancellation of a club that meets only monthly results in large time gaps between meetings. A longer time between meetings may result in lack of participation, as staff forget or become disinterested because the process of accumulating a specialized knowledge base takes too long.

Scheduling of journal article presentations can be carefully planned or "drop-in" versions where staff bring articles that they view as relevant to their practice. The former involves preselection and assignment of articles. Advanced preparation is more desirable, as complex studies may take several readings to interpret and time is needed to frame questions in preparation for the meeting. Planned presentations are also preferable because there generally is not enough time, particularly in the early stages of journal club development, to both read and critique a peer-reviewed article during a single meeting.

The choice of articles will depend on the primary aims of participants and level of membership commitment. A discussion with members at the outset of club formation will determine how to proceed. A new journal club may want to make the process of article reviews their primary objective. The group will need to target articles that address different types of research designs, perhaps beginning with randomized control trials (RCTs) as RCTs are the accepted standard for intervention studies.

One way to ensure that varied research methods are discussed is to preselect articles and have members sign up to prepare and lead the group discussion. Another approach is to post methodologies that need to be reviewed and have members search for topics that demonstrate use of these methodologies. A less ambitious approach would be to allow the staff to choose articles that they view as relevant to their practice and make the distinction regarding levels of evidence pertaining to each article presented. The latter approach would be more suitable if the duration of membership commitment is questionable.

Accessing articles from complex Web-based information systems is a learning exercise in itself. Staff who are unfamiliar with computer technology may become overwhelmed by having to search online databases. If learning to access the literature is a primary aim of the journal club, then resources and club time need to be shifted to this skill well before analysis of studies begins. Staff who are competent at searching for evidence can work with either informatics staff or in some cases a librarian to provide live online access. University librarians may also be amenable to providing live classes on how to find evidence to answer specific clinical questions.

If technical access issues are not the first priority (although a very essential skill for future independent access of the evidence), a nurse educator or other group coordinator may furnish articles for journal members. In this case the search would be conducted in advance, using the selection parameters previously mentioned. For example, if the group is interested in learning about evidence related to the prevention of deep vein thrombosis, then a randomized controlled trial on the use of a new pneumatic compression device would be preselected by the group's designated expert in advance of the session. Once more, health care institutions and university librarians may be helpful in this process.

Preestablished questions or criteria can guide members to evaluate the quality of the research journals used. A number of sources can be referenced to assist in this process. For example, the Greenhalgh (1997) Web-based *British Medical Journal* series provides a good foundation for evaluating the quality of published research. The first article in the series furnishes a list of general questions that apply to the evaluation of the methodological quality of published papers (Box 18.1). Subsequent articles in the series target more specific research methods, for example, how to interpret epidemiological study statistics. Goodfellow (2004) also provides a list of review guidelines for critiquing a quantitative research article.

These journals as well as published texts, for example, the handbooks developed by Sackett, Strauss, Richardson, Rosenberg, and Haynes (2000) and Gelbach (2002), and mentorship by nurse scholars, can

Box 18.1
Questions for Assessing Methodological Quality of Published Papers.

Who was the study about?

- How were the subjects recruited?
- Who was included? Who was excluded?
- Were the subjects studied in real-life circumstances?

Was the design of the study sensible?

- What specific intervention was being considered and what was it being compared with?
- What outcome was measured and how?

Was systematic bias avoided or minimized?
What is the study design?
Was assessment "blind"?
Were preliminary statistical questions dealt with?
Was the study large enough and continued long enough to make the results credible?

From: "How to Read a Paper: Assessing the Methodological Quality of Published Papers" by Trisha Greenhalgh, 1997. Copyright *British Medical Journal*.

provide journal club leaders with a point of reference for planning journal club discussion. The basic review criteria common to all sources are as follows:

- Establish the research question.

- Articulate researcher(s) study aim(s).

- Articulate the research design appropriate to answer the question.

- Describe methodology including sample selection and controls for internal validity.

- Describe data collection.

- Describe data analysis.

- State and interpret statistical results.

- Address strengths and limitations including external validity and clinical significance.

NURSING PRACTICE COUNCIL

The shared method of governance built into a professional practice model encourages and requires collective participation in order to attain mutual goals and objectives. The forum used for creating, revising, and endorsing standards of nursing practice provides an obvious and logical venue for learning about EBP. Staff nurses are regular participants in standards development specific to their respective areas of expertise and work together to develop nursing standards, procedures, and protocols. Concerns such as feasibility of proposed practice changes are freely expressed and addressed by both management and staff in the best of circumstances. Nursing practice working groups also approve standards through consensus building, provided there is evidence to support proposed practice innovations. Standards development structures present a prospect for introducing EBP knowledge. Staff can be educated and encouraged not only to use research findings to substantiate practice but also to determine best practices, using levels of evidence as a guide.

The education process for accessing evidence is the same as was described for journal club and for that matter any of the other shared-governance structures proposed in this chapter. The best-case scenario is training provided by a librarian and interpretation afforded by a doctorally prepared scholar. Ideally, expertise provided directly at practice development sessions will go a long way toward upgrading internal policy formation. Compromised methods to infuse EBP may include consultation with off-site experts or communication through e-mail. The e-mail alternative requires a basic level of experience with research review. It is reasonable to ask for clarity by e-mail to interpret a statistic, but teaching concepts such as odds ratios would require a more elaborate online learning mechanism.

Practice councils generally include nurses with clinical expertise who enjoy standards development and are skilled in composing standards. This group of professionals has the potential to champion evidence-based learning. Special efforts to train this group both during and apart from standards development meetings can groom experts to be emissaries of evidence-based learning throughout the organization.

PERFORMANCE IMPROVEMENT

Interventions targeted at improving specific nursing care processes measured by positive outcomes should ideally be evidence-based. The ability to access, implement, and measure the effects of an evidence-based solution is critical to any performance improvement model. Quality management through performance improvement has become embedded in most health care organizations as an approach to improve care delivery and performance. The circular paradigm developed by Shewhart and further developed by Deming (Brown, 1999) is routinely used in collaborative efforts to study and improve existing processes and their resultant outcomes to provide an analytical platform suitable to the application of best evidence to practice. The structure, process, and outcome components of the performance improvement (PI) model are derived from theory and mirror the systems elements of inputs, throughputs, and outputs described by von Bertalanffy (1968). In the application of this theory, the performance improvement effort focuses predominately on the process or throughput of a system to generate a desired outcome. Processes are sequentially related steps to produce outcomes (Goonan, 1993) Most nurses working in hospitals today have had some exposure to performance improvement methodology either by participating actively in a performance improvement team/project or passively by listening to reports of institutionally selected performance improvement endeavors.

The pertinence of evidence-based interventions is relative to the problem or process of care chosen for improvement. A search for evidence that focuses on processes of care linked to an established nurse-sensitive outcome such as pressure ulcers is likely to find considerable research evidence that will require systematic review. In some cases, there may not be much research published on a selected topic, particularly if it has appeared only recently on the health care horizon. Nonetheless, accessing lower levels of evidence, for example, a shared experience of professionals who practice at cohort medical centers, can be an equally important skill to develop.

Much like the Plan-Do-Check-Act (PDCA) cycle of quality management (Brown, 1999), the Population-Intervention-Comparison-Outcome (PICO) evidence-based learning strategy for formulating clinical questions is rooted in the scientific method. Figure 18.2 illustrates the congruence between the PDCA and PICO systematic approach to analysis.

The planning phase of PDCA requires assessment of the problem or process that is targeted for improvement. It is during this time that key process and outcome variables are chosen for data collection. Data are

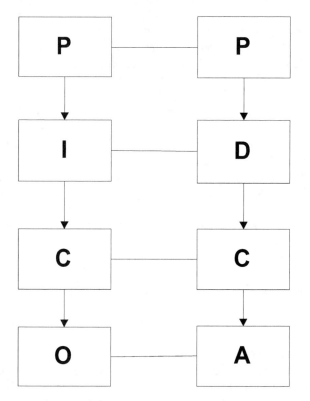

FIGURE 18.2 The population-intervention-comparison-outcome format for evidence-based queries complements the plan-do-check-act cycle of quality management and can enhance improvement initiatives.

then reviewed to better understand and evaluate the process under study. The population identification step of a PICO question for evidence-based queries is also a planning step to organize subsequent analysis around a targeted group.

In the planning phase of PDCA, variable data are collected and examined for variation within the data set as well as external performance benchmarks. For example, when exploring systems related to nosocomial wound infections, internal prevalence and incidence data as well as data from published epidemiological studies of targeted populations are appraised to determine and contrast internal versus national average incidence. The search for comparative evidence is certainly in keeping with the skills necessary to the application of a PICO strategy. Once a performance improvement (PI) project team understands the relative magnitude of a systems issue or problem, a search and analysis of the levels of published research is completed to find potential interventions most optimally through review of meta-analyses. This activity is congruent with the intervention-comparison phase of the PICO format. (The PI project team also determines effectiveness measures or desired outcomes for a chosen intervention during this time.) The selection and implementation of synthesized evidence-based interventions demonstrate application of the "do" phase of the PDCA cycle. This phase provides a final opportunity for learning through application of EBP. Measurement of preselected outcome data is similar to the outcome phase of the PICO format that evaluates the effectiveness of the evidence-based intervention employed in the field and supplies new evidence about whether or not the intervention improved selected outcomes. If improvement is noted, the project team will "act" to hold the gain that was measured during evaluation. Should outcome measurement data show no improvement, it may be necessary to revisit the literature, recheck the trustworthiness of the application process, or review other factors that contribute to process variation, which may have led to negative findings.

The resources needed to implement an evidence-based intervention through PI methods are likely to be less burdensome than those needed to establish and maintain a journal club because the PI team is already organized and functioning. Time to access the literature would need to be built into project activities. Available expertise at evidence retrieval and interpretation phases of the project also would be critical, as it would be in all the various models of implementation described in this chapter.

The benefits of EBP education within the performance improvement framework are twofold. A project supported by high levels of evidence is likely to be more sophisticated and credible than one based on a literature review in which all types of evidence are considered equal. Also, incorporating evidence retrieval, review, and implementation within the framework of a "learn-by-doing" project helps nurses to hold on to the procedural information, for example, how to search for Web-based journals and interpret levels of evidence.

There are limitations to the quality improvement approach to learning about EBP. As previously indicated some of the problems that generate projects are new and have not yet been or may never be published in peer reviewed literature, for example, issues pertaining to work-space design and technology (Institute of Medicine, 2003). The exploration of other types of research, however, is an important skill. A second limitation pertains to PI project timelines. PI projects tend to span several months or more. A single project with a few focused questions may not afford the ability to look at a broad range of research designs.

NURSING PEER REVIEW

Peer review is a vital part of any nursing practice model. Depending on the organizational structure, peer review may be conducted through a formal committee or a less structured case-study program. Peer review promotes excellence in professional practice by demonstrating that nurses hold themselves accountable for the services they provide. Herein lies another opportunity to learn about EBP. A good source of data for peers is nurse-sensitive indicators. Criteria for case selection within the nurse-sensitive outcomes data set can lead to identifying potential areas for safety and quality intervention as well as keeping the case volume manageable. An example of a criterion for case selection is a patient who falls, resulting in injury. Traditionally, peer reviewed case presentations are analyzed for adherence to practice standards. For example, a review may find that the nursing protocol for falls was not implemented or that there is too much variation in the patient admission process, leading to missed opportunities to assess for patient risk. It is at this point that the research literature should be consulted to make sure review determinations are based on the most current and scientifically sound evidence available. The process of evidence review might also uncover that a risk factor specific to the case under review was not included in the protocol, or perhaps best practice for patient admission processes and assessment of falls risk may be found.

Depending on the peer reviewed finding, a course of action is recommended. The course of action to address a failure to implement the falls protocol could range from remedial review of the nursing protocol, or if a pattern of repeated failure is noted, a more aggressive remedial action such as close provisional observation of practice. An action targeted at improvement of the patient admission process may result in the appointment of a performance improvement team. Whatever the course of action, it is important that review determinations or recommendations are founded on the best evidence because inaccurate determinations could potentially result in unjust disciplinary action. Additionally, recommendations for potential system change can impact on safety and resource use at a time when efficiency is considered an important tenet of quality.

Interventions generated from peer review activities often require the expertise of nurses with different perspectives. Clinical specialists may be consulted for education, quality specialists for data or systems improvement strategies, or managers for mentorship and personal direction. Effectiveness of interventions generated by this process can be measured through continued monitoring of nursing-sensitive indicators, observation, or documentation review.

The case study format is a peer review process that affords an appropriate setting for learning about evidence-based nursing. As previously stated, the support of EBP expertise will drive the agenda. Case studies can be organized similar to the journal club design. Case selection can be based on peer review findings, for example, a medication error, wherein an opportunity to share lessons learned is identified or simply becomes a clinical topic of interest. A suggested method is to assign inpatient units to host a breakfast or lunch where they present a case review that illustrates choice of evidence-supported interventions. This approach appeals to the self-esteem of unit staff and provides them with an opportunity to showcase their clinical knowledge and leadership talents, thus making a contribution to the overall nursing division.

The presenting unit staff in this scenario leads an open discussion for the entire division. Interdisciplinary attendance and participation are also applicable to this method of learning. Having a pharmacist, for example, present information specific to pharmacological aspects of case management can facilitate collaboration. The presenting unit then can moderate an open discussion of applied evidence with an interdisciplinary panel of invited experts.

BEYOND STRUCTURE

Organizational culture and leadership are central factors in setting the conditions for teaching and evaluating the practice of evidence-based nursing in the workplace. The intense work of nursing practice provides little time for focused traditional learning, especially during work hours.

Although the published literature outlines methods to teach evidence-based nursing and medicine, there is little evidence that teaching with the use of traditional methods leads to sustained behavior change (Holloway et al., 2004). Therefore, if the alternative structures proposed are to be successful, organizational and nurse leadership must internalize management practices that facilitate cooperation and staff engagement (Stetler, 2003).

In her review of organizational progress with translational research, Stetler (2003) outlines a framework that best sustains EBP. Key components of this framework are leadership support, capacity to engage in EBP, and an infrastructure to support and maintain an EBP culture. A primary aim of EBP is patient safety. In its report *Keeping Patients Safe*, the Institute of Medicine (2003) outlines these key practices for creating better and safer work environments:

- Balance the tension between production efficiency and reliability.

- Create and sustain trust.

- Manage the process of change.

- Involve workers in decision making.

- Use management practices that foster learning.

Though most of these practices are targeted to administrative leadership, nurse educators as leaders are best advised to inculcate these recommendations. As previously mentioned, flexibility and perseverance are essential necessities for teaching in today's work environment. Educators need to be responsive to change. For example, if a club meeting time is cancelled, an alternate time should be considered; also, food can be offered to entice busy participants. Though flexibility in scheduling can result in real inconvenience, the payoff is worth the effort. Nurses appreciate leaders who put them and their patients first. Intelligent nurses come to meetings prepared by their experiences. As with other professionals, they need administrative support. The nurse educator or coordinator can provide staff with the forum and materials to do what nurses do naturally and competently, that is, critically appraise what they observe and read. The educator's role is to raise the bar so that nurses may reach for the best evidence and provide the means to get there. This means pushing nurses to focus more on thinking rather than doing (i.e., homework) in the initial processes of learning evidence-based nursing. Scholarly expectations are worthwhile future goals for the nursing profession, but the educator may be needed to ignite the passion for this pursuit. Evidence-based nursing integrated through educator-steered, determined, and adaptable structural designs may be the bridge to creating a greater appreciation for lifelong learning.

Acknowledgments

The mentorship of Patricia Stone, PhD, MPH, RN, has been invaluable to understanding the learning needs of students with respect to EBP. Dr. Stone's high regard and respect for nurses is evident in the manner in which she has developed a clinically sophisticated and progressive style of teaching EBP at the graduate and postgraduate nurse level. As a nurse leader, Jacqueline Kostic, MS, RN, has created an organizational environment that has all of the structures detailed in this chapter as well as a climate of shared governance and collaboration. To be able to practice in this environment under such talented leadership is a special privilege.

REFERENCES

Anthony, M. (2004). Shared governance. *Online Journal of Issues in Nursing, 1*(4), 1–16.

Brown, J. (1999). *The healthcare quality handbook: A professional resource and study guide* (14th ed.). Pasedena, CA: Managed Care Consultants.

Gelbach, S. (2002). *Interpreting the medical literature* (4th ed.). New York: McGraw-Hill.

Goodfellow, L. (2004). Can journal club bridge the gap between research and practice? *Nurse Educator, 29*(3), 107–110.

Goonan, K. (1993). *Clinical quality and total quality management.* Wilton, CT: Juran Institute.

Greenhalgh, T. (1997). How to read a paper: Assessing the methodological quality of published papers. *British Medical Journal, 315,* 305–308.

Hess, R. (2004). From bedside to boardroom: Nursing shared governance. *Online Journal of Issues in Nursing, 9*(1), Manuscript 1. Retrieved from www.nursingworld.org/ojin/topic23/tpc23_1.htm.

Holloway, R., Nesbit, K., Bordley D., & Noyes K. (2004). Teaching and evaluating first and second year medical student's practice of evidenced based medicine. *Medical Education, 38*(8), 869–878

Institute of Medicine. (2003). *Keeping patients safe: Transforming the work environment of nurses* [Prepublication copy of book]. Washington, DC: National Academies Press.

Porter-O'Grady, T. (2003). Researching shared governance: A futility of focus. *Journal of Nursing Administration, 33*(4), 251–252.

Potter, P., Boxerman, S., Wolf, L., Marshall J., Grayson D., Sledge, J., et al. (2004). Mapping the nursing process. *Journal of Nursing Administration, 34*(2), 101–109.

Sackett, D., Strauss, S., Richardson, W., Rosenberg, W., & Haynes, R. (2000). *Evidence based medicine* (2nd ed.). Edinburgh, Scotland: Churchill Livingstone.

Stetler, C. (2003). Role of the organization in translating research into EBP. *Outcomes Management, 7*(3), 97–103.

von Bertalanffy, L. (1968). *General systems theory: Foundations, development and applications.* New York: Braziller.

Chapter 19

Making EBP Part of Clinical Practice: The Iowa Model

Linda Q. Everett and Marita G. Titler

> Learning and innovation go hand in hand. The arrogance of
> success is to think that what you did yesterday will be sufficient
> for tomorrow.
>
> —William Pollard

"The stark reality [is] that we invest billions in research to find appropriate treatments, we spend more than $1 trillion on healthcare annually, we have extraordinary capacity to deliver the best care in the world, but we repeatedly fail to translate that knowledge and capacity into clinical practice" (Institute of Medicine [IOM], 2003, p. 2). For example, failure to rescue, decubitus ulcers, and postoperative sepsis accounted for 60% of all patient safety incidents among Medicare patients hospitalized from 2000 through 2002; during this same time period decubitus ulcers accounted for $2.57 billion in excess inpatient costs to Medicare and postop pulmonary embolism, or deep vein thrombosis (DVT), account for $1.4 billion in excess inpatient costs to Medicare (Health Grades, 2004). When EBPs are effectively implemented, patient outcomes improve and resource use declines (Lubarsky, Glass, Ginsberg, De L. Dear, Dentz, Gan, Sanderson, Mythen, Dufore, Pressley, Gilbert, White, Alexander, Coleman, Rogers & Reves, 1997; McCormick, Cummings, & Kovner, 1997; Newman, Pyne, Leigh, Rounce, & Cowling, 2000; Schneider & Eisenberg, 1998; Titler, 1998; Titler, Hill, & Matthews, 1999). There is no guarantee, however, that the evidence is used in practice (Berg, Atkins, & Tierney, 1997; Dickersin & Manheimer, 1998; Kamerow, 1997), and the use of evidence by health care professionals is sporadic at best (Atkins, Kamerow, & Eisenberg, 1998; Bostrom & Suter, 1993; Carroll et al., 1997; Cronenwett, 1995; Eddy, 2005; Herr et al., 2004; Kirchhoff, 2004; McCurren, 1995; Pettengill, Gilles, & Clar, 1994; Rutledge, Greene, Mooney, Nail, & Ropka, 1996; Schneider & Eisenberg, 1998; Titler et al., 2003). It is the responsibility of all nurses to use the current best research evidence in care delivery. This chapter describes the process of implementing EBP in the clinical setting.

MODELS OF EVIDENCE-BASED PRACTICE

A number of models have been used in implementing EBP (Berwick, 2003; Doebbeling et al., 2002; Farquhar, Stryer, & Slutsky, 2002; Jones, 2000; Lavis et al., 2003; Lomas et al., 1991; Nutley & Davies, 2000; Nutley, Davies, & Walter, 2003; Rogers, 1995, 2003; Rycroft-Malone et al., 2002; Titler & Everett, 2001; Titler et al., 2003). Using a model to implement EBP helps organize the strategies being used and elucidates the barriers and facilitators that may influence adoption (e.g., organizational size, characteristics of users).

The Iowa Model of EBP

The Iowa Model of EBP is overviewed here as an example of an EBP *practice* model (Figure 19.1). This model has been widely disseminated and adopted in academic and clinical settings (Estabrooks, Winther, & Derksen, 2004; Titler et al., 2001). An organizational, collaborative model, it incorporates conduct of research, use of research evidence, and other types of evidence (Titler et al., 2001). Authors of the Iowa model adopted the definition of EBP as the conscientious and judicious use of current best evidence to guide health care decisions (Sackett, Rosenberg, Gray, Haynes, & Richardson, 1996). Best evidence may range from randomized clinical trials to case reports and expert opinion, depending on the availability of such evidence. Knowledge- and problem-focused "triggers" lead staff members to question current nursing practice and

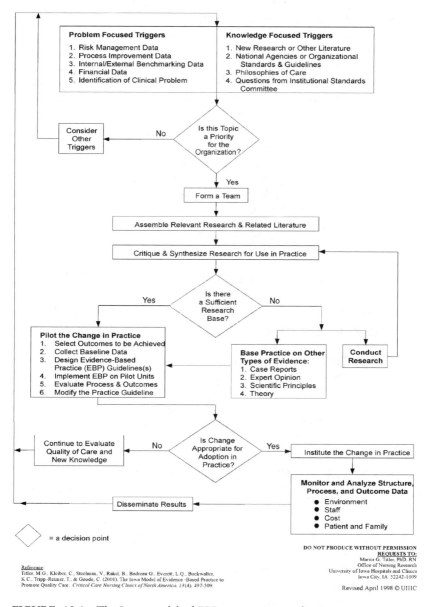

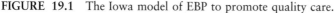

FIGURE 19.1   The Iowa model of EBP to promote quality care.

From "The Iowa Model of Evidence-Based Practice to Promote Quality Care," by M. Titler et al., 2001, *Critical Care Nursing Clinics of North America, 13*, pp. 497–502. Copyright 2001. Used with permission of author.

whether patient care can be improved through the use of research findings or other types of evidence. If literature review and critique of studies results in an insufficient number of scientifically sound studies to use as a base for practice, consideration is given to conducting a study. Nurses in practice collaborate with scientists in nursing and other disciplines to conduct clinical research that addresses practice problems encountered in the care of patients. Findings from such studies are then combined with findings from existing scientific knowledge to develop and implement these practices. If there is insufficient research to guide practice and conducting a study is not feasible, other types of evidence (e.g., case reports, expert opinion, scientific principles, or theory) are used or combined with available research evidence to guide practice. Priority is given to projects in which a high proportion of practice is guided by research evidence. Practice guidelines usually reflect research and nonresearch evidence and therefore are called EBP guidelines.

IMPLEMENTING EVIDENCE-BASED PRACTICE

The Iowa Model of Evidence-Based Practice to Promote Quality Care (see Figure 19.1) in conjunction with Rogers' diffusion of innovation model (Rogers, 2003; Titler & Everett, 2001) provide guiding steps in actualizing EBP. A team approach is recommended, with one person in the group providing the leadership for the project (Titler, 2002, in press).

Selecting a Topic

Ideas for EBP come from several sources categorized as problem- and knowledge-focused triggers. *Problem-focused triggers* are those identified by staff through quality improvement, risk surveillance, benchmarking data, financial data, or recurrent clinical problems. An example of a problem-focused trigger is increased incidence of deep venous thrombosis in postoperative patients. *Knowledge-focused triggers* are ideas generated when staff read research, listen to scientific papers at research conferences, or encounter EBP guidelines published by federal agencies or specialty organizations. Examples initiated from knowledge-focused triggers include pain management, prevention of skin breakdown, and checking placement of nasogastric tubes in adults. Sometimes topics arise from a combination of problem- and knowledge-focused triggers such as managing hydration in long-term care. It is critical that the staff members who will implement the potential practice changes are involved in selecting the topic and view it as contributing significantly to the quality of care (Titler, in press).

Is the Topic a Priority for the Organization?

When selecting a topic, it is necessary to consider how it fits with organization, department, and unit priorities in order to garner support from organizational leaders and the necessary resources to complete successfully and sustain the practice improvement. Indicators of fit between clinical topic and organizational priorities can be gleaned from strategic plans, quality improvement program objectives, and trends in types of patient volumes in specified units. For example, implementing flexible visiting practices in the ICU may not be a priority if the philosophy and leadership for family-centered critical care practice is missing. If a particular topic is selected and it is not an organizational fit, other problem- or knowledge-focused triggers should be considered.

Forming a Team

The next step is forming a team that is responsible for developing, implementing, and evaluating EBP. The team or group may be an existing committee, such as the quality improvement committee, the practice council, or the research committee; or a task force may be appointed to address a specific practice issue and use research findings or other evidence to improve practice. Team composition is directed by the topic selected and includes interested stakeholders in the delivery of care. For example, a team working on evidence-based pain management is interdisciplinary and includes pharmacists, nurses, physicians, and psychologists. In contrast, a team working on the EBP of bathing might include a nurse expert in skin care (e.g., GNP), assistive nursing personnel, and staff nurses. In addition to forming a team, key stakeholders who can facilitate the EBP project or put up barriers against successful implementation are identified. A stakeholder is a key individual or group of individuals who will be directly or indirectly affected by implementation of the EBP. Some of these stakeholders are likely to be team members. Others may not be team members but are key individuals within the organization or unit and can adversely or positively influence adoption of the EBP. An example of a key stakeholder in an acute care setting is the director of nursing (formal/positional power) or a staff nurse who is seen as an informal leader by his or her peer group (informal power) (Titler, in press). Questions to consider in identification of key stakeholders include the following:

- How are decisions made in the practice areas where the EBP will be implemented?

- What types of system changes will be needed (e.g., electronic documentation systems)?

- Who is involved in decision making?

- Who is likely to lead and champion implementation of the EBP?

- Who can influence the decision to proceed with implementation of an EBP?

- What type of cooperation do you need from which stakeholders to be successful?

- Who is likely to facilitate sustainability of the change in practice?

- What system changes are necessary to sustain the change in practice?

An important early task for the EBP team is to formulate the EBP question. This helps set boundaries around the project and assists in retrieval of the evidence. A clearly defined question specifies the types of people/patients (e.g., adults older than 65 years of age with acute pain), interventions or exposures (e.g., pain assessment), outcomes (e.g., less pain intensity; early ambulation), and relevant study designs that are likely to provide reliable data to address the clinical question (e.g., descriptive designs; randomized controlled trials) (Alderson, Green, & Higgins, 2003).

Retrieval, Critique, and Synthesis of the Evidence

Retrieving the evidence includes clinical studies, meta-analyses, integrative literature reviews, synthesis reports, and EBP guidelines. As more evidence is available to guide practice, professional organizations and federal agencies are developing and making available EBP guidelines and synthesis reports (Titler, in press). It is important that these are accessed as part of the literature retrieval process. Information about locating the evidence is available from other sources (DiCenso, Ciliska, Cullum, & Guyatt, 2004; LoBiondo-Wood & Haber, in press; Sackett, Straus, Richardson, Rosenberg, & Haynes, 2000).

Critiquing the evidence encompasses critique of research, synthesis reports, and EBP guidelines. There is no consensus among professional organizations or across health care disciplines regarding the best system to use for denoting the type and quality of evidence, or the grading schemas to denote the strength of the body of evidence (West et al., 2002). In "grading the evidence" two important areas are essential to address: (1) the quality of the individual research, and (2) the strength of the body of evidence (West et al., 2002). The critique process is a shared responsibility, using the same methodology. It is helpful, however, to have one individual provide leadership for the critique of the evidence, and design strategies for completing critiques. A group approach is recommended because it distributes the workload, helps those responsible for implementing the changes to understand the scientific base for the change in practice, arms nurses with citations and research-based sound bites to use in effecting practice changes with peers and other disciplines, and provides novices an environment to learn critique and application of evidence.

Based on a critique and synthesis of the evidence, EBP recommendations are set forth. The type and strength of evidence used to support the practice needs to be clearly delineated. The following are examples of practice recommendation statements:

- Older people who have recurrent falls should be offered long-term exercise and balance training (Strength of recommendation = B) (American Geriatrics Society, British Geriatrics Society, American Academy of Orthopaedic Surgeons, & Panel on Falls Prevention, 2001).

- Apply dressings that maintain a moist wound environment. Examples of moist dressings include, but are not limited to, hydrogels, hydrocolloids, saline moistened gauze, transparent film dressings. The ulcer bed should be kept continuously moist (Evidence Grade = B) (Folkedahl, Frantz, & Goode, 2002).

Can the Evidence Be Applied to Practice?

After the evidence is critiqued and EBPs are set forth, the next step is to decide if findings are appropriate for use in practice (Eddy, 2005). Criteria to consider in making these decisions include the following:

- Relevance of evidence for practice, particularly research evidence

- Consistency in findings across studies and guidelines

- A significant number of studies or EBP guidelines with sample characteristics (e.g., age, gender, type of illness) similar to those to which the findings will be used

- Consistency among evidence from research and other nonresearch evidence

- Feasibility for use in practice

- The risk/benefit ratio (risk of harm; potential benefit for the patient)

Practice changes should be based on knowledge and evidence derived from several sources (e.g., several research studies) that demonstrate consistent findings. Synthesis of study findings and other evidence may result in supporting current practice, making minor practice modifications, undertaking major practice changes, or developing a new area of practice.

Piloting and Trying the Change in Practice

If there is sufficient research or other types of evidence, the adoption of the evidence in practice is first piloted (see Figure 19.1) and thus, necessitates writing an evidence-based standard (e.g., policy, procedure, guideline) specific to the health care setting, using the grading schema that has been agreed upon (Haber et al., 1994). This is necessary so that individuals in the setting know (1) that the practices are based on evidence and (2) the type of evidence (e.g., randomized clinical trial, expert opinion) used in developing the evidence-based (EB) standard. Several different formats can be used to document the evidence base of the standard; use a consistent approach to writing EBP standards and referencing the research and related literature.

Clinicians (e.g., nurses, physicians, pharmacists) who adopt EBP are influenced by the perceived participation they have had in developing and reviewing the EBP standard (Baker & Feder, 1997; Bauchner & Simpson, 1998; Bero et al., 1998; Shortell et al., 1995; Soumerai et al., 1998; Timmermans & Mauck, 2005; Titler, 2004). Therefore, it is imperative that key stakeholders have an opportunity to review the written EBP standard and provide feedback. Focus groups are a useful way to provide discussion about the EB standard and to identify key areas that may be potentially troublesome during the implementation phase.

Other components of the pilot include collecting, prior to implementation, selected process and outcome measures to determine the effectiveness of the change in practice (see section on Evaluation), implementing the changes (see next section *Implementing EBP Changes*) in one or two units or for a circumscribed period of time (trying/piloting the change in practice), collecting follow-up process and outcome indicators, and modifying the organizational evidence-based policy, procedure, and standard as necessary.

Implementing the EBP Changes

Implementing EB changes in practice goes beyond writing a policy or procedure that is evidence-based; it requires interaction among direct care providers to champion and foster evidence adoption, leadership support, and system changes. Discussed in the following sections are strategies for implementation, organized by Rogers' seminal work on diffusion of innovations (Rogers, 2003). These strategies are useful for the pilot and in instituting the changes in practice in other areas of the clinical agency. Adoption of EBP is influenced by the nature of the clinical topic and the manner in which it is communicated (disseminated) to members (nurses) of a social system (organization, nursing profession) (Rogers, 1995; Titler & Everett, 2001) (see Figure 19.2).

Nature of the EBP Topic

The strength of the evidence alone does not guarantee that the EBP will be adopted (Grimshaw et al., 2004). Implementation processes that encourage practitioner adaptation or reinvention of EBP guidelines for use in their local agency increase adherence to the guideline (Bero et al., 1998; Berwick, 2003; Titler & Everett, 2001). To move evidence "from the book to the bedside," information from EBP must have perceived benefits for patients, nurses, physicians, and administrators; be "reinvented" and integrated into daily patient care processes; impart evidence in a readily available format; and make EB practices observable for practitioners (Berwick, 2003; Rogers, 2003). One way to impart the EBP actions is use of practice prompts, decision support systems, and quick reference guides. An example of a quick reference guide is shown in Figure 19.3.

Methods of Communication

Methods of communicating the EBP to those delivering care affects adoption of the practice (Carroll et al., 1997; Funk, Tornquist, & Champagne, 1995; Rogers, 2003; Wells & Baggs, 1994). Education of staff, use of opinion leaders, change champions, core groups, and consultation by experts in the content area are essential components of the implementation process. *Continuing education* alone does little to change practice behavior (Thomson O'Brien, Freemantle et al., 2004). Interactive and didactic

304

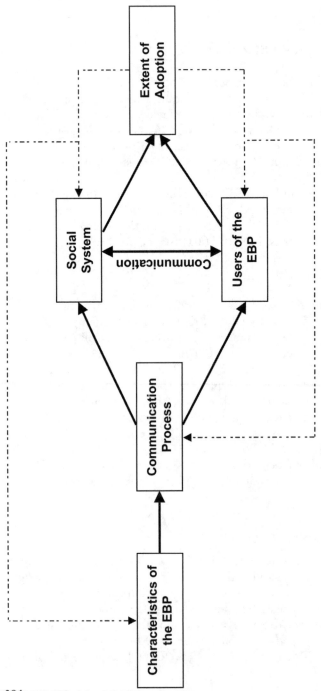

FIGURE 19.2   Implementation model.

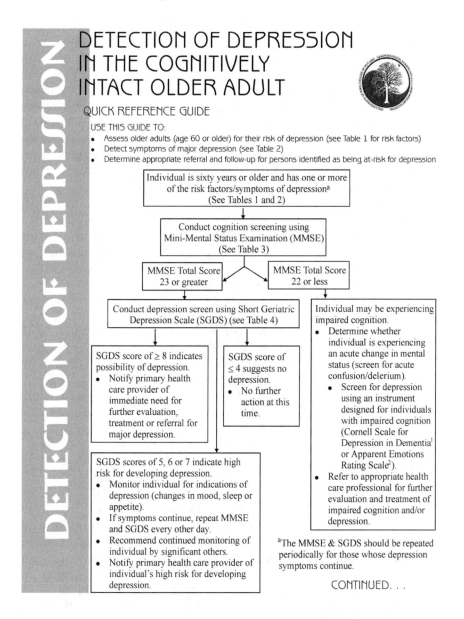

FIGURE 19.3   Quick reference guide: Detection of depression in the cognitively intact older adult.

From "Detection of Depression in the Cognitively Intact Older Adult," by M. Piven. 2001.

education, used in combination with other practice-reinforcing strategies, have more positive effects than education alone (Bero et al., 1998; Schneider & Eisenberg, 1998; Thomson O'Brien, Freemantle et al., 2004). It is important that staff know the scientific basis for the changes in practice as well as the improvements in quality of care that are anticipated by the change. Disseminating this information to staff needs to be done creatively, using various educational strategies. A staff in-service may not be the most effective method and it may not reach the majority of the staff. Although it is unrealistic for all staff to have participated in the critique process or to have read all studies used to develop the EBP, it is important that they know evidence-based myths and realities of the practice. Education of staff also must include ensuring that they are competent in the skills necessary to carry out the new practice. For example, if a pain assessment tool is being implemented to assess pain, it is essential that caregivers have the knowledge and skill to use the tool in their practice setting.

One method of communicating information to staff is through use of colorful posters that identify myths and realities or describe the essence of the change in practice (Titler et al., 2001). Visibly identifying those who have learned the information and are using the EBP (e.g., with buttons, ribbons, pins) stimulates interest in others who may not have internalized the change. As a result, the "new" learner may begin asking questions about the practice and be more open to learning. Other educational strategies such as train-the-trainer programs, computer-assisted instruction, and competency testing are helpful in education of staff (Titler, in press).

Several studies have demonstrated that *opinion leaders* are effective in changing behaviors of health care practitioners (Berner et al., 2003; Bero et al., 1998; Cullen, in press; Locock, Dopson, Chambers, & Gabbay, 2001; Oxman, Thomson, Davis, & Haynes, 1995; Soumerai et al., 1998; Thomson O'Brien et al., 2002), especially in combination with (a) outreach or (b) performance feedback. Opinion leaders are from the local peer group, viewed as a respected source of influence, considered by associates as technically competent, and trusted to judge the fit between the EBP and the local situation (Oxman et al., 1995; Soumerai et al., 1998; Thomson O'Brien, Oxman et al., 2004). They use the EBP, influence peers, and alter group norms (Collins, Hawks, & Davis, 2000; Rogers, 2003). The key characteristic of an opinion leader is that he or she is trusted to evaluate new information in the context of group norms. To do this, an opinion leader must be considered by associates as technically competent and a full and dedicated member of the local group (Oxman et al., 1995; Rogers, 2003; Soumerai et al., 1998). Social interactions such as hallway chats, one-on-one discussions, and addressing questions are important yet often overlooked components of translation (Berwick, 2003; Rogers, 2003). Thus, having local opinion leaders (early adopters) discuss the EBP with members of their peer group is necessary to translate research into practice. For example, in changing assessment practices for return of GI motility following abdominal surgery, the staff nurse leader of the EBP project functioned as the opinion leader. She changed her own practice, worked one-on-one with other staff nurses to change their practices and understand the evidence base for the change, and discussed the changes with physician colleagues who questioned the change (Madsen et al., in review). If the EBP change that is being implemented is interdisciplinary in nature (e.g., pain management), it is recommended that an opinion leader be selected for each discipline (nursing, medicine, pharmacy).

Change champions are also helpful for implementing EBP changes in practice (Rogers, 2003; Shively et al., 1997; Titler, 2004; Titler & Mentes, 1999). They are practitioners within the local group setting (e.g., clinical; patient care unit) who are expert clinicians, passionate about the clinical topic, committed to improving quality of care, and have a positive working relationship with other health professionals (Harvey et al., 2002; Rogers, 2003; Titler, 1998; Titler & Mentes, 1999). They circulate information, encourage peers to align their practice with the best evidence, arrange demonstrations, and orient staff to the EBP (Shively et al., 1997; Titler, 2004). The change champion believes in an idea, will not take no for an answer, is undaunted by insults and rebuffs, and above all, persists (Greer, 1988). For potential research-based changes in practice to reach direct care, it is imperative that one or two change champions be identified for each patient care unit or service where the change is being made (Titler, 2003). Staff nurses are some of the best change champions for EBP.

Using a *core group* in conjunction with change champions is also helpful for implementing the practice change (Barnason, Merboth, Pozehl, & Tietjen, 1998; Schmidt, Alpen, & Rakel, 1996; Titler et al., 2001). A core group is a select group of practitioners with the mutual goal of disseminating information regarding a practice change and facilitating the change in practice by other staff in their unit or peer group. Success of the core group approach requires that core group members work well with the change champion and represent various shifts, days of the week, and tenure in the practice setting. Core group members become knowledgeable about the scientific basis for the practice, assist with disseminating the EB information to other staff, and reinforce the practice change on a daily basis. The change champion educates the core group members and assists them in changing their practices. In turn, each member of the core group takes the responsibility for effecting the change in two or three of their peers. Core group members provide positive feedback to their assigned staff who are changing their practices and encourage those who are reluctant to change to try the new practice. Core group members also are able to assist the change champion in identifying the best way to teach staff about the practice change and to solve proactively issues that arise (Schmidt et al., 1996; Titler et al., 2001). Using a core group approach in conjunction with a change champion results in a critical mass of practitioners promoting adoption of the EBP (Rogers, 2003).

Outreach and consultation by an expert promotes positive changes in practice behaviors of nurses and physicians (Hendryx et al., 1998; Thomson O'Brien et al., 2003b). *Outreach (academic detailing)* is an expert who meets one-on-one with practitioners in their setting to provide information about the EBP and feedback on provider performance (Davis. Thomson, Oxman, & Haynes, 1995; Hendryx et al., 1998; Hulscher et al., 1997; Oxman et al., 1995; Thomson O'Brien et al., 2003a, 2003b). This strategy alone or in combination with other strategies results in positive changes in health care practices (Davis et al., 1995; Hendryx et al., 1998; Jiang, Fieselmann, Hendryx, & Bock, 1997; Pippalla, Riley, & Chinburapa, 1995; Thomson O'Brien et al., 2003a, 2003b; White, 1999). Advanced practice nurses (APNs) can provide one-on-one consultation to staff regarding use of the EBP with specific patients, assist staff in troubleshooting issues in application of the practice, and provide feedback on provider performance regarding use of the EBPs. Studies have demonstrated that when advanced practice nurses are used as facilitators of change, adherence to the EBP is promoted (Bauchner & Simpson, 1998; Hendryx et al., 1998; Titler, 2003; Watson, 2004). In application of the Iowa model, we have found it very helpful to have the staff nurse champion or opinion leader (or both) paired with a clinical specialist or advanced practice nurse that can facilitate the work of getting the changes integrated into day-to-day care delivery.

Users of EBP

Members of a social system influence how quickly and widely EBPs are adopted (Rogers, 2003). Audit and feedback, performance gap assessment (PGA), and trying the EBP are strategies that have been tested (Berwick & Coltin, 1986; Lomas et al., 1991; Rogers, 2003; Thomson O'Brien et al., 2003a; Titler, 2003, 2004; Titler et al., 2001). PGA and audit and feedback have consistently shown a positive effect on changing practice behavior of providers (Berwick & Coltin, 1986; Lomas et al., 1991; McCartney,

Macdowall, & Thorogood, 1997; Thomson O'Brien et al., 2003a). Baseline practice performance informs members at the *beginning* of change about a practice performance and opportunities for improvement. Specific practice indicators selected for performance gap assessment are related to the practices that are the focus of EBP change, such as every-4-hour pain assessment for acute pain management.

Audit and feedback are ongoing, with auditing of performance indicators (e.g., every-4-hour pain assessment) throughout the implementation process and discussing the findings with practitioners *during* the practice change (Jamtvedt, Young, Kristoffersen, Thomson O'Brien, & Oxman, 2004; Titler, 2004). This strategy helps staff know and see how their efforts to improve care and patient outcomes are progressing throughout the implementation process. Audit and feedback should be done at regular intervals throughout the implementation process (e.g., every 4 to 6 weeks) (Jamtvedt et al., 2004; Thomson O'Brien et al., 2003a). Performance gap assessment and audit and feedback data can be provided in run charts, statistical process control charts, or bar graphs (Carey, 2002).

Characteristics of users, such as educational preparation, practice specialty, and views on innovativeness influence adoption of an innovation (Retchin, 1997; Rogers, 2003; Rutledge et al., 1996; Salem-Schatz, Gottlieb, Karp, & Feingold, 1997; Schneider & Eisenberg, 1998; Shively et al., 1997). Users of an innovation usually try it for a period of time before adopting it in their practice (Meyer & Goes, 1988; Rogers, 2003). When "trying" an EBP, that is, piloting the change, is incorporated as part of the implementation process, users have the opportunity to use it for a period of time, provide feedback to those in charge of implementation, and modify the practice if necessary. Piloting the EBP as part of implementation has a positive influence on the extent of adoption of the new practice (Rogers, 2003; Shively et al., 1997; Titler, 2003; Titler et al., 2001).

Social System

Clearly, organizational context matters when implementing EBP (Ciliska, Hayward, Dobbins, Brunton, & Underwood, 1999; Denis, Hebert, Langley, Lozeau, & Trottier, 2002; Fleuren, Wiefferink, & Paulussen, 2004; Fraser, 2004a, 2004b; IOM, 2001; Morin et al., 1999; Rogers, 2003; Thompson, 2001; Vaughn et al., 2002). For example, investigators have demonstrated the effectiveness of prompted voiding for urinary incontinence in nursing homes, but sustaining the intervention in day-to-day practice was limited when the responsibility of carrying out the intervention was shifted to nursing home staff (rather than to the investigative team) and required staffing levels in excess of those currently extant in a majority of nursing home settings (Engberg, Kincade, & Thompson, 2004).

Leadership support is critical for promoting the use of EBP (Antrobus & Kitson, 1999; Baggs & Mick, 2000; Berwick, 2003; Carr & Schott, 2002; Jadad & Haynes, 1998; Katz, 1999; Morin et al., 1999; Nagy, Lunby, McKinley, & Macfarlane, 2001; Omery & Williams, 1999; Retsas, 2000; Stetler, 2003), and is expressed verbally by providing necessary resources, materials, and time to fulfill assigned responsibilities (Omery & Williams, 1999; Rutledge & Donaldson, 1995). Additional organizational variables that influence adoption include (1) access to inventers/researchers, (2) authority to change practice, and (3) support from and collaboration with peers, other disciplines, and administrators to align practice with the evidence base (Bach, 1995; Barnason et al., 1998; Crane, 1995; Funk, Champagne, Tournquist, & Wiese, 1995; Funk, Tornquist, & Champagne, 1995; Leatt, Baker, Halverson, & Aird, 1997; Nutley & Davies, 2000; Rodgers, 1994; Shortell et al., 1995; Thomson O'Brien et al., 2002; Titler, 1998; Tranmer, Coulson, Holtom, Lively, & Maloney, 1998; Walshe & Rundall, 2001). As part of the work of implementing the change, it is important that the social system—unit, service line, or clinic—ensure that policies, procedures, standards, clinical pathways, and documentation systems support the use of the EBPs (Rutledge & Donaldson, 1995; Titler, 2004). Documentation forms or clinical information systems may need revision to support changes in practice; documentation systems that fail to readily support the new practice thwart change. For example, if staff members are expected to reassess and document pain intensity within 30 minutes following administration of an analgesic agent, then documentation forms must reflect this practice standard. It is the role of upper and middle level leadership to ensure that organizational documents and systems are flexible and supportive of the EBPs.

Evaluation

Evaluation is a critical component of EBP; it provides information to determine if the EBP should be retained, modified, or eliminated. A desired outcome achieved in a more controlled environment, when a researcher is implementing a study protocol with a homogeneous group of patients (conduct of research), may not result in the same outcome when the practice is implemented in the natural clinical setting, by several caregivers, to a more heterogeneous patient population. Steps of the evaluation process are summarized in Table 19.1.

Evaluation should include both process and outcome measures (Lepper & Titler, 1999; Rosswurm & Larrabee, 1999; Titler, in press). The process component focuses on use of the EBP by staff in care delivery. Evaluation of the process should also note (1) barriers that staff encounter in carrying out the practice (e.g., lack of information, skills, or necessary equipment); (2) differences in opinions among health care providers; and (3) difficulty in carrying out the steps of the practice as originally designed (e.g., shutting off tube feedings 1 hour before aspirating contents for checking placement of nasointestinal tubes). Process data can be collected from staff or patient self-report or both, medical record audits, or observation of clinical practice. Examples of process and outcome questions are shown in Table 19.2.

Outcome data are equally important to evaluation to assess whether the patient, staff, and expected fiscal outcomes are achieved. Outcome variables measured should be those that are projected to change as a

TABLE 19.1   Steps of the Evaluation Process

1. Identify process and outcome variables of interest.
   Example: Process variable—Patients > 65 years of age will have a Braden scale completed upon admission.
   Outcome variable—Presence/absence of nosocomial pressure ulcer; if present, determine stage as I, II, III, IV.
2. Determine methods and frequency of data collection.
   Example: Process variable—Chart audit of all patients > 65 years old, 1 day a month.
   Outcome variable—Patient assessment of all patients > 65 years old, 1 day a month.
3. Determine number of patient assessments and chart audits for baseline and follow-up.
4. Design data collection forms.
   Example: Chart audit abstraction form (process).
   Outcome variable—pressure ulcer assessment form.
5. Establish content validity of data collection forms.
6. Educate data collectors.
7. Assess interrater reliability of data collectors.
8. Collect data at specified intervals.
9. Provide on-sight feedback to staff regarding the progress in achieving the practice change.
10. Provide feedback of analyzed data to staff.
11. Use data to assist staff in modifying or integrating the EBP change.

TABLE 19.2 Examples of Evaluation Measures

EXAMPLE PROCESS QUESTIONS

NURSES' SELF-RATING	SD	D	NA/D	A	SA
1. I feel well prepared to use the Braden Scale with older patients.	1	2	3	4	5
2. Malnutrition increases patient risk for pressure ulcer development.	1	2	3	4	5

EXAMPLE OUTCOME QUESTION

PATIENT
1. On a scale of 0 (no pain) to 10 (worst possible pain), how much pain have you experienced over the past 24 hours?   _____ (pain intensity)

SD, strongly disagree; D, disagree; NA/D, neither agree nor disagree; A, agree; SA, strongly agree
From "Developing an Evidence-Based Practice" by M. Titler, in G. LoBiondo-Wood and J. Haber (Eds.), *Nursing Research* (5th ed.), 2005. Copyright 2005, Mosby-Year Book. Used with permission.

result of changing practice (Rosswurm & Larrabee, 1999; Soukup, 2000; Titler, in press). It is important that baseline data be used for a pre/post comparison (Cullen, in press; Titler et al., 2001). Outcomes should be measured before the change in practice is implemented, after implementation, and at least every 6 to 12 months thereafter. Findings must be provided to clinicians to reinforce the impact of the change in practice and to ensure that they are incorporated into quality improvement programs. Feedback to staff includes verbal or written appreciation for the work and visual demonstration of progress in implementation and improvement in patient outcomes. The key to effective evaluation is to ensure that the EB change in practice is warranted (e.g., that it will improve quality of care) and that the intervention does not bring harm to patients (Lepper & Titler, 1999). For example, when instituting a change in practice for assessing return of bowel motility following abdominal surgery in older adults, it was important to inform staff that using other markers for return of bowel motility, rather than bowel sound assessment, did not result in increased paralytic ileus or bowel obstruction (Madsen et al., in review).

Beyond the Pilot

Following the pilot (which necessitates use of the aforementioned implementation and evaluation strategies), it is important to determine if changes should be made in other patient care units, services, or clinics. This decision is based on the evaluation results of the pilot, the applicability to other patient populations and care, and the potential benefits for patient care. For example, removing auscultation as an indicator of return of GI motility in adults following abdominal surgery cannot be applied automatically to medical patients, because the evidence reviewed, implemented, and evaluated focused on postoperative abdominal surgery patients, not medical patients. If the evidence is applicable to other units or patient populations, instituting the EBPs in these other areas requires planning implementation and evaluation activities, based on the techniques and lessons learned during the pilot. Clarity in planning a widespread practice change is essential for implementation across a department or service. For example, plans for implementing our fall-prevention interventions across adult inpatient units after piloting the change required (1) educating staff on all units, (2) selecting and educating unit-based champions, (3) finalizing the EB policy and procedures with the professional practice committee, (4) modifying of electronic documentation system to reflect the standards, (5) collecting process and outcome data, (6) providing data feedback at regular intervals, and (7) assigning accountability for rounding in the units to address adherence to the evidence-based practices. This has resulted in reduction of falls, and is part of the ongoing quality improvement process.

NURSING ROLES IN EBP IMPLEMENTATION

Sample performance criteria for various nursing roles are shown in Table 19.3. Chief nurse executives and their leadership staff set the stage and culture for EBP in their settings by explicating role expectations regarding the knowledge, skills, and behaviors necessary to promote adoption of EBPs. Enactment of the CNE role includes providing resources for EBP, such as easy access to EBP Web sites, retaining personnel with expertise in EBP, supporting programs that develop a critical mass of staff nurses with expertise in EBP (e.g., Evidence-Based Practice Staff Nurse Internship Program) (Cullen & Titler, 2004), providing access to assistance with analysis of data and transforming data into information, and assuring staffing ratios that promote use of the EBP. Providing this leadership is a continuous process that involves the following (Titler, Cullen, & Ardery, 2002):

TABLE 19.3   Sample EBP Performance Criteria for Nursing Roles

Staff Nurse (RN)	Advanced Practice Nurse (APN)	Nurse Manager (NM)	Associate Director for Clinical Services	Chief Nurse Executive
• Questions current practices • Participates in implementing changes in practice based on evidence • Participates as a member of an EBP project team • Reads evidence related to one's practice • Participates in QI initiatives • Suggests resolutions for clinical issues based on evidence	• Serves as coach and mentor in EBP • Facilitates locating evidence • Synthesizes evidence for practice • Uses evidence to write/modify practice standards • Role-models use of evidence in practice • Facilitates system changes to support use of EBP	• Creates a microsystem that fosters critical thinking • Challenges staff to seek out evidence to resolve clinical issues and improve care • Role-models EBP • Uses evidence to guide operations and management decisions • Uses performance criteria about EBP in evaluation of staff	• Hires and retains NMs and APNs with knowledge and skills in EBP • Provides learning environment for EBP • Uses evidence in leadership decisions • Sets strategic directions for EBP • Provides resources for EBP • Integrates EBP processes into division/service line governance	• Ensures that governance reflects EBP if initiated in the councils and committees • Assigns accountability for EBP • Ensures explicit articulation of organizational and department commitment to EBP • Modifies mission and vision to include EBP language • Provides resources to support EBP by direct-care providers • Articulates value of EBP to CEO and governing board • Role-models EBP in administrative decision making

- Incorporating EBP terminology into the mission, vision, strategic plan, and philosophy of care delivery;

- Establishing explicit performance expectations about EBP for staff at all levels of the organization;

- Integrating the work of EBP into the governance structure of nursing departments and the health care system;

- Recognizing and rewarding EBP behaviors.

Performance expectations of nurses in advanced practice roles (e.g., APN, GNP) include leading a team, finding the evidence, and synthesizing evidence for practice. Advanced practice nurses assist staff with focusing their clinical question about improving practice, finding and evaluating the research evidence, and maneuvering through governance structures to implement and sustain the changes in practice. Nurses in advanced practice roles (e.g. GNPs, APNs) are critical to helping staff retrieve and critique the studies and other evidence on the selected topic. Although staff nurses are often willing to participate, nurses in advanced practice roles provide significant leadership in the process by facilitating synthesis of the research and other evidence, critically analyzing what practices should be changed, assisting staff in communicating these changes to their peers, and role modeling changes in practice (Titler, in press).

Nurse managers set the tone, value, and work culture for the microsystems they lead. The role of the nurse manager is critical in making EBP changes a reality for staff providing direct care. Performance expectations include creating a culture that fosters interdisciplinary quality improvement based on evidence. Nurse managers must expect that staff will participate in EBP activities, role model the change in their practice, and provide written and verbal support for the practice change. When selecting a potential topic, it is important that the nurse manager values the idea and supports the potential changes. Nurse managers also foster EBP in their units by allocation of resources, which is an important element for staff nurse enactment of EBP. Staff migrate to microsystems that foster professional growth, professional nursing practice, data-based decision making, and innovative practices, which are all characteristics of cultures that promote adoption of EBP (Titler, in press).

Associate directors of nursing who hire, retain, and value via performance appraisals nurse managers and advanced practice nurses skilled in EBP are more likely to observe development of clinical innovations, and adoption of EBPs in the multiple units and sites of care delivery for which they are responsible. They must expect that their direct reports will foster EBP in their roles and reward these behaviors through performance appraisals and other forms of recognition (Titler, in press).

Staff nurses are essential to improving care delivery through use of evidence, and they serve key roles in influencing their peers in implementation of EBP standards. The role of staff nurses in EBP includes challenging the status quo of care delivery, asking clinical questions, bringing forward problem- and knowledge-focused triggers that might be addressed through the use of evidence, serving as change champions, and learning the evidence-based knowledge and skills to carry out EBP. Additionally, staff nurses should keep abreast of new knowledge generated through research and think critically about application of this evidence in practice (Cullen & Titler, 2004; Titler, in press).

The role of nursing assistants and assistive personnel is less well developed and little attention has been given to engaging nursing assistants in EBP work (Frantz, Xakellis, Harvey, & Lewis, 2003; Jones et al., 2004; Watson, 2004). To date, role expectations of nursing assistants for EBP are not available nor do EBP experts agree on their role. It is imperative, however, that nursing assistants have basic knowledge and skills to carry out EBP and that leadership staff work with them to clarify their role. For example, nursing assistants may do initial screening for pain assessment and work with licensed personnel to develop an effective, evidence-based plan of care.

Educators in clinical practice are important resources for teaching components of the EBP process, and for the evidence base of specific clinical topics. In addition, staff educators should think critically about the content they teach in orientation and staff education programs to determine if it is evidence-based. They should also be using evidence-based educational strategies.

CONCLUSIONS

Making an EB change in practice involves a series of steps and a process that is often nonlinear. Implementing change will take several weeks to months, depending on the nature of the practice change. It is important that senior leadership and those leading the project are aware of change as a process and continue to encourage and teach peers about the change in practice. The new practice must be continually reinforced and sustained or the practice change will be intermittent and soon fade, allowing more traditional methods of care to return (Titler, in press). We must also communicate and integrate the expectation that it is the professional responsibility of every nurse to read and use research in their practice;

redesign health care work to have evidence readily available for direct care providers; and provide human and monetary resources that support EBP. Given the limited number of resources available, it seems likely that decision makers will need to prioritize which EBP guidelines to implement, based on considerations of local burden of disease, availability of effective and efficient health care interventions and local evidence of suboptimal performance (Grimshaw et al., 2004). As federal agencies such as CMS start expecting and reimbursing for care based on evidence, EBP will no longer be an option but an expectation.

REFERENCES

Alderson, P., Green, S., & Higgins, J. P. T. (2003). *Cochrane reviewers' handbook* 4.2.1. Retrieved March 30, 2004, from http://www.cochrane.org/resources/handbook/handbook.pdf

American Geriatrics Society, British Geriatrics Society, American Academy of Orthopaedic Surgeons, and Panel on Falls Prevention. (2001). Guideline for the prevention of falls in older persons. *Journal of the American Geriatrics Society, 49*(5), 664–672.

Antrobus, S., & Kitson, A. (1999). Nursing leadership: Influencing and shaping health policy and nursing practice. *Journal of Advanced Nursing, 29*(3), 746–753.

Atkins, D. M., Kamerow, D. M., & Eisenberg, J. M. M. (1998, March–April). Evidence-based medicine at the Agency for Health Care Policy and Research. *ACP Journal Club, 128,* A1214.

Bach, D. M. (Ed.). (1995). *Implementation of the Agency for Health Care Policy and Research postoperative pain management guideline* (Vol. 30). Philadelphia: Saunders.

Baggs, J. G., & Mick, D. J. (2000). Collaboration: A tool addressing ethical issues for elderly patients near the end of life in intensive care units. *Journal of Gerontological Nursing, 26*(9), 41–47.

Baker, R., & Feder, G. (1997). Clinical guidelines: Where next? *International Journal for Quality in Health Care, 9*(6), 399–404.

Barnason, S., Merboth, M., Pozehl, B., & Tietjen, M. J. (1998). Utilizing an outcomes approach to improve pain management by nurses: A pilot study. *Clinical Nurse Specialist, 12*(1), 28–36.

Bauchner, H., & Simpson, L. (1998). Specific issues related to developing, disseminating, and implementing pediatric practice guidelines for physicians, patients, families, and other stakeholders. *Health Services Research, 33,* 1161–1177.

Berg, A. O., Atkins, D., & Tierney, W. (1997, April). Clinical practice guidelines in practice and education. *Journal of General Internal Medicine, 12*(Suppl. 2), S25–S33.

Berner, E. S., Baker, C. S., Funkhouser, E., Heudebert, G. R., Allison, J. J., Fargason, C. A., et al. (2003). Do local opinion leaders augment hospital quality improvement efforts? A randomized trial to promote adherence to unstable angina guideline. *Medical Care, 41*(3), 420–431.

Bero, L. A., Grilli, R., Grimshaw, J. M., Harvey, E., Oxman, A. D., & Thomson, M. A. (1998). Closing the gap between research and practice: An overview of systematic reviews of interventions to promote the implementation of research findings. *British Medical Journal, 317,* 465–468.

Berwick, D. M. (2003). Disseminating innovations in health care. *Journal of the American Medical Association, 289*(15), 1969–1975.

Berwick, D. M., & Coltin, K. L. (1986). Feedback reduces test use in a health maintenance organization. *Journal of the American Medical Association, 255,* 1450–1454.

Bostrom, J., & Suter, W. (1993). Research utilization: Make the link to practice. *Journal of Nursing Staff Development, 9*(1), 28–34.

Carey, R. A. (2002). *Improving healthcare with control charts: Basic and advanced SPC methods and case studies.* Milwaukee, WI: American Society for Quality.

Carr, C. A., & Schott, A. (2002). Differences in evidence-based care in midwifery practice and education. *Journal of Nursing Scholarship, 34*(2), 153–158.

Carroll, D. L., Greenwood, R., Lynch, K. E., Sullivan, J. K., Ready, C. H., & Fitzmaurice, J. B. (1997). Barriers and facilitators to the utilization of nursing research. *Clinical Nurse Specialist, 11*(5), 207–212.

Ciliska, D., Hayward, S., Dobbins, M., Brunton, G., & Underwood, J. (1999). Transferring public-health nursing research to health-system planning: Assessing the relevance and accessibility of systematic reviews. *Canadian Journal of Nursing Research, 31*(1), 23–36.

Collins, B. A., Hawks, J. W., & Davis, R. L. (2000, July). From theory to practice: Identifying authentic opinion leaders to improve care. *Managed Care,* 56–62.

Crane, J. (1995). The future of research utilization. In M. G. Titler & C. J. Goode (Eds.), *The nursing clinics of North America* (Vol. 30, pp. 566–579). Philadelphia: Saunders.

Cronenwett, L. R. (1995). Effective methods for disseminating research findings to nurses in practice. In M. G. Titler & C. Goode (Eds.), *The nursing clinics of North America* (Vol. 30, pp. 429–438). Philadelphia: Saunders.

Cullen, L. (in press). Evidence-based practice: Strategies for nursing leaders. In D. Huber (Ed.), *Leadership and nursing care management* (3rd ed.). Philadelphia: Elsevier.

Cullen, L., & Titler, M. G. (2004). Promoting evidence-based practice: An internship for staff nurses. *Worldviews on Evidence-Based Practice, 1*(4), 215–223.

Davis, D. A., Thomson, M. A., Oxman, A. D., & Haynes, R. B. (1995). Changing physician performance: A systematic review of the effect of continuing medical education strategies. *Journal of the American Medical Association, 274*(9), 700–705.

Denis, J.-L., Hebert, Y., Langley, A., Lozeau, D., & Trottier, L.-H. (2002). Explaining diffusion patterns for complex health care innovations. *Health Care Management Review, 27*(3), 60–73.

DiCenso, A., Ciliska, D., Cullum, N., & Guyatt, G. (2004). *Evidence-based nursing: A guide to clinical practice.* St. Louis, MO: Mosby.

Dickersin, K., & Manheimer, E. (1998). The Cochrane collaboration: Evaluation of health care and services using systematic reviews of the results of randomized controlled trials. *Clinical Obstetrics and Gynecology, 41*(2), 315–331.

Doebbeling, B. N., Vaughn, T. E., Woolson, R. F., Peloso, P. M., Ward, M. M., Letuchy, E., et al. (2002). Benchmarking Veterans Affairs medical centers in the delivery of preventive health services: Comparison of methods. *Medical Care, 40*(6), 540–554.

Eddy, D. (2005). Evidence-based medicine: A unified approach. *Health Affairs, 24*(1), 9–17.

Engberg, S., Kincade, J., & Thompson, D. (2004). Future directions for incontinence research with frail elders. *Nursing Research, 53*(Suppl. 6), S22–S29.

Estabrooks, C. A., Winther, C., & Derksen, L. (2004). Mapping the field: A bibliometric analysis of the research utilization literature in nursing. *Nursing Research, 53*(5), 293–303.

Farquhar, C. M., Stryer, D., & Slutsky, J. (2002). Translating research into practice: The future ahead. *International Journal for Quality in Health Care, 14*(3), 233–249.

Fleuren, M., Wiefferink, K., & Paulussen, T. (2004). Determinants of innovation within health care organizations: Literature review and Delphi study. *International Journal for Quality in Health Care, 16*(2), 107–123.

Folkedahl, B., Frantz, R., & Goode, C. (2002). *Evidence-based protocol: Treatment of pressure ulcers.* (M. G. Titler, Series Ed.) Iowa City: Research Dissemination Core, Gerontological Nursing Interventions Research Center, University of Iowa College of Nursing (P30 NR03979; PI: T. Tripp-Reimer).

Frantz, R. A., Xakellis Jr, G. C., Harvey, P. C., & Lewis, A. R. (2003). Implementing an incontinence management protocol in long-term care: Clinical outcomes and costs. *Journal of Gerontological Nursing, 29*(8), 46–53.

Fraser, I. (2004a). Organizational research with impact: Working backwards. *Worldviews on Evidence-Based Nursing, 1*(S1), S52–S59.

Fraser, I. (2004b). Translation research: Where do we go from here? *Worldviews on Evidence-Based Nursing, 1*(S1), S78–S83.

Funk, S. G., Champagne, M. T., Tornquist, E. M., & Wiese, R. A. (1995). Administrators' views on barriers to research utilization. *Applied Nursing Research, 8*(1), 44–49.

Funk, S. G., Tornquist, E., M., & Champagne, M. T. (1995). Barriers and facilitators of research utilization: An integrative review. In M. Titler & C. Goode (Eds.), *The nursing clinics of North America* (Vol. 30, pp. 395–408). Philadelphia: Saunders.

Greer, A. L. (1988). The state of the art versus the state of the science. *International Journal of Technology Assessment in Health Care, Vol. 4,* 5–26.

Grimshaw, J. M., Thomas, R. E., MacLennan, G., Fraser, C., Ramsay, C. R., Vale, L., et al. (2004). Effectiveness and efficiency of guide dissemination and implementation strategies. *Health Technology Assessment, 8*(6), i–xi, 1–72.

Haber, J., Feldman, H. R., Penney, N., Carter, E., Bidwell-Cerone, S., & Hott, J. R. (1994). Shaping nursing practice through research-based protocols. *Journal of the New York State Nurses Association, 25*(3), 4–12.

Harvey, G., Loftus-Hills, A., Rycroft-Malone, J., Titchen, A., Kitson, A., McCormack, B., et al. (2002). Getting evidence into practice: The role and function of facilitation. *Journal of Advanced Nursing, 37,* 577–588.

Health Grades Inc. (2004). *Health Grades quality study: Patient safety in American hospitals.* Health Grades, Inc.

Hendryx, M. S., Fieselmann, J. F., Bock, M. J., Wakefield, D. S., Helms, C. M., & Bentler, S. E. (1998). Outreach education to improve quality of rural ICU care. Results of a randomized trial. *American Journal of Respiratory and Critical Care Medicine, 158*(2), 418–423.

Herr, K., Titler, M. G., Schilling, M. L., Marsh, J. L., Xie, X., Ardery, G., et al. (2004). Evidence-based assessment of acute pain in older adults: Current nursing practices and perceived barriers. *Clinical Journal of Pain, 20*(5), 331–340.

Hulscher, M. E., van Drenth, B. B., van der Wouden, J. C., Mokkink, H. G., van Weel, C., & Grol, R. P. (1997). Changing preventive practice: A controlled trial on the effects of outreach visits to organise prevention of cardiovascular disease. *Quality in Health Care, 6*(1), 19–24.

Institute of Medicine. (2001). *Crossing the quality chasm: A new health system for the 21st century.* Washington, DC: National Academy Press.

Institute of Medicine. (2003). *Priority areas for national action: Transforming health care quality.* Washington, DC: National Academy Press.

Jadad, A. R., & Haynes, R. B. (1998). The Cochrane collaboration: Advances and challenges in improving evidence-based decision making. *Medical Decision Making, 18*(1), 2–9.

Jamtvedt, G., Young, J. M., Kristoffersen, D. T., Thomson O'Brien, M. A., & Oxman, A. D. (2004). Audit and feedback: Effects on professional practice and health care outcomes (Cochrane Review). *The Cochrane Library,* Issue 1, Chichester, UK: Wiley.

Jiang, H. J., Fieselmann, J. F., Hendryx, M. S., & Bock, M. J. (1997). Assessing the impact of patient characteristics and process performance on rural intensive care unit hospital mortality rates. *Critical Care Medicine, 25*(5), 773–778.

Jones, J. (2000). Performance improvement through clinical research utilization: The linkage model. *Journal of Nursing Care Quality, 15*(1), 49–54.

Jones, K. R., Fink, R., Vojir, C., Pepper, G., Hutt, E., Clark, L., et al. (2004). Translation research in long-term care: Improving pain management in nursing homes. *Worldviews on Evidence-Based Nursing, 1*(S1), S13–S20.

Kamerow, D. B. (1997). Before and after guidelines. *Journal of Family Practice, 44*(4), 344–346.

Katz, D. A. (1999). Barriers between guidelines and improved patient care: An analysis of AHCPR's unstable angina clinical practice guideline. *Health Services Research, 34*(1), 337–389.

Kirchhoff, K. T. (2004). State of the science of translational research: From demonstration projects to intervention testing. *Worldviews on Evidence-Based Nursing, 1*(S1), S6–S12.

Lavis, J. N., Robertson, D., Woodside, J. M., McLeod, C. B., Abelson, J., & Knowledge Transfer Study Group. (2003). How can research organizations more effectively transfer research knowledge to decision makers? *Milbank Quarterly, 81*(2), 221–248.

Leatt, P., Baker, G. R., Halverson, P. K., & Aird, C. (1997). Downsizing, reengin-
eering, and restructuring: Long-term implications for health care organizations.
Frontiers of Health Services Management, 13(6), 3–37.

Lepper, H. S., & Titler, M. G. (1999). Program evaluation. In M. A. Mateo &
K. T. Kirchhoff (Eds.), *Using and conducting nursing research in the clinical
setting* (2nd ed., pp. 90–104). Philadelphia: Saunders.

LoBiondo-Wood, G., & Haber, J. E. (Eds.). (in press). *Nursing research* (5th
ed.). St. Louis, MO: Mosby-Year Book.

Locock, L., Dopson, S., Chambers, D., & Gabbay, J. (2001). Understanding the
role of opinion leaders in improving clinical effectiveness. *Social Science and
Medicine, 53,* 745–757.

Lomas, J., Enkin, M., Anderson, G. M., Hannah, W. J., Vayda, E., & Singer, J.
(1991). Opinion leaders vs. audit and feedback to implement practice guidelines: Delivery after previous cesarean section. *Journal of the American Medical
Association, 265,* 2202–2207.

Lubarsky, D. A., Glass, P. S. A., Ginsberg, B., de L. Dear, G., Dentz, M. E., Gan,
T. J., et al. (1997). The successful implementation of pharmaceutical practice
guidelines: Analysis of associated outcomes and cost savings. *Anesthesiology,
86*(5), 1145–1160.

Madsen, D., Sebolt, T., Cullen, L., Folkedahl, B., Mueller, T., Richardson, C.,
et al. (in review). Why listen to bowel sounds? Report of an evidence-based
practice project. *American Journal of Nursing.*

McCartney, P., Macdowall, W., & Thorogood, M. (1997). Feedback to general
practitioners increased prescribing of aspiring to patients with ischaemic heart
disease. *British Medical Journal, 315,* 35–36.

McCormick, K. A., Cummings, M. A., & Kovner, C. (1997). The role of the
Agency for Health Care Policy and Research in improving outcomes of care.
Nursing Clinics of North America, 32(3), 521–542.

McCurren, C. (1995). Research utilization: Meeting the challenge. *Geriatric Nursing, 16*(5), 132–135.

Meyer, A. D., & Goes, J. B. (1988). Organizational assimilation of innovations: A
multilevel contextual analysis. *Academy of Management Journal, 31,* 897–923.

Morin, K. H., Bucher, L., Plowfield, L., Hayes, E., Mahoney, P., & Armiger, L.
(1999). Using research to establish protocols for practice: A statewide study
of acute care agencies. *Clinical Nurse Specialist, 13*(2), 77–84.

Nagy, S., Lumby, J., McKinley, S., & Macfarlane, C. (2001). Nurses' beliefs
about the conditions that hinder or support evidence-based nursing. *International Journal of Nursing Practice, 7*(5), 314–321.

Newman, K., Pyne, T., Leigh, S., Rounce, K., & Cowling, A. (2000). Personal
and organizational competencies requisite for the adoption and implementation
of evidence-based healthcare. *Health Services Management Research, 13,*
97–110.

Nutley, S., Davies, H., & Walter, I. (2003). *Evidence based policy and practice:
Cross sector lessons from the UK.* Keynote paper for the Social Policy Research
and Evaluation Conference, Wellington, NZ.

Nutley, S., & Davies, H. T. O. (2000, October–December). Making a reality of
evidence-based practice: Some lessons from the diffusion of innovations. *Public
Money and Management,* 35–42.

Omery, A., & Williams, R. P. (1999). An appraisal of research utilization across the United States. *Journal of Nursing Administration, 29*(12), 50–56.

Oxman, A. D., Thomson, M. A., Davis, D. A., & Haynes, R. B. (1995). No magic bullets: A systematic review of 102 trials of interventions to improve professional practice. *Canadian Medical Association Journal, 153*(10), 1423–1431.

Pettengill, M., Gilles, D., & Clar, C. (1994). Factors encouraging and discouraging the use of nursing research. *Image: Journal of Nursing Scholarship, 26*(2), 143–147.

Pippalla, R. S., Riley, D. A., & Chinburapa, V. (1995). Influencing the prescribing behavior of physicians: A metaevaluation. *Journal of Clinical Pharmacy and Therapeutics, 20,* 189–198.

Piven, M. (2001). *Detection of depression in the cognitively intact older adult with QRG and consumer insert.* Iowa City: Research Dissemination Core of the Gerontological Nursing Interventions Research Center, University of Iowa College of Nursing.

Retchin, S. M. (1997). The modification of physician practice patterns. *Clinical Performance and Quality Health Care, 5,* 202–207.

Retsas, A. (2000). Barriers to using research evidence in nursing practice. *Journal of Advanced Nursing, 31*(3), 599–606.

Rodgers, S. (1994). An exploratory study of research utilization by nurses in general medical and surgical wards. *Journal of Advanced Nursing, 20,* 904–911.

Rogers, E. M. (1995). *Diffusion of innovations.* New York: Free Press.

Rogers, E. M. (2003). *Diffusion of innovations* (5th ed.). New York: Free Press.

Rosswurm, M. A., & Larrabee, J. H. (1999). A model for change to evidence-based practice. *Image: Journal of Nursing Scholarship, 31*(4), 317–322.

Rutledge, D. N., & Donaldson, N. E. (1995). Building organizational capacity to engage in research utilization. *Journal of Nursing Administration, 25*(10), 12–16.

Rutledge, D. N., Greene, P., Mooney, K., Nail, L. M., & Ropka, M. (1996). Use of research-based practices by oncology staff nurses. *Oncology Nursing Forum, 23*(8), 1235–1244.

Rycroft-Malone, J., Kitson, A., Harvey, G., McCormack, B., Seers, K., Titchen, A., et al. (2002). Ingredients for change: Revisiting a conceptual framework. *Quality and Safety in Health Care, 11,* 174–180.

Sackett, D., Rosenberg, W., Gray, J., Haynes, R., & Richardson, W. (1996). Evidence based medicine: What it is and what it isn't. *British Medical Journal, 312,* 71–72.

Sackett, D. L., Straus, S. E., Richardson, W. S., Rosenberg, W., & Haynes, R. B. (2000). *Evidence-based medicine: How to practice and teach EBM.* London: Churchill Livingstone.

Salem-Schatz, S. R., Gottlieb, L. K., Karp, M. A., & Feingold, L. (1997). Attitudes about clinical practice guidelines in a mixed model HMO: The influence of physician and organizational characteristics. *HMO Practice, 11*(3), 111–117.

Schmidt, K. L., Alpen, M. A., & Rakel, B. A. (1996). Implementation of the Agency for Health Care Policy and Research Pain Guidelines. *AACN Clinical Issues, 7*(3), 425–435.

Schneider, E. C., & Eisenberg, J. M. (1998). Strategies and methods for aligning current and best medical practices: The role of information technologies. *Western Journal of Medicine, 168*(5), 311–318.

Shively, M., Riegel, B., Waterhouse, D., Burns, D., Templin, K., & Thomason, T. (1997). Testing a community level research utilization intervention. *Applied Nursing Research, 10*(3), 121–127.

Shortell, S. M., O'Brien, J. L., Carmen, J. M., et al. (1995). Assessing the impact of continuous quality improvement/total quality management: Concept versus implementation. *Health Services Research, 30,* 377–401.

Soukup, S. M. (2000). The center for advanced nursing practice evidence-based practice model. *Nursing Clinics of North America, 35*(2), 301–309.

Soumerai, S. B., McLaughlin, T. J., Gurwitz, J. H., Guadagnoli, E., Hauptman, P. J., Borbas, C., et al. (1998). Effect of local medical opinion leaders on quality of care for acute myocardial infarction: A randomized controlled trial. *Journal of the American Medical Association, 279*(17), 1358–1363.

Stetler, C. B. (2003). Role of the organization in translating research into evidence-based practice. *Outcomes Management, 7*(3), 97–105.

Thompson, C. J. (2001). The meaning of research utilization: A preliminary typology. *Critical Care Nursing Clinics of North America, 13*(4), 475–485.

Thomson O'Brien, M., Freemantle, N., Oxman, A., Wolf, F., Davis, D., & Herrin, J. (2004). Continuing education meetings and workshops. (Systematic review). *Cochrane Effective Practice and Organisation of Care Group Cochrane Database of Systematic Reviews, 4.*

Thomson O'Brien, M., Oxman, A., Haynes, R., Davis, D., Freemantle, N., & Harvey, E. (2004). Local opinion leaders: effects on professional practice and health care outcomes (Cochrane Review). *Cochrane Library(4).*

Thomson O'Brien, M. A., Oxman, A. D., Davis, D. A., Haynes, R. B., Freemantle, N., & Harvey, E. L. (2003a). Audit and feedback versus alternative strategies: effects on professional practice and health care outcomes. *Cochrane Library,* Issue 2. Oxford, UK: Update Software.

Thomson O'Brien, M. A., Oxman, A. D., Davis, D. A., Haynes, R. B., Freemantle, N., & Harvey, E. L. (2003b). Educational outreach visits: Effects on professional practice and health care outcomes. *Cochrane Library,* Issue 2.

Thomson O'Brien, M. A., Oxman, A. D., Haynes, R. B., Davis, D. A., Freemantle, N., & Harvey, E. L. (2002). Local opinion leaders: effects on professional practice and health care outcomes (Cochrane Review). *Cochrane Library* (2).

Timmermans, S., & Mauck, A. (2005). The promises and pitfalls of evidence-based medicine. *Health Affairs, 24*(1), 18–28.

Titler, M. (2003, July). *TRIP Intervention saves healthcare dollars and improves quality of care* (Abstract/Poster). Paper presented at session of Translating Research Into Practice: What's Working? What's Missing? What's Next? Sponsored by the Agency for Healthcare Research and Quality, Washington, DC.

Titler, M. G. (1998). Use of research in practice. In G. LoBiondo-Wood & J. Haber (Eds.), *Nursing research* (4th ed.). St. Louis, MO: Mosby-Year Book.

Titler, M. G. (2002). *Toolkit for promoting evidence-based practice.* Iowa City: Department of Nursing Services and Patient Care, University of Iowa Hospitals and Clinics.

Titler, M. G. (2004). Methods in translation science. *Worldviews on Evidence-Based Nursing, 1*, 38–48.

Titler, M. G. (in press). Developing an evidence-based practice. In G. LoBiondo-Wood & J. Haber (Eds.), *Nursing research* (5th ed.). St. Louis, MO: Mosby-Year Book.

Titler, M. G., Cullen, L., & Ardery, G. (2002). Evidence-based practice: An administrative perspective. *Reflections of Nursing Leadership, 28*(2), 26–27, 46.

Titler, M. G., & Everett, L. Q. (2001). Translating research into practice: Considerations for critical care investigators. *Critical Care Nursing Clinics of North America, 13*(4), 587–604.

Titler, M. G., Herr, K., Schilling, M. L., Marsh, J. L., Xie, X., Ardery, G., et al. (2003). Acute pain treatment for older adults hospitalized with hip fracture: Current nursing practices and perceived barriers. *Applied Nursing Research, 16*(4), 211–227.

Titler, M. G., Hill, J., & Matthews, G. (1999). *Development and validation of an instrument to measure barriers to research utilization.* Paper presented at the 16th Annual AHSR Conference. Research to Action: The Role of Health Services Research, Chicago, IL.

Titler, M. G., Kleiber, C., Steelman, V. J., Rakel, B. A., Budreau, G., Buckwalter, K. C., et al. (2001). The Iowa model of evidence-based practice to promote quality care. *Critical Care Nursing Clinics of North America, 13*(4), 497–509.

Titler, M. G., & Mentes, J. C. (1999). Research utilization in gerontological nursing practice. *Journal of Gerontological Nursing, 25*(6), 6–9.

Tranmer, J. E., Coulson, K., Holtom, D., Lively, T., & Maloney, R. (1998). The emergence of a culture that promotes evidence based clinical decision making within an acute care setting. *Canadian Journal of Nursing Administration, 11*(2), 36–58.

Vaughn, T. E., McCoy, K. D., Bootsmiller, B. J., Woolson, R. F., Sorofman, B., Tripp-Reimer, T., et al. (2002). Organizational predictors of adherence to ambulatory care screening guidelines. *Medical Care, 40*(12), 1172–1185.

Walshe, K., & Rundall, T. G. (2001). Evidence-based management: From theory to practice in health care. *Milbank Quarterly, 79*(3), 429–457.

Watson, N. M. (2004). Advancing quality of urinary incontinence evaluation and treatment in nursing homes through translation research. *Worldviews on Evidence-Based Nursing, 1*(S2), S21–S25.

Wells, N., & Baggs, J. G. (1994). A survey of practicing nurses' research interests and activities. *Clinical Nurse Specialist, 8*, 145–151.

West, S., King, V., Carey, T. S., Lohr, K. N., McKoy, N., Sutton, S. F., et al. (2002). *Systems to rate the strength of scientific evidence.* Evidence Report/Technology Assessment No. 47 (Prepared by the Research Triangle Institute-University of North Carolina Evidence-based Practice Center under Contract No. 290-97-0011). AHRQ Publication No. 02-E016. Rockville, MD: Agency for Healthcare Research and Quality.

White, C. L. (1999). Changing pain management practice and impacting on patient outcomes. *Clinical Nurse Specialist, 13*(4), 166–172.

Chapter 20

Using Journal Clubs to Introduce Evidence-Based Practice

Ellen Fineout-Overholt

> The only person who is educated is the one who has learned how to learn—and change.
>
> —Carl Rogers

Journal clubs are a teaching/learning strategy to facilitate clinicians' and students' understanding of the EBP process and increase their use of best evidence for clinical decision making. Journal clubs have been around for more than 100 years. William Osler is reported to have started the formal tradition in 1875 at McGill University in Montreal, Canada (Forsen, Hartman, & Neely, 2003); however, health care professionals have shared ideas about how to provide care to their patients for centuries.

What is it about a journal club that makes it worth trying? Ebbert, Montori, and Schultz (2001) conducted a systematic review of evidence about the effectiveness of journal clubs with postgraduate physicians, using Cochrane Collaboration methodology for their study. They found seven studies that met their rigorous inclusion criteria: one randomized controlled trial, three cohort studies, one pre/post study, and two cross-sectional studies. They concluded that how a journal club is conducted is essential to its success. Using a structure and assessment tools that enhance participants' satisfaction with the process and outcome is important (Berstein, Hollander, & Barlas, 1996). Ebbert and colleagues further concluded that conducting journal clubs may improve the use of evidence in clinical practice, but that more research is necessary to establish this notion. There is little research on the effectiveness of journal clubs in nursing. Nevertheless, journal clubs can be used successfully to introduce health care providers to the concepts and principles of EBP. This chapter focuses on the purposes and proposed benefits of a journal club, infrastructure essentials for conducting a journal club, methods for conducting a journal club, and evaluation of outcomes associated with the effectiveness of a journal club.

OVERALL PURPOSES AND PROPOSED BENEFITS OF A JOURNAL CLUB

The primary purpose of a journal club is to assist clinicians who want to improve the application of research into their practices. Journal clubs are perfect forums in which novices and experts in clinical practice can strategize to overcome challenges they encounter as they investigate evidence to answer their clinical questions and begin to implement EBP. There is a role for every level of practitioner who chooses to participate in a journal club, for example, facilitator/discussion leader, planner, and learner. Using a guided approach to evidence, facilitators of journal clubs provide opportunities for dialogue around clinical issues and the scientific evidence that addresses them, and in doing so, practitioners' knowledge bases about care options can be built. In a journal club, health care providers also can gain skills in asking clinical questions, finding relevant evidence, critical appraisal of scientific evidence, and outcomes and recommendations from evidence.

Other specific purposes of a journal club include introducing students to health care professions, preparing for licensure or credentialing exams, debating clinical issues, and acting as a catalyst for cultural and educational change (Sierpina, 1999). Journal clubs also can serve as a launching pad for research or quality improvement ideas. A journal club can provide opportunities for participants to hone many skills, including those needed for implementing EBP, as well as interpersonal interaction and presentation skills. In addition, journal clubs can add to the critically appraised topic (CAT) database for an institution. (The following Web sites provide more information about CATs: http://www.cebm.net/cats.asp and http://

www.bii.a-star.edu.sg/docs/mig/CAT.pdf) Applying for continuing education credits for those who actively participate in a journal club can be an added bonus, as can the social networking afforded by the club (Ebbert et al., 2001).

CHAMPIONS, MOTIVATED LEARNERS, AND COMMITTED FACILITATORS/MENTORS

Part of the infrastructure necessary for successful EBP initiatives is champions at multiple levels: administrators, educators, and learners (Fineout-Overholt, Cox, Robbins, & Gray, 2005). Champions are those participants, facilitators, and supporters who believe in EBP and in the purposes of journal clubs and can communicate the worth of EBP and journal clubs to the group. They provide the energy, time, money, and other resources necessary to make the journal club happen. Administrative champions are important as supporters with access to resources. Educator champions support the journal club facilitators and reinforce the knowledge and skills gained in the journal club through other learning opportunities (Edwards, Woolf, & Hetzler, 2002). In addition, some educator champions may be mentors to journal club facilitators, coaching them through the journal club process. Learner champions provide the contagion for the rest of the club; they set the tone through their enthusiasm and motivation (Goodfellow, 2004). For journal clubs to be successful, learners must be motivated.

Champions can occur serendipitously; however, most often they are cultivated. For example, I have found that champions can arise through discussing EBP with colleagues, fostering opportunities to experience successful EBP initiatives for learners, or demonstrating successful initiatives for administrators.

CONSIDERATIONS FOR THE *BEST* JOURNAL CLUB

There are several points that need to be considered and addressed for journal clubs to be successful. When beginning a journal club, a clearly articulated purpose is critical. Knowing what the facilitator expects to accomplish through the journal club can help potential participants determine the investment they want to make in the process. Facilitators need to consider the given goals of the journal club and determine beforehand who the participants will be; for example, will membership be interdisciplinary, multidisciplinary, nursing only, medicine only, or include laypersons. The specific purpose of the club will drive these types of decisions. Knowing when the club is going to meet and any predetermined format will assist participants to accomplish the goals they set for themselves. A facilitator who can determine which persons have demonstrated interest in learning or teaching the EBP process can provide opportunities for them to fulfill those roles in the journal club. When facilitators are considering which participants should attend the journal club, they must remember that the most important characteristic of a participant is a hearty desire to learn and a willingness to work.

Committed leadership is essential to the *best* journal club. Without committed facilitators, the journal club can become an academic exercise. Mentors can be facilitators of the journal club or they can be seasoned EBP experts who can provide journal club facilitators with experiential wisdom on how to conduct, troubleshoot, and maintain a journal club. There may be many types of facilitators, including educators, researchers, performance improvement coordinators, or clinician experts. The purpose of the journal club will drive which kind of facilitator would be the best to address the defined issues. A group of facilitators may guide the journal club and rotate in leadership according to the expertise they can provide to address a given topic or series. Although the journal club is conducted by the participants, an educator-mentor who is knowledgeable in EBP can validate the journal club's importance. The facilitator can mentor the group and move the group forward in the EBP process. The role of the mentor/facilitator cannot be overstated.

The facilitator can provide guidance for the journal club participants and make the club clinically meaningful for learners. In addition, the facilitator can provide an overall purpose for the club that meets a greater need, such as preparing participants for upcoming exams, by focusing on the latest and best evidence for a clinical problem. In successful journal clubs, participating practitioners along with the facilitator exhibit a commitment to excellent patient care, excellent clinical skills, excellent clinical judgment, and diligence.

Another marker for success is the involvement of medical or reference librarians who are experts at retrieving evidence to answer questions. The perspective offered by these seasoned data gatherers can lead to healthy discussions about the benefit of evidence and the recommendations that can be made from the research.

Another consideration is the meeting time for a journal club. Participants' schedules must drive the meeting time frame. Some participants want to attend lunch meetings, whereas others prefer early evening meetings. Fineout-Overholt and others (2005) further indicated that, "Whatever the time, food and camaraderie are great incentives to increase attendance" (p. 428) and Phillips and Glasziou (2004) stated that a sense of humor is a definite asset to a successful journal club and to the challenges that are associated with attending or leading it.

Finally, when establishing a journal club, computer access and access to evidence databases cannot be ignored. Some *a priori* thinking by administrators and faculty who lead the journal club are required to ensure that these essential resources that are central to the EBP process are present. The final consideration mentioned here—time—is certainly not the least important. The time to conduct and to participate in the journal club must be contemplated. Administrators at different levels have the capacity for allocating time for the journal club, and participants must budget their time to attend the club and learn from this method. Attending to the aforementioned considerations before embarking on a journal club endeavor will increase the likelihood of success.

ESSENTIAL STEPS TO DEVELOPING A JOURNAL CLUB

To achieve success with a journal club, certain steps need to be taken. The first step toward success is to establish qualified, invested leadership for the journal club. This key activity ensures that those leading will exhibit commitment and thus be able to establish a club and maintain its momentum. The second step is that the facilitator must define goals and purposes for the group. A structured plan for where the club is going gives potential participants a clear picture of what the club is about and what to expect if they join. The third step is for learners/participants to identify themselves and become invested in the process. The fourth step is to demystify the purpose of the club and provide clear directions on where and when the club will meet.

There are other steps that one can take to ensure success when conducting a journal club:

- Make it mandatory.
- Recruit homogeneous learners.
- Have basic didactic exchange to even the playing field.
- Serve food.
- Start with basic, original single studies.
- Select relevant research.
- Don't be too ambitious.

When faculty or managers make the journal club mandatory, a facilitator can depend on attendance and a consistent approach to learning can be assured. The facilitator can build on prior meetings, and skills can be honed and polished. With inconsistent attendance, learners are usually at different levels of understanding and skill and it is difficult to build on prior knowledge and skill attainment. Having learners with common goals narrows the scope of the journal club and enables attendees to delve deeper into the evidence. Passion for the topic is also a great impetus for participants in the journal club. With a varied or heterogeneous learner group, interests are divided and less depth of study can be achieved. If there is a heterogeneous group that decides to convene a journal club, however, there are options and strategies that could be used, such as determining common issues of interest or rotating topics.

To enable all learners to begin at the same level of knowledge, the initial meeting needs to start with a basic educational exchange, for example, a short slide presentation and discussion on the steps of EBP and the process of the journal club, and an assessment to determine what is known and what needs to be known regarding the journal club topic. Inevitably, there will be learners for whom the initial meeting will be a review, but to many it will represent clarification or new material. After teaching about how to formulate a question and find the evidence to answer it, the next step in the EBP process, critical appraisal, is best begun with basic, original single studies; then the group can build up to the skills needed for critical appraisal of evidence syntheses. In addition, it is essential that the evidence selected for critical appraisal be relevant to a meaningful patient scenario. Patient scenarios that are only academic exercises are not the best choice for making the search and critical appraisal of evidence relevant. Being mindful not to be too ambitious in setting the goals for the journal club will facilitate goal accomplishment. Trying to accomplish more than is truly possible makes the journal club a pressured learning environment and stymies the opportunity to absorb EBP principles.

GENERAL FORMAT FOR JOURNAL CLUB

Consistent use of a structured instrument has been shown to be the best choice for participant satisfaction (Berstein et al., 1996). Box 20.1 contains a rapid critical appraisal format for randomized controlled trials. (Other instruments can be found online at http://www.phru.nhs.uk/casp/appraisa.htm and http://www.med.ualberta.ca/ebm/cpg.htm.) Role-modeling of the chosen problem-solving approach is helpful to participants,

Box 20.1
Rapid Critical Appraisal Check List
for a Randomized Clinical Trial (RCT)

Name of Study: _____   Date: _____

1. Are the study findings valid?

   A. Were the subjects randomly assigned to the experimental and control groups?

                          Yes   No   Unknown

   B. Were the follow-up assessments conducted long enough to fully study the effects of the intervention?

                          Yes   No   Unknown

   C. Did at least 80% of the subjects complete the study?

                          Yes   No   Unknown

   D. Was random assignment concealed from the individuals who were first enrolling subjects into the study?

                          Yes   No   Unknown

   E. Were the subjects analyzed in the group to which they were randomly assigned?

                          Yes   No   Unknown

   F. Was the control group appropriate?

                          Yes   No   Unknown

   G. Were the subjects and providers kept blind to study group?

                          Yes   No   Unknown

   H. Were the instruments used to measure the outcomes valid and reliable?

                          Yes   No   Unknown

   I. Were the subjects in each of the groups similar on demographic and baseline clinical variables?

                          Yes   No   Unknown

(continued)

Box 20.1 (continued)

---

2. What are the results of the study and are they important?

   A. How large is the intervention or treatment effect (NNT, NNH, effect size, level of significance)? _____

   B. How precise is the intervention or treatment confidence interval)? _____

3. Will the results help me in caring for my patients?

   A. Are the results applicable to my patients?

      Yes   No   Unknown

   B. Were all clinically important outcomes measured?

      Yes   No   Unknown

   C. What are the risks and benefits of the treatment? _____

   D. Is the treatment feasible in my clinical setting?

      Yes   No   Unknown

   E. What are my patient's/family's values and expectations for the outcome that is trying to be prevented and the treatment itself? _____

---

particularly when the evidence is ambiguous. Facilitators may need to foster learner feedback actively. Group leaders have the privilege of creating a culture that encourages continued insight into the EBP process and growth in EBP skills. Providing frequent, constructive feedback to learners is helpful in creating a positive, productive environment. Making the journal club culture one that emphasizes growth and accomplishment is essential to its success and to successful evidence-based practitioners. Fostering a spirit of clinical inquiry and comfort with uncertainty will promote a journal club culture of continuous learning and practice improvement. To achieve this, facilitators must communicate that there is no forbidden question and that the journal club is designed for evidence-users, not experts in research methodology.

CHOOSING A JOURNAL CLUB THAT'S RIGHT FOR YOU

Once a journal club has been planned, and considerations have been addressed, it is time to determine what type of journal club is needed or desired. The *topic-based* journal club provides an environment that is conducive to debate, as the goal is to determine the best intervention for a given clinical condition. These journal clubs do not necessarily encompass the entire EBP process and may focus only on the critical appraisal of evidence. How the evidence is found may not be a primary focus and thus the expectation of participants of this type of journal club may be that their skills in asking questions and finding evidence have already been honed. In a topic-based journal club, the facilitator may present the clinical scenario, the question, and the search strategy to find the evidence to address the question. In addition, critical appraisal of the evidence may also be presented, if the goal is to devise a plan for addressing the stated clinical issue. The final outcome of a topic-based journal club is to determine the evidence-based recommendations for a predefined clinical issue.

The *teaching-based* journal club focuses on a specific concept or strategy. For example, honing searching skills would be a good topic for a teaching-based journal club. The emphasis would be placed on skill building. Getting through an allotted amount of content is not the purpose of this type of journal club. The teaching-based journal club must be within a clinically meaningful context. Participants will find the skill-building sessions more valuable if they are able to immediately use the skills in their practice.

The third type of journal club is the *EBP-skills-focused* journal club. The purpose of this type of journal club is to move participants sequentially through each step of the EBP process. As with other journal clubs, beginning with a meaningful clinical scenario is essential. The focus of the first journal club meeting in this series could be to assist participants in formulating the clinical question derived from the scenario. The second session may focus on devising the search strategy based on the clinical question. The third session may involve the actual search and determination of relevant evidence and may need to be held in a computer lab. The fourth session may be critical appraisal of the relevant evidence. The final two sessions will be discussions about application of evidence and the evaluation of clinical outcomes. These are simply examples of how the journal club sessions and formats could be structured. Combinations of these formats may best meet the needs of the participants. It is important for the facilitator and the participants to determine in partnership the structure of the sessions for a journal club.

MEASURING THE EFFECTIVENESS OF A JOURNAL CLUB

Evaluation of a journal club is as essential as determining whether or not a medication had the expected effect; however, there is no one measure of success. It has been said that the "see one, do one, teach one" approach can assist facilitators in evaluation of skills; however, this still requires some decisions about mechanisms for evaluation. To build participants' presentation skills and also evaluate their EBP knowledge and skills, designating certain topics or skills for them to teach allows for direct observation evaluation. To further test knowledge retention, pre- and posttesting often work well. The best way to evaluate integration of EBP skills and knowledge is to observe the skills being used in a clinical setting and the application of the evidence to practice. Notwithstanding that all of these mechanisms for evaluation are somewhat challenging and require commitment from the facilitator, the data received about the measure of success the journal club afforded its participants is invaluable. More efforts need to be focused on research about the process and monitoring of journal club outcomes. Despite the need for further scientific evidence to support the effectiveness of journal clubs, this mechanism provides an opportunity for those who wish to learn and implement EBP to disseminate and gain knowledge.

REFERENCES

Berstein, J., Hollander, J., & Barlas, D. (1996). Enhancing the value of journal club: Use of a structured review instrument. *American Journal of Emergency Medicine, 14*(6), 561–563.

Ebbert, J., Montori, V., & Schultz, H. (2001). The journal club in postgraduate medical education: A systematic review. *Medical Teacher, 23*(5), 455–461.

Edwards, K., Woolf, P., & Hetzler, T. (2002). Pediatric residents as learners and teacher of evidence-based medicine. *Academic Medicine, 77*(7), 748.

Fineout-Overholt, E., Cox, J., Robbins, B., & Gray, Y. (2005). Teaching evidence-based practice. In B. M. Melnyk & E. Fineout-Overholt (Eds.), *Evidence-based practice in nursing and healthcare: A guide to best practice* (pp. 407–442). Philadelphia: Lippincott, Williams & Wilkins.

Forsen, J., Hartman, J., & Neely, J. (2003). Tutorials in clinical research, pt. 8: Creating a journal club. *Laryngoscope, 113*(3), 475–483.

Goodfellow, L. (2004). Can a journal club bridge the gap between research and practice? *Nursing Educator, 29*(3), 107–110.

Phillips, R., & Glasziou, P. (2004). What makes evidence-based journal clubs succeed? *ACP Journal Club, 140*(3), A11–A12.

Sierpina, V. (1999). The journal club: A forum for cultural change and the study of alternative and integrative medicine at a university health science center. *Integrative Medicine, 2*(1), 31–34.

Chapter 21

Traveling Posters: Communicating on the Frontlines

Priscilla Sandford Worral

> An idea that is developed and put into action is more important than an idea that exists only as an idea.
>
> —Buddha

Sackett (2000) identifies failure to gain grassroots commitment as one reason why randomized controlled trials "fail" frontline patient care. Experimental trials are characterized by the tight control over confounding variables necessary to demonstrate efficacy of an intervention as causing a specific outcome. Frontline patient care, however, is anything but controlled. Patients are more diverse than alike and are not always willing or able to follow the treatment regimen prescribed for them. Nursing staff differ in patient care experience, skill level, and educational background. How, then, are direct-care nurses supposed to base their practice decisions on evidence derived from studies that do not reflect what they see in everyday patient care, that they rarely read, and that they do not understand?

CLINICAL CONTEXT

Barriers and facilitators to use of research findings to make practice decisions have been the focus of a number of studies in recent years (Hutchinson, & Johnston, 2004; LaPierre, Ritchey, & Newhouse, 2004; McCaughan, Thompson, Cullum, Sheldon, & Thompson, 2002). Nurses cite lack of awareness of available research literature, lack of time to review the literature or implement an evidence-based change, lack of skill to critically review studies, lack of organizational support or authority to make practice changes, and lack of clinical credibility of study results as reasons for not using research as a basis for clinical decision making. Facilitators for using research findings have been identified to include organizational supports such as availability of time, access to expertise, and user-friendly presentation of research findings that are relevant for practice.

Hired by the chief nursing officer (CNO) to facilitate integration of research conduct and use into nursing practice, a doctorally prepared coordinator of nursing research faced the challenge of bringing EBP to the "coal-face" of frontline patient care. Many barriers to research use cited in the literature were present in the coordinator's own setting. At that time, more than 80% of registered nurses (RNs) providing direct patient care in the 325-bed urban academic medical center were graduates of diploma or associate degree programs with no formal research education. Confronted by the same problems of short staffing and inexperience faced by most hospitals during a time of nursing shortage, nurses at the bedside focused on making it through the shift. Few bedside nurses had even heard of the phrase "EBP."

Compared with staff nurses, a larger percentage of nurse managers had completed at least a baccalaureate degree in nursing. Almost all of these individuals, however, had taken a traditional research course directed more toward research conduct than research use. A majority of the nurse managers viewed research as uninteresting and unrelated to practice. As was the case with staff RNs, these managers had little understanding of EBP.

Organizational support has been a key facilitator to overcoming these barriers. Committed to creating a professional nursing environment, the CNO has led the development of a shared governance councilor structure in which RNs have authority for making decisions relevant to nursing care. To provide staff nurses the opportunity to participate in councilor work without leaving patient care units short of staff, the CNO has added 40 full-time equivalent positions to the number of staff nurses employed by the institution. Staff nurses who are council members are scheduled for one shift of professional practice time each month. Staff nurses who serve as council co-chairs are scheduled for one shift of professional practice time each week.

Included in the councilor structure is the Nursing Research Council (NRC), comprised primarily of staff nurses who have volunteered to represent their service lines. Two of these RNs serve as council co-chairs. The CNO supports a full-time salaried position for the doctorally prepared coordinator of nursing research who serves as coach to support NRC research and EBP activities. The CNO also supports a salary offset for a medical librarian to serve as liaison to the NRC. Ad hoc members of the NRC include the dean of the College of Nursing, a nurse member of the hospital Ethics Committee, and a master's-prepared nurse epidemiologist.

DISCIPLINED CLINICAL INQUIRY AS AN ORGANIZING FRAMEWORK

As described by Sanares and Heliker (2002), disciplined clinical inquiry (DCI) is a stakeholder-driven model based on the theoretical framework of critical social theory and employing a participatory action research design. Participatory action research is characterized by collaboration between stakeholders and researcher to solve a problem that has been identified by the stakeholders themselves. Consistent with this method, the purpose of the DCI model in nursing is to empower nurses to collaborate in identification and solution of problems affecting their practice (Sanares & Heliker).

Three empowering processes in the DCI model focus on language, leadership, and locus. The process of communication or language is to transform research terms into a format more consistent with EBP that is more meaningful to the direct care nurse. The leadership process is one of coaching and collaboration among clinicians, patients, educators, and researchers. Locus relates to the process of creating a professional culture and transformed environment of care in which decisions are made on the basis of best evidence, patient preferences and needs, and expert clinical judgment. Nursing judgments are themselves the outcomes of reflective thinking, knowledge synthesis, and systematic inquiry (Sanares & Heliker, 2002).

The use of DCI as an organizing framework for the hospital's NRC EBP activity was a natural fit because many of the components of DCI were already in place. Consistent with the organizational commitment to staff nurse authority for their practice, the NRC addresses those clinical issues identified by staff nurse representatives on the council or brought to them by other staff nurses or nursing councils. Because a majority of NRC representatives have little or no formal research education, the coordinator of nursing research initially led discussions of how to reframe clinical issues into questions that included population and intervention of interest, current practice comparison, and outcome(s) of interest. These questions, called PICO questions in the language of EBP (Sackett, Richardson, Rosenberg, & Haynes, 1998), were—and still are—used by the coordinator of nursing research to help NRC members search the literature for best evidence on which to base support of current practice or identify the need for practice change. Discussion of search results during NRC meetings includes use of reflective thinking, inquiry, and synthesis led by staff nurse co-chairs and coached by the coordinator of nursing research.

Within the NRC, members were primary stakeholders in making an EBP change and the coordinator of nursing research served as coach. Within the broader context of nursing services, the nurse, unit or council that first brought their clinical question to the NRC was the primary stakeholder in directly affecting any practice change; NRC members served as coaches for those staff they represented. Consequently, the NRC made a concerted effort to provide results of their evidence review in a practice-relevant format. Components of the results report included (1) a one-page summary that would provide primary points for use by busy nursing staff; (2) a report table detailing each study included in the review for use by those interested in more detail; and (3) a reference list of all articles. Evidence-review summary-page content is specified in Box 21.1. Details for each study included in the NRC evidence-review report table are depicted in Figure 21.1.

Box 21.1
Content Information Included in Evidence Review Summaries

- Specific statement of the issue identified
- Literature search procedure
- Synthesis of studies critically reviewed
- Recommendations for practice change OR statement of insufficient evidence

Authors (Year)	Primary Variables and Design	Study Sample/ Size	Major Findings	Strengths/ Weaknesses
	Research variables: *Design:*			*Strengths:* *Weaknesses:*

FIGURE 21.1   Study detail included in NRC evidence-review table.

TRAVELING POSTERS

In nursing, the "coal face" of patient care is wherever that care is delivered. As staff nurses themselves, NRC members were well aware that engaging their peers in discussion of evidence upon which to base practice change would gain little support unless those discussions were held on the unit. Additionally, structuring review of results as traditional in-service programs would have little effect on actual practice change if staff viewed themselves as passive recipients of information rather than active participants in dialogue about how evidence might be integrated appropriately into nursing care. Therefore, NRC members were interested in developing a mechanism not only for bringing results of evidence reviews directly to the nursing units, but also for allowing meaningful dialogue. Although NRC members were gaining confidence in their ability to critically review research articles with support from the coordinator of nursing research, they were unsure of their ability to coach their fellow staff nurses.

After discussion with their peers, NRC members decided to use posters in the unit nurses' lounge to display results of evidence reviews. Posters would include highlights of information included on the summary page. Accompanying handouts would include the table of individual study reviews and the list of references. NRC members introduced the posters at monthly unit staff meetings and engaged other staff members in dialogue on the poster display while waiting for shift report to start or during breaks. One poster was created for each evidence review completed and a schedule was developed for moving the poster from one unit to the next every 5 to 7 days. One NRC member with strong interest in the idea of traveling posters volunteered to oversee the process of moving the posters between units and reminding other members when units in their service line[1] were scheduled for the poster display.

---

[1] Service lines are comprised of one to seven inpatient units plus ambulatory care areas serving a common patient population, for example, the hematology/oncology service line, included an inpatient adult hematology/oncology unit, bone marrow transplant unit, apheresis care area, and regional oncology center.

EVALUATION AND PROCESS REFINEMENT

During the first year of traveling posters, feedback from unit staff indicated mixed success of the process. Although nurses on those units initiating the question or issue that had prompted NRC review demonstrated interest in findings, others varied in their level of interest. Because studies selected for review were those in which specific patient populations were sampled, findings and recommendations were not of equal practice relevance across all units in the hospital. Additionally, because not all nurses' lounges had adequate space to display the poster on a table or wall-mounted display board, the posters themselves did not always survive in one piece during the 5- to 7-day stay on a unit.

Based on their dialogue with fellow staff nurses, NRC members consistently found that although those nurses who had initiated a clinical question and request for NRC support were interested in results of the evidence review, most had little understanding of EBP. This lack of understanding was especially evident on those units and those shifts on which an NRC member was not included among the staff as well as on units from which no NRC request for support had been generated.

As a council, the NRC agreed that their first step in addressing these problems would be to create a poster on the basics of EBP. To engage nurses in active participation in learning about EBP, an NRC member volunteered to develop a brief cognitive test that nurses could complete after reading the poster and could deposit in a box set up next to the display. As an additional incentive, the NRC discussed applying for continuing-education credit for those nurses who correctly answered 80% of test questions. Poster content and NRC EBP cognitive test items are displayed in Figure 21.2 and Box 21.2, respectively.

To resolve the problem of where to display the poster so that it would remain intact and would not inconvenience staff by taking up space on tables or display boards intended for other purposes, the NRC agreed to request assistance from the Nursing Professional Development Council (NPDC). The NPDC had recently created the Wisdom Wagon, a stand-alone cart that could be wheeled from unit to unit to display information on such topics as new equipment, Joint Commission on Accreditation of Healthcare Organizations (JCAHO) requirements, and so forth, determined by that council to be of hospital-wide importance. The NPDC agreed to include the NRC EBP poster in their schedule for display on nursing units over a 1-month period.

CURRENT STATUS AND NEXT STEPS

In the 2 years since the NRC poster on EBP was displayed on nursing units, anecdotal reports of NRC members indicate that some success has

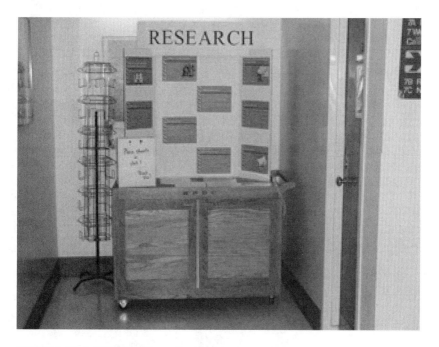

FIGURE 21.2 NRC EBP traveling poster.

been achieved in increasing nurses' awareness and understanding of EBP. As before, the greatest increase in nurse understanding has taken place on those units and shifts where NRC members are included among patient care staff. Among the 60 nurses who completed the test included with the poster, all achieved a score of 80% or higher, indicating that those nurses who did read the poster and complete the test were able to demonstrate adequate point-in-time understanding of the basics of EBP.

Celebration of the success of NRC efforts to bring EBP to the coalface of patient care might best be described as celebrating incremental changes. For example, during the first year of staff nurse participation on the NRC in 1996, only one clinical issue was brought to the council with a request for an evidence review. Over the next several years, the number of requests increased annually from one to two or perhaps three. Today, the council receives more than 10 requests per year that are appropriate for an evidence review. Examples of issues identified by staff nurses for evidence review are presented in Box 21.3. In an effort to improve timeliness of response to those requests, several NRC members have initiated evidence reviews independently, asking for assistance from the coordinator of nursing research to review their work. Only a few years

Box 21.2
NRC EBP Test Items

Name: _____ Unit: _____

RESEARCH-BASED PRACTICE QUESTIONS

1. Name one resource for finding research articles.

2. Who comprises the multidisciplinary team for changing practice?

3. Refer to the following scenario to answer the question:

   There is a question as to whether or not TEDS stockings provide the same level of DVT prophylaxis as sequential compression devices (SCDs). You found three articles on this topic.

   (a) The first article stated TEDS are as effective and less expensive, and is a meta-analysis of multiple controlled studies.

   (b) The second article stated SCDs are more effective and is a case report.

   The third article is an article on opinions of respected authorities and stated SCDs on patients decrease the prevalence of DVTs when compared with TEDs.

   Which change is practice would you recommend, the use of TEDs or the use of SCDs? (Remember that the level of evidence shows the strength of scientific merit.)

After answering the questions please return this sheet to the box on the Wisdom Wagon or your clinical educator's mailbox. Thank you!

Box 21.3
Staff Nurse Issues for NRC Evidence Review

- Relative effectiveness of sequential compression devices to decrease incidence of deep vein thrombosis in post-procedure adult inpatients

- Relative effectiveness of incentive spirometry to decrease post-procedure pulmonary complications in adult inpatients

- Effectiveness of salt pork for treatment of epistaxis in hospitalized children and adults

- Incidence of bacteriuria among children and adults with neurogenic bladders who are reusing clean straight catheters for intermittent catheterization versus sterile catheters for intermittent catheterization for bladder management

---

earlier, members had depended on the coordinator of nursing research to initiate these efforts.

The NRC currently is in the process of developing a user-friendly Web-based format for displaying results of evidence reviews on the institutional intranet council Web site. Members still intend to use the Wisdom Wagon for future display of results of evidence reviews, but have decided to include only those reviews with wide-scale practice relevance.

Use of traveling posters to bring EBP to the coal-face of patient care delivery has met with some success. Disciplined clinical inquiry has demonstrated effectiveness as a model for engaging NRC members in systematic and reflective inquiry guided by the coordinator of nursing research. As NRC members become more confident and competent in their ability to retrieve and apply evidence to guide practice change, disciplined clinical inquiry has the potential to demonstrate similar effectiveness on nursing units where engagement of staff nurses is guided by their NRC representative.

REFERENCES

Hutchinson, A. M., & Johnston, L. (2004). Bridging the divide: A survey of nurses' opinions regarding barriers to, and facilitators of, research utilization in the practice setting. *Journal of Clinical Nursing, 13,* 304–315.

LaPierre, E., Ritchey, K., & Newhouse, R. (2004). Barriers to research use in the PACU. *Journal of Perianesthesia Nursing, 19*(2), 78–83.

McCaughan, D., Thompson, C., Cullum, N., Sheldon, T., & Thompson, D. R. (2002). Acute care nurses' perceptions of barriers to using research information in clinical decision-making. *Journal of Advanced Nursing, 39*(1), 46–60.

Sackett, D. L. (2000). Why randomized controlled trials fail but needn't: Failure to gain "coal-face" commitment and to use the uncertainty principle. *Canadian Medical Association Journal, 162*(9), 1311–1314.

Sackett, D. L., Richardson, W. S., Rosenberg, W., & Haynes, R. B. (1998). *Evidence-based medicine: How to practice and teach EBM.* Edinburgh, Scotland: Churchill Livingston.

Sanares, D., & Heliker, D. (2002). Implementation of an evidence-based nursing practice model: Disciplined clinical inquiry. *Journal for Nurses in Staff Development, 18*(5), 233–238.

Glossary of Selected Terms in EBP*

Audit and Feedback

Audit and feedback is monitoring of critical indicators of practice (e.g., meperidine use) and providing the data/information back to those responsible for patient care (Davis, Thomson, Oxman, & Haynes, 1995; Oxman, Thomson, Davis, & Haynes, 1995; Schoenbaum et al., 1995). Audit and feedback is an ongoing process that is done periodically (e.g., every 3 months) during the implementation, evaluation, and sustainability phases of translating evidence into practice. Feedback reports can use data aggregated at different levels, such as the individual provider, patient care unit, service line, organization, or health system. It is helpful to provide data that compares indicators over time to demonstrate improvements (or lack thereof) in the EBPs (Jamtvedt, Young, Kristoffersen, Thomson O'Brien, & Oxman, 2004).

Change Champions

Change champions are practitioners from the local peer group who continually promote the EBP. They impart information about the EBP, encourage peers to align their practice with the evidence, demonstrate skills and knowledge necessary to carry out the EBP, and teach new and existing personnel about the EBP (Titler & Everett, 2001).

Clinical Practice Guideline

A systematically developed statement designed to assist the practitioner and patient make decisions about appropriate health care for specific

---

*Note: Contributed, in part, by Marita Titler, PhD, RN, FAAN

clinical circumstances (NHS Research and Development: Centre for Evidence Based Medicine [NHS], 2001).

Clinical Significance

A judgment about the interpretation of the statistical results (that the difference or relationship has meaning for patient care) (Mateo & Kirchhoff, 1999).

Confidence Interval (CI)

Quantifies the uncertainty in measurement. It is usually reported as a 95% CI, which is the range of values within which we can be 95% sure that the true value of an effect for a whole population lies within a range. For example, for an NNT (number needed to treat) of 10 with a 95% CI of 5 to 15, we would have 95% confidence that the true NNT value lies between 5 and 15 (Mount Sinai Hospital-University Health Network: Centre for Evidence-Based Medicine, 2001).

Cost-Effectiveness Analysis

Converts effects into health terms and describes the costs for some additional health gain (e.g., cost per additional MI prevented) (NHS, 2001).

Effect Size

A statistic that indicates the efficacy of a treatment or intervention. For example, when a study employs a correlational analysis, the correlation coefficient is informative of the effect size. When employing a t test, Cohen's d (a derivative of standardized and unstandardized mean differences) is the pertinent index of effect size. Other statistics used to determine an effect for dichotomous variables are relative risk and odds ratio (see definitions below).

Efficacy

Efficacy describes research that is designed to test interventions under tightly controlled conditions (e.g., dedicated person to deliver the intervention in a controlled clinical setting) with a homogenous patient population (e.g., women 65 to 80 years of age with osteoporosis). Efficacy studies are done prior to application of the intervention in the real world (Brown, 2002).

Effectiveness

Effectiveness is determining if an intervention or treatment works in the real world without controls of an efficacy study.

Evidence-Based Guideline

A written guide of evidence-based health care practices/actions. The recommendations for practice should be referenced and identify the strength of the evidence for each of the practice recommendations. Component parts of evidence-based guidelines vary but usually include a brief description of the practice topic (e.g., acute pain), the types of patients that the guideline can be used for (e.g., elders, hospitalized elders, children, or adults), the assessment and interventions used to carry out the EBPs and the risk/benefits of the EBP.

Macrosystem

This term is used interchangeably with organizational context to convey the organization or health system "at large" in which the EBP is being implemented. Macrosystems are composed of multiple microsystems.

Meta-analysis

An overview that uses quantitative methods to summarize results *or* a mathematical summary of results of several studies (Mateo & Kirchhoff, 1999; NHS, 2001).

Meta-synthesis

A method of summarizing qualitative findings so that they may be viewed in a larger interpretive context and presented in an accessible and usable form for practicing nurses (Sandelowski, Docherty, & Emden, 1997).

Microsystem

Microsystem is used to convey the patient care unit(s), ambulatory clinic(s), or other specific patient-care areas within the macrosystem in which the EBP is implemented. For example, an EBP on acute pain management may be first implemented in two or three patient care units or microsystems prior to being "rolled out" across the entire organization or macrosystem. Microsystems are composed of the unit culture, leadership, nature of the personnel, and manner in which people in the unit relate to one another in delivery of services/patient care, and routine monitoring of performance within the specified patient care unit.

Number Needed to Treat (NNT)

The number of patients who need to be treated to prevent one bad outcome. It is the inverse of the absolute relative risk (ARR): NNT = 1/ARR. (NHS, 2001).

Odds-Ratio

The odds-ratio is an effect size statistic that compares two groups in terms of the relative odds of a status of an event (e.g., death, illness, successful outcome, receipt of treatment, gender, or exposure to a toxin). The dependent variables are inherently dichotomous (e.g., good outcome or bad outcome).

Opinion Leaders

Opinion leaders are informal leaders from the local health care setting who are viewed as important and respected sources of influence among their peer group (e.g., nurses, physicians). A key characteristic of opinion leaders is that they are trusted to evaluate new information in the context of group norms. Opinion leaders are evaluators who are trusted to judge the fit between a technology or new practice and the local situation (Titler & Everett, 2001).

Organizational Context

The organizational context is the health system environment in which the proposed EBP is to be implemented. This may be an acute care, home health care or long-term-care system. The core elements that help describe the organizational context include the prevailing culture of the system (e.g., patient centered), the nature of human relationships in the system including the leadership styles that are operational (e.g., team work; clear role delineation), and the organization's approach to routine monitoring of performance of systems and services within the organization (e.g., routine use of audit and feedback) (Kitson, Harvey, & McCormack, 1998).

Outcomes Effectiveness

The ability of an intervention or care processes to produce (or fail to produce) desired outcomes (e.g., decreased pain intensity, decreased length of stay) in the typical practice environment with a variety of patients, many of whom have other factors that may affect the amount of benefit or outcome of the intervention (Brown, 2002). This often is used to denote the application of an intervention in the real world of practice. Evaluation of an EBP project is a type of outcome effectiveness. Evaluation of an EBP is important to determine (1) if the intervention can be used successfully in day-to-day practice and (2) if application of interventions in the real world of practice results in outcomes similar to those achieved in efficacy studies of the intervention.

Outcome Evaluation

A quality improvement technique that monitors outcomes, usually of patients, to determine if the outcomes from application of the EBP are similar to those intended, such as a decrease in pain intensity scores. Staff and fiscal outcomes also might be used in outcomes evaluation.

Outreach/Academic Detailing

Outreach and academic detailing are terms often used synonymously to convey the use of a trained individual who meets one-on-one with practitioners in their setting to provide information about the EBP. Information conveyed during outreach may include data on provider performance, information about the EBP, and consultation regarding specific issues in use of the EBP. Studies have demonstrated that outreach visits alone or used in combination with other translation interventions result in positive changes in practice behaviors of nurses and physicians (Titler, 2002).

Performance Gap Assessment

Performance gap assessment is baseline evaluation of practice performance that informs members of an organization about a particular practice, and opportunities for improving performance related to a specific indicator (e.g., frequency of acute-pain assessment) or set of indicators (e.g., acute-pain management of hospitalized elders) (Oxman et al., 1995; Schoenbaum et al., 1995). This is a data-driven strategy/intervention used early in the implementation phase of translating evidence into practice to convey to individuals the congruency or incongruency between their current clinical practice and recommended practices from evidence-based guidelines, EBP reports, or systematic reviews.

Point Estimation

A mean of a sample is only a guess of the true population mean. As such, it has a degree of error associated with using it, because we are only using a fraction of the elements of the population in deriving it. So if we were to calculate the mean of a sample and the answer was 35, we would say that our best guess of the population mean is 35, but realize that it probably is slightly higher or lower than 35. This guess is called a point estimation.

Process Evaluation

Process evaluation is a quality improvement technique that monitors specific indicators directly related to the EBP. Monitoring nurses' use of a standard pain intensity scale for pain assessment is a type of process monitor to determine if nurses' processes of acute-pain management are aligned with the evidence on this topic. Process evaluation is usually undertaken to determine if the EBP is being used and implemented consistently by care providers.

Protocol

"A detailed plan of scientific or medical experiment, treatment, or procedure" (Merriam-Webster, 1996, p. 939). A protocol may be even more specific than a guideline, as it is not only disease focused but can be tailored to a specific population and practice situation.

Randomized Controlled Clinical Trial

A group of patients is randomized into an experimental group and a control group. These groups are followed up for the variables/outcomes of interest (NHS, 2001).

Relative Risk Ratio

The relative risk ratio or index is just the opposite of the odds-ratio. This index relates to the probability of risk (or lack of success) to that of success. Therefore, the ideal value of this index is less than 1. In other words, we want the probability of failure (the numerator) to be less than the probability of success (the denominator). Therefore, we want a very small fraction of less than 1.

Strength of Evidence

This is an overall grade of the strength of evidence on a specific topic. Although various grading schemas are used, practice recommendations are usually graded using A, B, C, and so forth, with A being consistent findings from several randomized clinical trials and D or E grades used to convey conflicting research results, and/or use of expert opinion, case reports, or consensus (Agency for Healthcare Research and Quality [AHRQ], 2002).

Sustainability

The ability of an organization or individual to continue the use of EBP in routine clinical care following initial implementation.

Systematic Reviews

Systematic reviews are a summary of past research on a topic of interest. The summary is arrived at through a rigorous scientific process similar to methods used in primary research. The scientific process used in systematic reviews includes: the review question(s), how studies will be located, the methods used for critical appraisal of the primary studies, criteria for inclusion and exclusion of studies, synthesis methods (e.g., meta-analysis, narrative summary across studies), and summary recommendations for practice and future research. The final product is a summary of the best available scientific evidence following application of the aforementioned process (AHRQ, 2002; Joanna Briggs Institute, 2000, 2001).

Translation Research

Translation research is the scientific investigation of methods and variables that influence rate and extent of adoption of EBP by individuals and organizations to improve clinical and operational decision-making in the delivery of health care services. This includes testing the effect of strategies and interventions for promoting the adoption of EBP, with the outcomes being the rate and extent of health care providers' use of these practices. (Titler & Everett, 2001).

REFERENCES

Agency for Healthcare Research and Quality. (2002). *Systems to rate the strength of scientific evidence. Summary.* Bethesda, MD: U.S. Department of Health and Human Services. Agency for Healthcare Research and Quality, Evidence Report/Technology Assessment Report Number 47, Publication No. 02-E015.

Brown, S. J. (2002). Focus on research methods. Nursing intervention studies: A descriptive analysis of issues important to clinicians. *Research in Nursing and Health, 25,* 317–327.

Davis, D. A., Thomson, M. A., Oxman, A. D., & Haynes, R. B. (1995). Changing physician performance: A systematic review of the effect of continuing medical education strategies. *Journal of the American Medical Association, 274*(9), 700–705.

Jamtvedt, G., Young, J. M., Kristoffersen, D. T., Thomson O'Brien, M. A., & Oxman, A. D. (2004). Audit and feedback: Effects on professional practice and health care outcomes (Cochrane Review). *Cochrane Library, Issue 1,* Chichester, UK: Wiley.

Joanna Briggs Institute. (2000). Appraising systematic review. *Changing Practice, 1*(1).

Joanna Briggs Institute. (2001). An introduction to systematic reviews. *Changing Practice, 2*(1).

Kitson, A., Harvey, G., & McCormack, B. (1998). Enabling the implementation of evidence based practice: A conceptual framework. *Quality in Health Care, 7*(3), 149–158.

Mateo, M. A., & Kirchhoff, K. T. (1999). *Conducting and using nursing research in the clinical setting* (2nd ed.). Philadelphia: Saunders.

Merriam-Webster's Collegiate Dictionary (10th ed.). (1996). Springfield, MA: Merriam-Webster.

Mount Sinai Hospital-University Health Network: Centre for Evidence-Based Medicine. (2001). Retrieved http://www.library.utoronto.ca/medicine/ebm/glossary/NHS Research and Development: Centre for Evidence Based Medicine, 2001.

Oxman, A. D., Thomson, M. A., Davis, D. A., & Haynes, R. B. (1995). No magic bullets: A systematic review of 102 trials of interventions to improve professional practice. *Canadian Medical Association Journal, 153,* 1423–1431.

Sandelowski, M., Docherty, S., & Emden, C. (1997). Qualitative metasynthesis: Issues and techniques. *Research in Nursing and Health, 20,* 365–371.

Schoenbaum, S. C., Sundwall, D. N., Bergman, D., Buckle, J. M., Chernov, A., George, J., et al. (1995). *Using clinical practice guidelines to evaluate quality of care: Vol. 2. Methods.* Rockville, MD: U.S. Department of Health and Human Services, Public Health Service, Agency for Health Care Policy and Research.

Titler, M. G. (2002). Developing an EBP. In G. LoBiondo-Wood & J. Haber (Eds.), *Nursing research* (5th ed.). St. Louis, MO: Mosby-Year Book.

Titler, M. G., & Everett, L. Q. (2001). Translating research into practice: Considerations for critical care investigators. *Critical Care Nursing Clinics of North America, 13,* 587–604.

Annotated Bibliography

Relinie Rosenberg

Barratt, A., Wyer, P. C., Hatala, R., McGinn, T., Dans, A.L., Keitz, S., Moyer, V., & Guyatt, G. (2004a, August 17). Tips for learners of evidence based medicine: 1. Relative risk reduction, absolute risk reduction and number needed to treat. *Canadian Medical Association Journal, 171,* 353–358. Retrieved October 22, 2004, from http://www.cmaj.ca/cgi/reprint/171/4/353

> The article presents three measures of effect—relative risk reduction, absolute risk reduction, and number needed to treat (NNT)—in a fashion designed to help clinicians understand and use them as they seek to apply clinical evidence to the care of individual patients. The authors present a series of tips adapted from approaches developed by educators with experience in teaching evidence-based medicine skills to clinicians. The authors conclude that these tips will help clinicians overcome common pitfalls in learning to use relative risk reduction, absolute risk reduction, and NNT.

Barratt, A., Wyer, P. C., Hatala, R., McGinn, T., Dans, A. L., Keitz, S., Moyer, V., & Guyatt, G. (2004b, August 17). Tips for teachers of evidence based medicine: 1. Relative risk reduction, absolute risk reduction and number needed to treat. *Canadian Medical Association Journal, 171,* 347–352. Retrieved October 22, 2004, from http://www.cmaj.ca/cgi/data/171/4/353/DC1/1

> This article presents scripts that teachers of evidence-based medicine can use to help clinical learners understand the principles of relative risk reduction, risk difference (absolute risk reduction), and number needed to treat (NNT). The authors cover three tips

previously developed and used by experienced teachers of evidence-based medicine for the purpose of overcoming common pitfalls that learners experience in acquiring these skills. They provide guidance for each tip on when to use the tip, the teaching script for the tip, a bottom-line section, and a summary card. The authors conclude that the result of field-testing on these tips suggests that other educators may find this material useful in their own teaching.

Center for Evidence-Based Medicine. (2004). *Teaching EBM tips.* Retrieved October 18, 2004, from http://www.cebm.utoronto.ca/teach/materials/tips.htm

The University of Toronto, CEBM University Health Network Web site offers teaching tips for evidence-based medicine (EBM) and distinguishes identifying questions that are patient-based (arising out of the clinical problems of the patient under the learner's care) and learner centered (targeting the learning needs of the learner) as the challenge to teachers of EBM. The site describes the use of educational prescriptions and gives a sample prescription form for use in teaching EBM.

Center for Health Evidence (2004). *Evidence-based medicine: A new approach to teaching the practice of medicine. Evidence-users' guide to evidence based practice.* Retrieved October 24, 2004, from http://www.cche.net/usersguides/main.asp

This paper describes evidence-based medicine as a new paradigm for medical practice and how this approach differs from prior practice, and briefly outlines the building of a residency program in which a key goal is to practice, role-model, teach, and help residents become highly adept in evidence-based medicine. This paper presents some barriers educators and practitioners face in implementing the new paradigm as well as methods for scaling these barriers. The paper concludes that incorporating these practices into postgraduate medical education and continuing to work on their further development will result in more rapid dissemination and integration of evidence-based medicine into medical practice.

DiCenso, A., Ciliska, D., Marks, S., McKibbon, A., Cullum, N. & Thompson, C. (2004). EBM syllabi: Evidence-based nursing. Retrieved October 18, 2004, from http://www.cebm.utoronto.ca/syllabi/nur/

The article is part of evidence-based medicine (EBM) syllabi from University of Toronto CEBM that gives an introduction to evidence-based nursing. Resources to facilitate evidence-based nursing are described, such as evidence-based journals, systematic reviews, centers for evidence-based nursing, and EBP guidelines. The authors include sample scenarios, searches, completed worksheets, and critically appraised topics (CATs).

Fonteyn, M. (2002, January 5). Implementation forum print and online versions of Evidence-Based Nursing: Innovative teaching tools for nurse educators. *EBN, 5.* Retrieved November 23, 2004, from http://ebn.bmj-journals.com

> This article describes how nurse educators can use the print and online version of the journal EBN (Evidence-Based Nursing) as a tool to enhance student learning in using current clinical research. It provides examples of how nurse teachers can use print and online versions of EBN to augment and enhance the content of classroom-based courses, clinically based courses, and nursing research courses. The author concludes that EBN is a practical and effective tool to help students learn ways of quickly and efficiently locating and digesting current research findings for nursing practice.

Greiner, A. (n.d.). Educating health professionals to use an evidence base. Retrieved October 18, 2004, from http://www.iom.edu/Object.File/Master/10/474/0.pdf

> The paper explores the existing evidence base related to educating health professionals in EBP, the educational and regulatory barriers to integrating this topic area in the academic and continuing education settings, proposed actions for overcoming these barriers, and model schools or educational programs offering curricula in this topic area. The paper includes questions that serve to initiate the development of strategies for reform of health professions education.

Homer, C., & Leap, N. (2002, March). Teaching and learning evidence-based midwifery practice. *Nursing Review.* Retrieved November 25, 2004, from http://www.nmh.uts.edu.au

> This article describes the design and implementation of a new subject, evidence-based midwifery practice, in the Faculty of Nursing, Midwifery and Health at the University of Technology in Sydney, Australia. Their major strategy is designing the subject to ensure that research is incorporated into the practice. Employed teaching and learning strategies that maximized opportunities for participatory action and interaction are explained. The authors conclude that the subject of evidence-based midwifery seems to be an effective way to discuss research methods, the process of carrying out research, and the implications for practice, while at the same time informing students of the wide range of important studies that will inform their midwifery practice.

Ismach, R. B. (2004, June 16). Teaching evidence-based medicine to medical students. *SAEM Medical Educator's Handbook*, 1–8. Retrieved October 18, 2004, from http://www.saem.org/download/ Hand-6.pdf

> The paper describes evidence-based medicine (EBM) as a collection of tools used by clinicians to access and manage medical information, especially those published in the medical literature. The author discusses resources for teaching EBM, using Web-based tutorials, educational prescriptions, and critically appraised topics (CATs). The author concludes that faculty development is a prerequisite to teach EBM to medical students and that EBM is best taught at the bedside or in clinically oriented settings. The paper includes a table with the five steps in practicing EBM and a table of skills and concepts useful in EBM.

Long, J. D. (2000, September 22). Using the OJKSN as a teaching tool with RN/BSN students. *Online Journal of Knowledge Synthesis for Nursing*. Retrieved November 25, 2004, from http://www.stti.iupu-i.edu/VirginiaHendersonLibrary

> The article describes the use of *The Online Journal of Knowledge Synthesis for Nursing* (OJKSN) as a powerful teaching tool used in the RN/BS program in Lubbock Christian University in helping students to discover the link between research-based practice and client outcomes while making an immediate application to nursing practice. The teaching strategy is described as it is used in the introductory activity, group activity, and individual activity. The author evaluates the teaching strategy and concludes that using OJKSN as a teaching strategy is a valuable tool that offers a rich array of opportunities for adult learners to delve into the world of nursing research; students are able to see clearly the practical application of research to practice.

Montori, V. M., Kleinbart, J., Newman, T. B., Keitz, S., Wyer, P. C., & Guyatt, G. (2004, September 14). Tips for learners of evidence-based medicine: 2. Measures of precision (confidence intervals). *Canadian Medical Association Journal, 171*, 611–615. Retrieved October 22, 2004, from http://www.cmaj.ca/cgi/reprint/171/6/611

> This article describes two related but different statistical measures of an estimate's precision: p values and confidence intervals. The authors focus on confidence intervals and present a series of tips or exercises for clinicians to understand and interpret confidence intervals. The authors conclude that clinicians need to understand and interpret confidence intervals to use research results properly in making decisions.

Montori, V. M., Kleinbart, J., Newman, T. B., Keitz, S., Wyer, P. C., & Guyatt, G. (2004, September 14). Tips for teachers of evidence-based medicine: 2. Confidence intervals and p values. *Canadian Medical Association Journal, 171*(6). Retrieved October 22, 2004, from http://www.cmaj.ca/cgi/data/171/6/611/DC1/1

> This paper describes EBP as a new approach to teaching the integration of research and practice in gerontology. Based on the concept of evidence-based medicine, the paper teaches techniques that involve (a) precisely defining a problem and what is required to solve it; (b) conducting an efficient search of the literature; (c) selecting the best of the relevant studies; (d) applying rules of evidence to determine their validity; (e) identifying the strengths and weaknesses of the studies; and (f) extracting the practice message and applying it to the patient, client, or organization. The paper discusses barriers to, and evaluation of, this method of teaching. The author concludes that EBP has the potential to transform the education and practice of social and health service providers.

Steele, L. L. (2001, September 10). Incorporating research application into nurse practitioner education. *Online Journal of Knowledge Synthesis for Nursing.* Retrieved November 24, 2004, from

> This article shows how a systematic review of research literature was incorporated into a clinical course for NP (nurse practitioner) students to demonstrate the natural fit of research application in the advanced practice setting and provide evidence that using research is critical to clinical decision-making. A description and example of the teaching strategy is provided. The author concludes that the importance of the role of research in advanced practice and the utilization of research as a basis for evaluating interventions and outcomes must be valued by faculty involved in the education of nurse practitioners.

Stevens, K. R., & Long, J. D. (1998, November 17). Incorporating systematic reviews into nursing education. *Online Journal of Knowledge Synthesis for Nursing, 5*(7) 1E. Retrieved November 25, 2004, from http://www.nursingsociety.org/library

> This article provides a description of systematic reviews and focuses on the *Online Journal of Knowledge Synthesis for Nursing* (OJKSN) as a source of systematic reviews. The authors propose a strategy and research application projects for incorporating the use of OJKSN in teaching undergraduate and graduate students. They also provide a description of research application projects and instructions to students. The authors conclude that research

application projects provide a focal point for the study of research in both the undergraduate and graduate courses.

Taylor, R., Reeves, B., Mears, R., Keast, J., Binns, S., Ewings, P., Khan, & Khalid, (2001, June 1). Development and validation of a questionnaire to evaluate the effectiveness of EBP teaching. *Medical Education, 35*, 544–547. Retrieved October 18, 2004, from.

The focus of this study is to develop and validate a questionnaire to evaluate the effectiveness of EBP teaching. Health care professionals with a range of EBP experience—categorized as novice (little or no prior EBP education) and experts (health care professionals and academics currently teaching EBP)—completed 152 questionnaires. Moderate to good sensitivity index scores were observed for both knowledge and attitude scores as the result of comparing individuals before and after an EBP intervention. The authors conclude that the results of this validation study indicate that the developed questionnaire is a satisfactory tool with which to evaluate the effectiveness of EBP teaching interventions.

Index